examination SURGERY

A guide to passing the Fellowship Examination in General Surgery

examination SURGERY

A guide to passing the Fellowship Examination in General Surgery

Christopher J Young MBBS MS FRACS
Clinical Associate Professor, Central Clinical School, University of Sydney, Australia
Head of Unit, Royal Prince Alfred Hospital Colorectal Unit, Sydney, Australia
Visiting Medical Officer General and Colorectal Surgery, Royal Prince Alfred and Concord Hospitals
Chairman, Royal Australasian College of Surgeons Board In General Surgery

Marc A Gladman MBBS DRCOG DFFP PhD MRCOG MRCS (Eng) FRCS (Gen Surg, UK) FRACS
Professor of Colorectal Surgery, Concord Clinical School, School of Medicine, University of Sydney, Australia
Head of Academic Colorectal Unit and Consultant Colorectal Surgeon, Concord Hospital, Sydney, Australia
Director, Enteric Neuroscience & Gastrointestinal Research Group, ANZAC Research Institute, University of Sydney, Australia

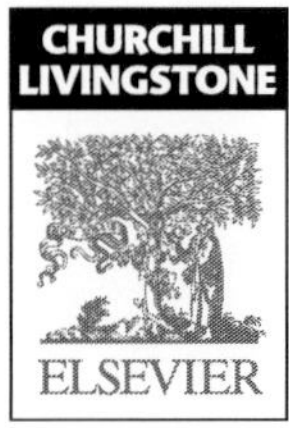

Sydney Edinburgh London New York Philadelphia St Louis Toronto

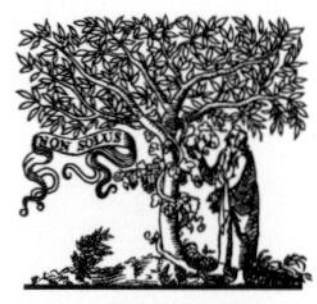

Churchill Livingstone
is an imprint of Elsevier

Elsevier Australia. ACN 001 002 357
(a division of Reed International Books Australia Pty Ltd)
Tower 1, 475 Victoria Avenue, Chatswood, NSW 2067

eISBN: 9780729581486

National Library of Australia Cataloguing-in-Publication Data

---

Examination surgery: a guide to passing the fellowship examination in general surgery / Christopher J Young, Marc A Gladman.

9780729541480 (paperback)

Surgery—Examinations—Study guides.

Young, Christopher J.
Gladman, Marc A.

617.0076

Publishing Director: Luisa Cecotti
Content Strategist: Larissa Norrie
Senior Content Development Specialist: Neli Bryant
Project Managers: Martina Vascotto, Rochelle Deighton and Nayagi Athmanathan
Edited by Jon Forsyth
Proofread by Fiona Forsyth
Cover and Internal design by Stan Lamond
Index by Robert Swanson
Typeset by Toppan Best-set Premedia Limited

Contents

Preface

Our life is what our thoughts make it.
(Marcus Aurelius Antonius, 121–180).

The fellowship examination in general surgery has a reputation for being one of the most difficult and rigorous postgraduate examinations. General surgery is, by necessity, a discipline that covers a broad range of surgical conditions incorporating a large number of topics. Consequently, trainees are expected to have acquired a tremendous amount of technical and non-technical knowledge at completion of training. Accordingly, the breadth and depth of basic and clinical science, clinical practice and operative surgical knowledge assessed in the fellowship examination is formidable. It is not surprising, therefore, that success rates in the examination consistently hover around the 50–60% mark. For most candidates, this examination is the most important of their life and represents the final barrier to independent practice as a specialist general surgeon, frequently reflecting the culmination of 25 to 35 years of education since childhood.

Examination surgery represents the synthesis of our collective experience of delivering tutorials, lectures and 'mock examinations' for over a decade to candidates preparing for the fellowship examination in general surgery. Whilst there can be no substitute in the examination for knowledge gained by hard work, clinical experience and appreciation of the published literature, the fellowship examination is designed to test clinical wisdom, judgment, insight and safe practice and not just encyclopaedic knowledge. Accordingly, the aim of this book is to use a practical approach to provide candidates with appropriate direction, focus and instruction on how to organise their studies and to prepare for each component of the examination with particular emphasis on examination *technique* to optimise performance. It is most certainly *not* intended to replace other reference textbooks for the various components of the examination.

One of the most significant challenges of embarking on a project such as this is to produce a book that is relevant and accurately reflects the material encountered in the examination. To this end, we have collected and catalogued past papers and questions from the last 10 years to assemble a list of the most frequently encountered topics. This information has been distilled into the respective sections of this book that mirror each of the individual components of the current fellowship examination, namely: (i) the written papers; (ii) the clinical examinations; and (iii) the *viva voce* examinations. Within each of the sections of the book, we will attempt to simplify and demystify the common questions and scenarios frequently encountered in the examination and present a structured approach, incorporating suitable techniques and strategies that we have developed and refined from our own experiences of preparing for examinations and from being involved with the education of postgraduate trainees in general surgery sitting the fellowship examination. Using sample 'model answers', the purpose of this approach is to equip candidates with the confidence to address common cases/topics, but it will also enable individual candidates to develop a reliable, systematic approach to successfully address any scenario that they may encounter in the examination.

It must be emphasised that we are most certainly not advocating that the model answers contained within this book are the only way to tackle examination questions. Indeed, you personally may have a different style or technique and you will certainly hear some of our recommendations challenged by your mentors. This epitomises surgical practice, where different general surgeons manage different conditions or perform different operations in different ways. *We are merely presenting one way of answering the questions that we, and our numerous students over the years, have found useful and successful in the fellowship examination.* We urge you to refrain from getting bogged down in the debate of which approach is right or wrong, but instead concentrate on understanding the arguments surrounding many of these key issues and incorporate different techniques and advice from your peers and mentors, as well as from this book, into your own answers.

While this book is aimed squarely at candidates preparing for the fellowship examination in general surgery of the Royal Australasian College of Surgeons, its contents will also be relevant to candidates preparing for the fellowship examination of the Royal Colleges of Surgeons in the UK and Ireland (Intercollegiate Specialty Examination), Canada, South Africa and Hong Kong, as well as having general application to all general surgeons, surgical residents and medical students.

Today's trainees are dependent on the enthusiasm and commitment of their trainers, supervisors and surgical mentors to mould them into tomorrow's surgeons. We sincerely hope that this book furnishes candidates with the appropriate tools to successfully negotiate the examination as they progress to becoming the future generation of specialist surgeons.

Good luck!

Christopher J Young
Marc A Gladman

Historical note

The fellowship in Australasia

The Royal Australasian College of Surgeons (RACS) was formed in 1927 to provide education, training, examination and the setting of standards for surgical practice and continuing professional development to surgeons in Australia and New Zealand. There are now nine surgical specialty areas within RACS of which general surgery is the largest, containing approximately one-third of the total number of fellows of the College. Until 1933, an application for Fellowship of the Royal Australasian College of Surgeons (FRACS) was considered by the credentials committee of each state or dominion and a report was sent to the College council once a candidate had completed a minimum of 5 years training in surgery. From 1933, the censor in chief would determine if a candidate had completed a satisfactory period of training, allowing the candidate to appear in person before a board of censors who were empowered to test the ability and knowledge of the candidate on a case-by-case basis, with no standardised form of assessment. Formal examination in the form of exam papers and vivas in general surgery did not begin until 1947.

Today, there are approximately 550 general surgical trainees throughout Australia and New Zealand, with approximately 120 new trainees accepted into general surgical SET each year, with an application ratio of 4 : 1. The RACS runs a primary exam, which must be completed at the SET 1 level. It comprises two multiple choice examinations, known as the surgical science examination (SSE) generic and specialty specific, and a clinical examination in the form of an OSCE. The Part II examination is now known as *the fellowship examination*. It is taken in the fifth year of surgical training and is an exit exam that assesses a candidate's proficiency and ability to practise independently as a general surgeon. The seven components of the fellowship examination have been subject to change and modification over the years, but the format currently consists of two written examinations, two clinical vivas, and three separate *viva voce* examinations in anatomy, operative surgery, and pathophysiology and critical care.

The Fellowship in the United Kingdom and Ireland

There are four Royal Colleges of Surgeons in the UK and Republic of Ireland involved in surgical education, training and examination of trainees. Fellowship of the Royal College of Surgeons (FRCS) is the professional qualification to practise as a surgeon and is bestowed by the Royal College of Surgeons of England, Royal College of Surgeons in Ireland, Royal College of Surgeons of Edinburgh and Royal College of Physicians and Surgeons of Glasgow. The original fellowship was taken between basic and higher surgical training and was available in general surgery and in certain specialties (ophthalmic or ENT surgery or obstetrics and gynaecology), although these were not formally specified in the initials. In 1995, the original fellowship examination was replaced by the Membership of the Royal College of Surgeons (MRCS) and Associate Fellowship of the Royal College of Surgeons (AFRCS), which continued to be taken between basic and higher surgical training, and a range of higher fellowship examinations taken at the end of higher specialist training. These 'exit' or part III examinations were specific to each of the subspecialties and were identified accordingly with additional abbreviations following 'FRCS', such that the fellowship in general surgery became 'FRCS (Gen Surg)'.

The Joint Committee on Intercollegiate Examinations (JCIE) is responsible, in line with the statutory requirements of the General Medical Council (GMC) Postgraduate Board, to the presidents and through them the councils of the four surgical royal colleges of Great Britain and Ireland, for the supervision of standards, policies, regulations and professional conduct of the intercollegiate specialty examinations (specialty fellowship examinations). Success in the examination is a mandatory requirement for surgical trainees working toward the award of Certificate of Completion of Training (CCT) by the GMC Postgraduate Board or for the award of Certificate of Specialist Doctor (CSD) or Specialist Registration with the Medical Council of Ireland.

Candidates who are successful in the intercollegiate specialty examination are eligible for election to, or award of, the fellowship of the College to which they are affiliated. Successful candidates who are not affiliated to one of the four surgical royal colleges of Great Britain and Ireland (i.e. who do not hold the MRCS/AFRCS) may apply to any one of these for election to, or award of, the fellowship.

The intercollegiate specialty examination in general surgery currently consists of two sections. Section 1 is a written test composed of a combination of multiple choice questions in single best answer (SBA) and extended matching items (EMI) format. Candidates must meet the required standard in section 1 in order to gain eligibility to proceed to the next part of the examination. Section 2 is the clinical component of the examination and consists of two clinical examinations and three separate oral examinations covering: (i) emergency surgery with critical care; (ii) general surgery and subspecialty; and (iii) academic surgery.

Authors

Christopher J Young MBBS MS FRACS
Clinical Associate Professor, Central Clinical School, University of Sydney, Australia
Head of Unit, Royal Prince Alfred Hospital Colorectal Unit, Sydney, Australia
Visiting Medical Officer General and Colorectal Surgery, Royal Prince Alfred and Concord Hospitals
Chairman, Royal Australasian College of Surgeons Board In General Surgery

Marc A Gladman MBBS DRCOG DFFP PhD MRCOG MRCS (Eng) FRCS (Gen Surg, UK) FRACS
Professor of Colorectal Surgery, Concord Clinical School, School of Medicine, University of Sydney, Australia
Head of Academic Colorectal Unit and Consultant Colorectal Surgeon, Concord Hospital, Sydney, Australia
Director, Enteric Neuroscience & Gastrointestinal Research Group, ANZAC Research Institute, University of Sydney, Australia

Contributors

The authors would like to pay special tribute and gratitude to Drs Jerome M Laurence and Naseem Mirbagheri for their significant contribution to this book. Their dedication, knowledge and input helped ensure the success of this project.

Jerome M Laurence MBChB MRCS FRACS PhD
Fellow in HPB Surgery, Royal Brisbane and Women's Hospital, Brisbane, Australia

Naseem Mirbagheri MBBS FRACS
Colorectal Research Fellow, Academic Colorectal Unit, Concord Hospital, Sydney, Australia

Reviewers

Sulman Ahmed, MBBS, MS, FRACS
VMO — General and hepatobiliary surgeon, Nepean & Nepean Private Hospitals, Sydney, Australia

Phillip Carson, MBBS, FRCS(Ed), FRACS, FRCS, FRCS (Glasg)
Associate Professor of Surgery, Royal Darwin Hospital and Flinders NT Medical Program, Darwin, Australia

Jane G Fox, MBBS, FRACS
Senior Lecturer, Monash University Department of Surgery, Director Breast Services, Monash Health, Melbourne, Australia

Alex Matthews, VMO
General Surgeon at POW/RHW Hospitals, Randwick, Sydney, Australia
Chairman of the NSW Regional Board in General Surgery, Royal Australasian College of Surgeons

Chris Pyke, PhD, FRACS, FACS
Senior Lecturer, University of Queensland, Mater Hospital, Brisbane, Australia

Akhtar Sayed-Hassen, BA, MACHA (UK), FRCS, FRACS
General Surgeon, Epworth Eastern Hospital, Melbourne, Australia

Jim Toouli, B(Med)Sci, MBBS, PhD FRACS
Emeritus Professor of Surgery, Flinders University, Adelaide, Australia

Bruce Philip Waxman, B(Med)Sci, MBBS, FRACS FACS FRACS
Director, Associate Professor, Academic Surgical Unit, Monash University, Dandenong Hospital, Monash Health, Melbourne, Australia

Foreword

The life of a surgeon is a complex mix of medical knowledge, technical skill and those non-technical attributes which recognise our mastery of the profession such as decision making, leadership, communication and advocacy to name a few. Nonetheless what defines us as a surgeon is our ability to undertake an operation safely. To this end the Surgical Education and Training Program (SET) provided by the Royal Australasian College of Surgeons and the Specialist Surgical Societies aims to produce a safe surgeon capable of independent practice. Training is competency based and assessment is undertaken throughout training. The Final Fellowship Examination provides a last objective assessment of a trainee's ability to practice independently.

As this final hurdle approaches, trainees need to concentrate on the core knowledge and essential clinical skills that will maximise their chances of passing this exam. Many trainees do not do themselves justice through poor preparation, nervous tension and poor technique. There is a need for a text to provide advice to trainees on how to optimise their chances of passing this final exam.

Examination Surgery, authored by Christopher Young and Marc Gladman, does just that. It provides a holistic approach to preparing for the exam. As the authors point out in Chapter 1.2, the exam is like a race, one needs to train for it and perform on the day. This book optimises a trainee's chances of doing so. The authors recommend the acronym PASS — plan, awareness, syllabus and structure. This is an excellent approach to training for the race. To ensure the trainee performs on the day this book addresses the content and structure of the exam, the marking system, and answers uncertainties about the exam process. Clinical material is covered by addressing the exam format of written papers and vivas. An extensive range of possible questions and model answers are also provided. These cover most of the clinical scenarios candidates are likely to encounter.

I commend this book to those trainees who are keen to ensure that years of hard work and hours of study are not wasted by a poor performance at the final hurdle.

Associate Professor Michael Hollands
President Royal Australasian College of Surgeons

Acknowledgments

The authors are most grateful and would like to extend their most sincere thanks to the following for assistance with the manuscript preparation and review: Drs Nabila Ansari, Kirk Austin, Chris Byrne, Peter Campbell, Kristenne Clement, Nagham Glenie, Jonathan Hong, Yu Xuan Kitzing, Cindy Mak, Farid Meybodi, Natasha Nassar, Raffi Qasabian, Rebecca Read, Charbel Sandroussi, Robyn Saw, Kerwin Shannon, Sanjay Warrier, and Danette Wright.

Abbreviations

ABPI	ankle brachial pressure indices
ACS	abdominal compartment syndrome
AD	autosomal dominant
ADP	adenosine phosphate
AFP	alpha-fetoprotein
AJCC	American Joint Committee on Cancer
ALND	axillary lymph node dissection
ALP	alkaline phosphate
ALT	alanine aminotransferase
APP	abdominal perfusion pressure
APTT	activated partial thromboplastin time
AST	aspartate aminotransferase
BCC	basal cell carcinoma
BMI	body mass index
BP	blood pressure
BSL	blood sugar level
CARS	compensatory anti-inflammatory response syndrome
CASH	chemotherapy-associated steatohepatitis
CBD	common bile duct
CC	cranio-caudal
CCF	congestive cardiac failure
CD	Crohn's disease
CEA	carcinoembryonic antigen
CFA	common femoral artery
CFV	common femoral vein
CHA	common hepatic artery
CHD	common hepatic duct
CLND	complete lymph node dissection
CMV	cytomegalovirus
CRC	colorectal cancer
CRP	C-reactive protein
CRS	clinical risk score
CT	computed tomography
DALM	dysplasia associated lesion/mass
DCIS	ductal carcinoma in situ
DIPJ	distal interphalangeal joint
DPA	dorsalis pedis artery
EBV	Epstein-Barr virus
ECF	epirubicin, cis-platin, 5FU
ELND	elective lymph node dissection
EMR	endoscopic mucosal resection
EPA	external pudendal artery
ERAS	enhanced recovery after surgery
ERCP	endoscopic retrograde cholangiopancreatography
ESLN	external branch of superior laryngeal nerve
ESR	erythrocyte sedimentation rate
ETT	endotracheal tube

EUS	endoscopic ultrasound
EUS-FNA	EUS-fine needle aspiration
FAP	familial adenomatous polyposis
FAST	focused assessment with sonography for trauma
FBC	full blood count
FCU	flexor carpi ulnaris
FDP	flexor digitorum profundus
FFP	fresh frozen plasma
FLR	future liver remnant
FNA	fine needle aspiration
FNAC	fine needle aspiration cytology
FOBT	faecal occult blood testing
FV	femoral vein
GB	gallbladder
GCS	Glasgow Coma Scale
GDA	gastro-duodenal artery
GGT	gamma-glutamyltransferase or gamma-glutamyl transpeptidase
GIST	gastrointestinal stromal tumour
GIT	gastrointestinal
GORD	gastro-oesophageal reflux disease
GSV	great saphenous vein
HBsAg	hepatitis B surface anitgen
HCV	hepatitis C virus
HITTS	heparin induced thrombosis thrombocytopenia syndrome
HIV	human immunodeficiency virus
HNPCC	hereditary non-polyposis colorectal CA
HRT	hormone replacement therapy
HSV	*herpes simplex virus*
HTN	hypertension
IAP	intra-abdominal pressure
IBD	inflammatory bowel disease
IDC	indwelling catheter
IFN	interferon
IMA	inferior mesenteric artery
IPAA	ileal J-pouch anal anastomosis
IPC	intermittent pneumatic compression
IPMN	intraductal papillary mucinous neoplasm
ITA	inferior thyroid artery
LAMN	low grade appendiceal mucinous neoplasm
lat.	latissimus
LBO	large bowel obstruction
LCIS	lobular carcinoma in situ
LMWH	low-molecular-weight heparin
LSV	long saphenous vein
LUQ	left upper quadrant
LVHR	laparoscopic ventral hernia repair
MAP	MUTYH-associated polyposis
MCPJ	metacarpophalangeal joint
MIBG	metaiodobenzylguanidine
MLO	mediolateral oblique

MMR	mismatch repair
MODS	multi-organ dysfunction syndrome
MRI	magnetic resonance imaging
MSI	microsatellite instability
NCCN	National Comprehensive Cancer Network
NGT	nasogastric tube
NSTI	necrotising soft tissue infection
OCP	oral contraceptive pill
OIS	organ injury scale grade
OPSI	overwhelming post-splenectomy infection
PBD	posterior belly of digastric
pec.	pectoralis
PFA	profunda femoris artery
PIPJ	proximal interphalangeal joint
PNMT	phenyl ethanolamine-N-Methyl-transferase
PNS	parasympathetic nervous system
PR	per rectum
PT	prothrombin time
PTA	percutaneous transluminal angioplasty
PTA	posterior tibial artery
PTC	papillary thyroid cancer
PTEN	pentaerythritol tetranitrate
PTH	parathyroid hormone assay
PTX	prothrombinex
PV	per vaginum
QPTH	quick parathyroid hormone assay
RCT	randomised control trial
RFA	radiofrequency ablation
RHA	right hepatic artery
RLN	recurrent laryngeal nerve
RPSD	right posterior sectoral duct
RRR	relative risk reduction
RTx	radiotherapy
RUQ	right upper quadrant
SBO	small bowel obstruction
SCC	squamous cell carcinoma
SCM	sternocleidomastoid muscle
SCPRT	short-course pre-operative radiotherapy
SEMS	self expanding metallic stents
SEPS	subfascial endoscopic perforator vein surgery
SFA	superficial femoral artery
SFJ	saphenofemoral junction
SIRS	systemic inflammatory response syndrome
SLN	sentinel lymph node
SLNB	sentinel lymph node biopsy
SMA	superior mesenteric arteries
SMN	submandibular
SMV	superior mesenteric vein
SNS	sympathetic nervous system
SOB	short of breath

SPJ	saphenopopliteal junction
SSV	short saphenous vein
STI	sexually transmitted infection
TAC	temporary abdominal closure
TBSA	total body surface area
TLND	therapeutic lymph node dissection
TNM cancer staging	T is based on depth of invasion through the wall of the oesophagus, N refers to the number of lymph nodes involved, M refers to presence of distant metastasis
TPN	total parenteral nutrition
TRAM	transverse rectus abdominal muscle
TSH	thyroid-stimulating hormone
UC	ulcerative colitis
ULAR	ultra-low anterior resection
US	ultrasound
UTI	urinary tract infection
UWSD	underwater seal drain
VNPI	Van Nuys prognostic index
VRE	vancomycin resistant enterococci
WBRT	whole brain radiotherapy
WCC	white cell count
WE	wide excision
WLE	wide local excision
YAG	yttrium aluminium garnet

Section 1

Examination information and preparation

Chapter 1.1

Basic examination requirements and organisation

If you think education is expensive, try ignorance.
(Derek Curtis Bok, b 1930)

The Fellowship in Australasia

Examination requirements

The eligibility requirements for the fellowship examination in general surgery are set out in the *Board In General Surgery Training Regulations Handbook*. (The Board in General Surgery is comprised of the Royal Australasian College of Surgeons, General Surgeons Australia and New Zealand Association of General Surgeons.) In summary, a trainee is eligible to present for the fellowship examination when each of the following criteria are fulfilled:

1. completion of at least six, 6-month accredited terms beyond SET 1;
2. completion of 600 major operative cases performed after SET 1, with satisfactory completion of the minimum number of upper gastrointestinal endoscopies and colonoscopies;
3. application is supported by the trainee's supervisor and the regional subcommittee.

Award of full fellowship of RACS requires satisfactory completion of eight, 6-month terms in accredited posts, and completion of 800 major operative cases beyond SET 1, with satisfactory completion of a number of courses, research requirements and attendance at trainee days.

International medical graduates on a pathway to general surgical fellowship, who after initial assessment by the college have been deemed to be 'partially comparable' to an Australasian General Surgeon, are usually required to complete 2 years of clinical oversight and may present for the fellowship examination after completing 9 months of satisfactory supervision.

Examination organisation

The fellowship examination is currently held twice per year in April/May and August/September with the written examination preceding the *viva voce* examinations. The May *viva voce* examinations alternate between Melbourne and Brisbane in Australia and Auckland and Wellington in New Zealand, whilst the location in September alternates between Adelaide and Sydney.

At present, the seven components of the fellowship examination in general surgery are as follows.

1. Written paper 1 — 25 spot test questions of equal value to be answered in 2 hours (4.8 minutes per question): 19/25 correct required to pass.
2. Written paper 2 — 8 short answer questions to be answered in 2 hours (15 minutes per question).
3. Clinical *viva voce* 1 — 2 'medium' cases are presented to the candidate over 40 minutes (approximately 20 minutes each).
4. Clinical *viva voce* 2 — 6 'short' clinical cases are presented to the candidate for clinical examination, discussion and comment over 40 minutes (approximately 6 minutes per case).
5. Surgical anatomy *viva voce* — a 25 minute examination comprising two sections:
   a. During the first 12.5 minutes, five images are shown to candidates as starting points for discussion. All candidates are shown the same images.
   b. In the second 12.5 minutes, five 'wet' specimens are examined.
6. Operative surgery *viva voce* — a 30 minute examination comprising two sections:
   a. 10 minutes is centred on a scenario (e.g. an operative cholangiogram).
   b. Then five computer images are shown over 20 minutes. These images serve as a 'primer' for the discussion, which may include pre-operative decision making and work up, operative technique and strategy or management of intra-operative and post-operative complications. All candidates are shown the **same** images.
7. Pathophysiology and critical care and clinical reasoning *viva voce* — a 40 minute examination comprising two sections:
   a. two computer-based scenarios, each of 10 minutes duration. The scenarios (e.g. pancreatitis) lead to a discussion which is directed towards clinical management.
   b. The second component comprises five computer images of pathology specimens examined over 20 minutes. All candidates are, once again, shown the same images.

In recent years, there have been great efforts to make the general surgery fellowship examination more structured and to incorporate questions and topics commonly encountered in general surgical practice. There has also been a strenuous attempt to ensure that the questions asked are the same for all candidates, although this is most challenging to achieve in the clinical *viva voce* examinations due to the variable inpatient and out-patient surgical population available at the time of the examinations.

Currently, the results of the fellowship examination are announced at an afternoon ceremony after the Court of Examiners have met and deliberated. The candidates are given an envelope informing them whether they have passed or failed, with successful candidates being introduced to the Court of Examiners. Non-attendees are informed by express post, and all candidates receive formal notification within 2 days. The senior examiner is responsible for constructing the feedback to unsuccessful candidates from the reports of the 14 examiners who assessed the candidate during the exam. This feedback can be of great help in redirecting an unsuccessful candidate towards a subsequent successful attempt at the fellowship examination.

Typically, the pass rate at each of the individual general surgical fellowship examinations is between 50 and 60%. In 2010, it was 62%, giving an overall annual pass rate of 76% when both sittings are taken into account. In 2009, the overall annual pass rate was 88%. The vast majority of candidates who enter are eventually successful in passing the fellowship examination in general surgery. Of those candidates who initially presented in 2005, 91.8% had passed the examination by 2010.

The Intercollegiate Specialty Examination in General Surgery in the UK and Ireland

Examination requirements

The examination regulations were opened out in November 2006 to allow those not in training positions in the UK to enter the examination and to use success in the examination as evidence when applying to the General Medical Council Postgraduate Board for entry to the Specialist Register under the Certificate of Eligibility for Specialist Registration route. The current regulations (January 2012) are as follows.

1. The applicant must hold a medical qualification recognised for registration by the General Medical Council of the United Kingdom or the Medical Council of Ireland. The applicant must have been qualified for at least 6 years.
2. The applicant must provide evidence of having reached the standard of clinical competence defined in the Intercollegiate Surgical Curriculum either for the award of the Certificate of Completion of Training (CCT) by the General Medical Council Postgraduate Board or for the award of Certificate of Completion of Specialist Training (CCST) by the Irish Surgical Postgraduate Training Committee (ISPTC). The required standard may have been achieved through training or qualifications, and experience considered together. The passing of the Intercollegiate Specialty Examination alone does not imply that the CCT, CCST (Ireland) or placement on the Specialist Register will be automatic; the examination will form only part of the evidence required.
3. This evidence must consist of three structured references in the format prescribed by the Joint Committee on Intercollegiate Examinations (JCIE). These references must be completed by the appropriate senior colleagues with direct experience of the applicant's current clinical practice in the appropriate specialty as defined in the Guidance Notes for Referees.

Examination organisation

The Intercollegiate Specialty Examination is comprised of two separate sections. Section 1 is a computer-based test that is held at numerous centres around the UK and Ireland in March, August and November each year. Section 2 is held in February, June and October each year. Candidates must meet the required standard in section 1 in order to gain eligibility to proceed to section 2.

At present, the format of the examination is as follows.

Section 1 is a written test composed of 2 papers:

1. Paper 1: Single Best Answer [SBA] (2 hours)
2. Paper 2: Extended Matching Items [EMI] (2 hours 30 mins)

There is ***no*** negative marking.

Section 2 is the clinical component of the examination and consists of a series of structured interviews (scenario- or patient-based) on clinical topics. It consists of clinical and oral examinations in all aspects of general surgery that include the relevant aspects of anatomy, physiology and pathology:

The examination consists of the following:

1. Clinical examination
   a. This consists of two sessions of short cases, each session lasting for 30 minutes. Candidates have the opportunity to discuss cases relevant to their subspecialty (if declared). However, the clinical examination covers the full range of general surgery.
2. Oral examination
   a. There are three oral examinations:
      i. Emergency surgery with critical care (30 minutes)
         This covers the subject of emergency and trauma surgery and the management of the critically ill; relevant pathology investigations and operative surgery are included.
      ii. General surgery and subspecialty (30 minutes)
         Part of this oral is directed toward the candidate's major subspecialty interest, if such an interest is declared.
      iii. Academic (20 minutes)
         This oral is designed to enquire into the critical abilities of the candidate. All candidates are given two papers (one in each of general surgery and nominated subspecialty interest) to read for 1 hour prior to the academic oral and are then examined for 20 minutes, with 10 minutes being allocated to each paper.

From 1 January 2012, candidates have up to a maximum of 7 years to complete the examination process as follows.

1. Section 1: Candidates have a 2-year period from their first attempt with a maximum of four attempts with no re-entry.
2. Section 2: Candidates will have a maximum of four attempts and up to one further exceptional attempt.

The overall pass rate for section 1 is typically 70–80%, although the success rates differ between trainees (approximately 90%) and non-trainees (approximately 30–50%). The overall pass rate for section 2 is typically between 60–80%, although the success rates again differ between trainees (approximately 70–90%) and non-trainees (approximately 20–50%).

Chapter 1.2

Preparation for the fellowship examination

We are what we repeatedly do. Excellence, therefore, is not an act, but a habit. (Aristotle, 384–322BC)

It is no exaggeration to say that this chapter is one of the most important in this book. We recommend that you repeatedly refer back to it during your preparations. Successful negotiation of the fellowship examination in general surgery requires adequate time, planning, energy and focus. In sporting terms, it represents a 'marathon' and not a 'sprint' and your preparation should reflect this. You would not contemplate attempting to run a marathon and expect to finish if you hadn't adequately trained or prepared for the event! There are two important components to get right if you are to be successful in the fellowship examination: (i) the preparation leading up to the exam ('the training') and (ii) performance within the exam ('the race'). All too often, candidates are unable to establish or maintain direction, focus or even motivation when preparing for the examination, especially as preparations often begin 6–12 months prior to the exam. Similarly, many 'otherwise good' candidates let themselves down by not performing to the best of their ability during the exam itself. Accordingly, this chapter aims to provide a basic approach and style to help you organise and maximise your preparations leading up to the exam and optimise your performance within it. Our intention is to furnish you with the necessary 'tactics' and 'strategies' to maximise your chances of success in the exam.

We are the first to acknowledge that there is more than one style or way to approach the exam to ensure success. Indeed, many candidates become quite confused by receiving varying opinions from different mentors that at times appear to be contrary. We advise candidates to adopt a style that incorporates as many of the tips and approaches learned from recent candidates and mentors as possible. Having *a* style and having thought about tactics for the exam is far more important than the specific nature of what is adopted. The approach and style employed in this chapter has proved valuable for the numerous candidates that we have successfully coached over the years and has the advantage of being reproducible and easy to recall during the pressure of the exam. We recommend the use of the acronym 'PASS' to shape your preparation and performance:

PASS the exam

Plan, prepare and practise

Awareness of aims, format and marking scheme of the examination

Syllabus

Structure

Plan, prepare and practise

Plan your studies

In general terms, planning for the examination relates to the assembly of all the necessary materials/resources required for study (as detailed within this chapter) and the subsequent creation of a study plan. The importance of having an appropriate study plan cannot be overemphasised. The breadth and depth of basic and clinical science, clinical practice and operative surgical knowledge assessed in the fellowship examination is formidable. A study plan will help break this formidable list of topics down into finite, manageable sections that can be learned in a systematic fashion. More importantly, it will impose 'deadlines' to work towards to ensure that your preparations stay 'on track'. It is easy to become disorientated and bogged down in the minutia of subspecialty practice and lose days/weeks of study time. However, demonstration of a good performance within each of the sections of the examination across the generality of surgery is necessary to pass. Accordingly, your timetable should cover the entire syllabus. Don't forget to 'reward' yourself to maintain motivation, as you successfully negotiate each of these sections, especially if achieved 'on time'.

In addition, most successful candidates manage to achieve a nice rhythm to their studies with acquisition and revision of pertinent facts at a constant pace, rather than cramming at the last minute. A plan will help pace your preparations and will avoid 'burn-out' and nonchalance. Optimum methods of learning will vary between candidates, so incorporate your preferred methods and play to your strengths when creating your plan. Don't forget to generate a plan for each of the seven components of the examination and devote an appropriate proportion of time to each. It is also important to work adequate breaks/holidays into your schedule; it is *unrealistic* to expect that you can work continuously for up to 12 months without a break!

Prepare

With an appropriate plan in place, preparations can begin in earnest. Frequently, it is a group pursuit rather than a solo exercise, especially when it comes to practising and rehearsing for the five *viva voce* examinations. Everyone has different styles and preferences for study. Some like covering the curriculum, including reading texts and journals, on their own, while others prefer to join a '*study group*'. Study groups typically consist of 2–7 candidates, depending on the region and hospital, and facilitate the sharing of information, resources and experiences and provide an excellent forum for 'mock *vivas*'. Additionally, as the members of a study group may be drawn from a number of hospitals across a city or region, there is increased access to mentors from each of these hospitals for practise *viva* sessions. By maximising the number of 'mock sessions' that you take part in, your performance in the exam will be enhanced through personal practise and by observing the techniques/mistakes of others being tested. You should also try to attend a 'preparation course'. Many regions have well organised courses for the fellowship examination. These are often an invaluable source of information that will make you appreciate the knowledge and verbal and clinical skills required to pass the exam.

Preparing for the examination clearly involves the acquisition/revision of knowledge and techniques for the examination, but it is also important to prepare psychologically. This is pertinent not only to the long run-up to the exam, but also performance within it. For most candidates, this examination is the most important of their life and represents the final barrier to independent practice as a specialist general surgeon, frequently reflecting the culmination of 25–35 years of education since childhood. Accordingly, most (honest!) candidates find it to be the most anxiety-provoking experience of their lives. The amount of pressure associated with this examination is unparalleled with so much riding on it. In addition, the preparation for this exam is longer and more intense than any other. Unsurprisingly, maintenance of psychological wellbeing and mental stamina is integral to allow studies/revision to progress. It can also prove very difficult balancing work, social and family commitments to allow productive study. However, it is important (and a relief) to realise that most (honest!) candidates consider the exam to be reasonably fair and 'very passable' upon reflection after the event.

An important factor in achieving success is to 'stay in shape' psychologically during those deep dark hours submerged in textbooks. We recommend two strategies, frequently employed in sports and corporate arenas, to achieve optimum 'psychological' performance in the run-up to and within the exam, respectively. Firstly, remain focused on the prize on offer in the run-up to the exam. It is a Fellowship in General Surgery. Use this as your motivation whenever your focus wanes, remembering that it is *the ultimate* prize that represents the culmination of your training and attainment of 'specialist status'. After years as a junior doctor, you will finally be able to work as a consultant general surgeon and to begin enjoying the clinical status and satisfaction, as well as the financial rewards that it affords. If contemplation of this 'intangible' reward proves insufficient to maintain your focus, consider rewarding yourself (and your family) with a more tangible prize, such as a well-earned holiday or expensive purchase. Secondly, remain focused on optimising your performance during the examination itself. Athletes and business entrepreneurs 'dream of winning' and rehearse the race/sales pitch a thousand times in their head prior to the 'big day' to ensure successful delivery. Similarly, there is no excuse for you to not be prepared to answer predictable and common questions that repeatedly come up in the examination. This doesn't necessarily mean memorising responses '*ad verbatim*' but you should have a 'standard patter' ready to roll out for trauma scenarios, dealing with intraoperative complications etc. We will aim to provide some of these approaches/model answers as we progress through this book.

Practise, practise, practise

Even with the most thorough intellectual and psychological preparations, candidates who haven't practised sufficiently will be unsuccessful in the exam. Drawing on our previous analogy, it is impossible to imagine an athlete presenting to a big event without having taken part in practise events. Further, the vast majority of the material encountered in the examination is predictable, as alluded to above, and thus can be practised ahead of the exam to guarantee a superior performance on the day. Candidates who are well-practised not only find themselves more at ease and comfortable during the exam, but they also score higher, as they run through their 'rehearsed' response/answer.

Indeed, you should be aiming to practise every component of the exam to such an extent that you find the majority of the cases/questions that you are presented with in the exam a 'gift'. When you are actually in the exam, you should barely be able to contain your eagerness to demonstrate your knowledge to the examiners when questioned on particular topics, just as you have practised on numerous occasions over the preceding months.

It is imperative that you prepare sample written answers and organise practise *viva* sessions with surgical tutors ahead of the exam. Even though everyone is different, a good rule of thumb is that you should be practising medium and short cases for 6–18 months prior to the examination. Many successful candidates have at least three 1-hour tutorials per week for 6–12 months prior to the fellowship examination. In fact, some have six tutorials per week in the last 3 months prior to examination. Do not be concerned about approaching your tutors, many of whom will be able to relate to the position that you are in and be willing to teach. Each candidate presenting for the exam will have 14 examiners in all, 10 of whom cover the *vivas*. To replicate the diversity of examiners, you will need a range of 'practise *viva*' tutors. Acquiring the knowledge from a book or journal to facilitate the construction of answers may be a solo pursuit, but the ability to verbalise your answers to simulate the *viva voce* is a completely separate activity that requires a different set of skills. This can only be practised by actually speaking in a group or in formal tutorial sessions that simulate the exam. Finding that you fall short of what is expected, at least initially, is an essential part of preparation. You must also practise the written examinations and submit them for critiquing. It is better to feel the pain during training than to suffer the pain of failing at the examination. Another useful strategy includes accessing the anatomy department at your local university to examine specimens. Such a session tends to be more productive if you set aside specific periods of time to attend with peers so that you can examine each other and try to coerce a mentor to come along to act as an examiner if possible.

You will be amazed at how your technique improves with practise. Nothing is more annoying for a candidate than to know an answer and not to be able to communicate it. Remember that you are likely to be judged very early on in a written or verbal answer by the content of your words. Smooth talking does not necessarily come naturally, and just like the ease of flow of music from a great concert pianist, great written and *viva* technique only comes from repetition and practise. Mock *vivas* will also enable you to develop the appropriate level of confidence and humility when answering exam questions.

A recent successful candidate noted:

> *From years gone by, there are also thousands of notes and useful presentations accumulated and passed on from trainee to trainee. They are useful for quick summaries. I found study group extremely helpful. It won't be useful if you haven't done any reading but it does motivate you to study. We had a schedule of topics to cover by a certain time to keep us on track. We did all the past written papers going back over the last 10 years. Study group also helps clarify things that you have learned. It is surprising how different people study and interpret things differently. It is important to remember that you don't have to all agree, there is often more than one way to approach problems, but you do have to be safe. It is unhelpful for the group to argue about the best way of doing something as there may be more than one way. The most important thing about study group is that it makes you talk, which is what happens in the exam. The ability to present, discuss and justify the information you have learned and the way you have chosen to do something is what the exam is all about and is something we don't do enough of during our training, especially in a structured, logical and succinct manner.*

Awareness of the aims, format and marking scheme of the examination

Most successful individuals in the examination, and in life in general, have an astute awareness and comprehensive appreciation of what will determine success. More importantly, they are able to distinguish factors that will lead to success from those that lead to failure. Frequently, this gives rise to an impressive, often uncompromising, focus to achieve certain aims/goals. With respect to the examination, to give you the very best chance of success, it is imperative that you are aware of:

- the required overall standard to pass
- what format the examination takes
- how the exam is marked.

Your chances of achieving a favourable outcome in the exam will be significantly improved with this awareness at the forefront of your mind whilst preparing and sitting the examination.

Awareness of the aim of the fellowship examination

It is important to appreciate that the expected standard at the fellowship examination is that equivalent to a surgeon fit to enter safe general surgical practice. Accordingly, the expectation is a level of knowledge that would be required of a competent general surgeon to safely look after his/her patients. It is not a test of subspecialist surgical practice as a colorectal, upper gastrointestinal or breast surgeon. All too often candidates overlook the fact that it is a *clinical* examination and in their desire to pass the examination they elect to take time away from clinical training and busy jobs. However, such candidates are less likely to be successful than those immersed in active, busy clinical practice. It is imperative that you keep this 'standard' in mind whilst you are preparing for and participating in the exam. Look at your bosses and try to 'talk the same language'. Consultant general surgeons tend to be logical, pragmatic, considered and decisive. All too often, candidates come across as being chaotic, unrealistic, ill-advised and too indecisive; the exact opposite of what the examiners are looking for. Present yourself as a safe, confident (but not arrogant) consultant general surgeon and you will have every chance of passing the examination.

Awareness of the examination format (FRACS only)

Refer to Chapter 1.1 for more detailed information relating to the format of the examination to pace your progression through the various components on the day. The RACS publication *General surgery fellowship examination candidate guide* is an excellent 27 page publication that describes the fellowship examination and what is expected of candidates. The examinations department of RACS also has documents it sends out to candidates to help familiarise themselves with the format of the examinations.

Awareness of the marking system/court process (FRACS only)

It is unimaginable to prepare for, or sit an examination without being aware of how you can accumulate sufficient marks to pass. Currently, the fellowship examination system employs a closed marking system using a Likert scale, with two examiners for each of the seven exam components. The two examiners decide, by consensus, whether to award a mark of either 8.0 (clear fail), 8.5 (borderline pass/fail), 9.0 (pass) or 9.5 (good pass). It is unlikely that a candidate who has scored an 8.0 in any component of the examination will pass the fellowship examination. After the seven examination components have been marked, the examiners in general surgery meet under the chairmanship of the senior examiner in the Specialty Court of General Surgery. Candidates who achieve a combined total score of 63 or more, and a score of 9 or more in both clinical exams, are automatically approved to pass. Those who receive a score of 62.5 or more, with a score of 9 or more in at least one clinical exam, may be discussed or may be approved to pass without discussion, according to the court's deliberations. All candidates who score 62.5 and 62.0 are discussed by the court, where all the seven exam components for each candidate are discussed. After explaining the allocation of marks for each component, examiners are not able to talk a candidate 'down', only talk a candidate 'up'. This has the effect that about 50% of those discussed with 62.5 and 25% of those with 62.0 end up passing the exam. Candidates who score 61.5 and below are usually failed without discussion, although occasionally candidates with 61.5 may be discussed but few will pass.

Many successful candidates remark that they felt that the examiners were trying to pass them and that the system was fair. The above process also tends to favour 'passing', rather than failing a candidate. It has been our observation over the years that generally unsuccessful candidates who blame the examiners or the exam process for their failure tend to lack a degree of insight into the purpose and mechanics of the exam and will only be successful once they are able to change their attitude and approach to the exam. If you fall into this category (and have enough insight to appreciate it!), enlist the help of objective, unbiased mentors/peers and be receptive to their criticisms and be prepared to radically overhaul your approach; this may be the only way that you will ever pass the exam.

Syllabus of the Fellowship exam (FRACS only)

It is essential that you adequately familiarise yourself with what you need to know. Many candidates experience uncertainty about this and can become overwhelmed and intimidated by the volume of potential topics. We recommend an initial five-step approach to circumvent this:

1. use Chapter 1.3 of this book to create a 'learning list'
2. obtain/review the General Surgery Curriculum of the Board in General Surgery
3. obtain previous written paper 2 papers from the RACS
4. liaise with recent candidates/supervisors
5. use the suggested reading list in Chapter 1.4 of this book.

There is no 'official' syllabus for the Fellowship examination. However, our scrutiny of previous examination questions has enabled us to establish that the examination content, perhaps not surprisingly, reflects the general surgery curriculum as produced and published by the Board in General Surgery. Therefore, it is essential that you obtain and review the content of the curriculum and organise your revision accordingly. To facilitate your studies, we have collected and catalogued past papers and questions from the last 10 years to compile a list of the most frequently encountered topics within each section of the exam. Chapter 1.3 provides a summary of this information and the ensuing sections of this book mirror the individual components of the current fellowship examination to provide model answers/suggested structures to address this content.

You should also obtain past written papers. The last 10 years of the second written paper (each consisting of eight questions) are available from the College. Many recent candidates and hospital supervisors will also have lists of what has been examined in the 'written paper 1'. However, you cannot obtain the actual papers. Many recent candidates and supervisors will also have lists of what is asked and expected in the five *viva voce* examinations. It is not the ability to regurgitate answers to 'past questions' that helps achieve success, moreover, it is the accumulation of the knowledge and 'know-how' required to answer these questions that leads to enhanced performance. Finally, you should peruse general surgical and allied texts to help identify any gaps or 'missed' topics that need to be addressed. Chapter 1.4 details some of the suggested resources to help your preparations.

Structure, structure, structure

Arguably, the most important factor in determining success in the fellowship examination is the ability to present a structured response. This is the one key distinguishing feature that separates 'good' from 'under-performing' candidates. It is so important and so commonly and regularly neglected by candidates in the exam that it justifies reemphasis; *always use a structure when answering questions*. Having 'inputted' and retained all that knowledge, do not compromise your performance in the exam by being unable to 'output' and communicate it to the examiners in a coherent, logical manner. The subsequent sections of this book will provide suggested structures and approaches to tackle different questions within each of the various components of the exam. It is important to appreciate the importance of structure for the following reasons:

The importance of structure

1. **Exemplifies the approach of a competent general surgical consultant — exactly what you are trying to demonstrate in the exam.**
2. **A key factor in distinguishing good from borderline/failing candidates — you don't want to be the latter.**
3. **Actually makes it easier for you to deliver the knowledge/information that is inside your head to the examiners to ensure that they award marks appropriately.**
4. **The most commonly neglected/forgotten principle of exam technique — observe how often you and your peers forget to structure your answers when practising mock examinations.**
5. **Allied to (4), providing unstructured (written/verbal) answers is the easiest way to annoy/frustrate examiners and get them offside!**
6. **Imperative when dealing with surgical emergencies/critical care — remember the acronyms of EMST/ATLS etc.**
7. **Buys you precious seconds to compose your thoughts when faced with seemingly difficult/unfamiliar scenarios, particularly under the extreme pressure of the exam.**

We advocate the use of the 'five Ss' (silence, say, succinct, schema, systematic) approach to structure the answer to any question/scenario.

1. Silence — pause for a second (or two) to (i) compose your thoughts and (ii) *ensure* that you answer the question that you *have* been asked, not the one you *hoped* you would have been asked. Always engage your brain before your pen or your mouth — another common mistake made by unsuccessful candidates.
2. Say 'it depends' — the answer to most questions is 'it depends'. Responses will be different in varying circumstances. Medicine is rarely static and predictable. Your

answer should acknowledge this. For example, management of common bile duct stones at laparoscopic cholecystectomy depends on: (i) patient factors; (ii) surgeons factors; (iii) institutional factors.

3. Succinct answer — do not be tempted to over embellish or make your response too verbose. Whilst it can be useful to try to control the exam and steer it in a preferred direction, be careful not to 'dig holes' for yourself or mention subjects/terms that you are not confident talking about. You should be aiming for a detailed and concise response that sufficiently answers the examiner's question to maximise the number of points scored. Producing succinct responses and avoidance of straying into 'dangerous territory' is only possible after extensive practise and again emphasises the need to immerse yourself in mock exam situations, as described above.
4. Schema for your answer — we advise candidates to frame their answer in terms of 'suburbs, streets and houses'. This means providing a general comment (the suburb), followed by the main subheadings next (the streets) and only then fill in the finer details (the houses) using a systematic approach (see below). There is no use giving the 15th most likely cause of pancreatitis first, if you have not mentioned alcohol and gallstones already. Similarly, if you are asked how to stage a particular cancer, do not jump straight into intricate details of the tumour classification without first stating which staging system you are using (the suburb), followed by its constituent details; for example, tumour, lymph node status and presence or absence of metastases (the streets). Only then should you expand the information within each (the houses).
5. Systematic approach — very often in the exam, and in real-life surgical practice, you need to think on your feet and have multiple options to succinctly and eloquently answer questions or to create lists of differential diagnoses, especially in the *viva voces*. This task is made substantially easier by structuring the answer using an appropriate system or classification. Commonly employed and successful methods include:
   a. most common to least common
   b. an anatomical approach, such as pre-hepatic, hepatic and post-hepatic causes of jaundice or anterior abdominal wall, intraperitoneal, retroperitoneal, back structures to stratify causes of abdominal pain/masses
   c. use of a surgical sieve approach using acronyms such as TIN CAN BED (traumatic, inflammatory/infective, neoplastic [primary/secondary], connective tissue, arteriovenous, nutritional, biochemical, endocrine, degenerative/drugs) or VITAMIN C (vascular, inflammatory, traumatic, autoimmune, metabolic, infective, neoplastic, congenital)
   d. use of tailored approaches relevant to specific scenarios making use of acronyms when appropriate, such as using CHIASMA (congestive, haematological, inflammatory/infective, autoimmune/alcohol, storage disorders [Wilsons/Gauchers], masses, amyloid) to classify the causes of hepatosplenomegaly.

Summary/key points

Ensure that you **PASS** the exam by:

- **p**lanning, **p**reparing and **p**racticing for the exam
- being **a**ware of the aims, format *and* marking scheme of the examination
- covering the entire **s**yllabus when studying
- using a **s**tructure when answering *every* question that incorporates the five Ss — silence, say, succinct, schema, systematic.

Chapter 1.3

Important topics for the fellowship examination

Using official College material and extensive feedback from previous candidates sitting the exam, we have collected and catalogued past papers and questions during the last 10 years to assemble the list of the *most frequently* encountered topics, which is provided in this chapter. This is provided for each of the seven sections of the current fellowship examination and the remainder of this book will be arranged in sections to mirror this format.

While this list covers approximately 80–90% of the content that may be examined in the examination, it is vital to appreciate that the list is not absolutely comprehensive as it is impossible to include every single topic that has ever been examined in the fellowship. Further, the content of the exam changes from year to year and will continue to do so in the future. The purpose of this chapter is to provide a list of common topics that serves as a 'checklist' of material to be learned. Use of this chapter will hopefully prevent you from spending too much time on 'preferred' topics and not enough time on 'less desirable' topics. The astute reader will note that the lists reflect the topics within the 13 modules that are outlined in the general surgery curriculum and formal reference to it is strongly encouraged.

Written paper 1
Spot test questions

Abdominal wall and retroperitoneum
Groin/scrotal swellings

Breast
Breast cancer image
Phylloides tumour image
Nipple discharge image

Colorectal
Rectal cancer endoscopic image
Colon cancer, screening, polyps, staging
Clostridium difficile colitis image
Large bowel obstruction AXR image
Rectal prolapse image
Appendicitis CT image
Fistula-in-ano image
Fissure-in-ano image
Anal squamous cell carcinoma image
Perianal warts image

Duodenum and small bowel
Small bowel obstruction CT image
Small bowel obstruction AXR image
Meckel's diverticulum image
Gastrointestinal stromal tumour (GIST) image

Endocrine
Sestamibi parathyroid scan (adenoma)
Adrenal tumour image — photo or CT scan

Head and neck
Parotid swelling image
Submandibular stone-sialogram image

Skin and soft tissue
Malignant melanoma image
Basal cell carcinoma image
Squamous cell carcinoma

Surgical oncology

Lymphoscintogram image

Trauma

Pelvic fracture CT scan image, plain x-ray image
Splenic trauma grade IV CT image
Seatbelt injury image

Upper gastrointestinal and hepatobiliary

Barium swallow image — achalasia /oesophageal cancer
Gastric ulcer image
ERCP image — choledochal cyst
Liver anatomy image — segments, sectional anatomy (CT)
Pancreas CT image — pseudocyst
Splenic artery aneurysm — angiogram
Arterial, venous and lymphatic systems
Diabetic foot image
Ischaemic leg image

Written paper 2
Short answer questions

Abdominal wall and retroperitoneum

Inguinal hernia repair

Breast

Pathology report/synoptic reporting
Breast cancer — staging, histological features, ER/PR, genetics, investigations, reconstruction
Prophylactic mastectomy
Paget's disease of the nipple

Colorectal

Inherited conditions/genetics
Rectal dissection/autonomic nervous system
Laparoscopic surgery — indications advantages/disadvantages
ERAS (enhanced recovery after surgery)
Large bowel obstruction — management
Stenting — indications and role
Colonoscopic complications
Appendicitis — investigations and management

Duodenum and small bowel

Small bowel obstruction — management
Enterocutaneous fistula — management
Problems post terminal ileal resection

Endocrine

Solitary thyroid nodules — investigation and management
Thyrotoxicosis — aetiology and pathology
Primary hyperparathyroidism — aetiology, investigation and management
Pancreas cystic lesion
Phaeochromocytoma — investigation and management

Head and neck

Lymph node drainage levels and tumour drainage

Sepsis and the critically ill or compromised patient

Abdominal compartment syndrome
VRE (vancomycin resistant enterococci)

Skin and soft tissue

Malignant melanoma — surgery, sentinel lymph node biopsy, role of regional lymph nodes

Transplantation

Renal transplantation — post-operative problems, anuria
Donor nephrectomy consent
Risk of malignancy in transplant patients

Trauma

Blunt and/or penetrating injury — initial management
Laparostomy
Crush and compartment syndrome
Head injury
Burns

Upper gastrointestinal and hepatobiliary

Dysphagia
Gastro-oesophageal reflux disease — investigations and management
Oesophageal malignancy and stents
Obesity and bariatric surgery — indications, management and publications
Bleeding duodenal ulcer/haematemesis and meleana
Laparoscopic cholecystectomy and post-operative complications
Cirrhosis
Liver metastases/solid liver lesion — investigations and management
Pancreas mass
OPSI (overwhelming post-splenectomy infection)

Arterial, venous and lymphatic systems

Leg ulcers — causes and management
Measures to minimise lymphoedema

Other general topics

Post-operative complications — give list of principles
Causes/management of anaemia
Radiation hazard — how to decrease or minimise
Needle stick injury
Low post-operative urine output management

Clinical viva 1

Medium cases

Breast

Breast cancer

Colorectal

Rectal cancer
Colon cancer
Ulcerative colitis, +/– ileal pouch
Crohn's disease

Endocrine

Total thyroidectomy for papillary carcinoma or multinodular goitre

Upper gastrointestinal and hepatobiliary

Gastro-oesophageal reflux disease
Oesophageal cancer
Chronic stomach ulcer disease
Chronic liver disease, usually in conjunction with conditions such as hernia
Post-operative liver resection from colorectal metastases or HCC
Pancreatic tumour — insulinoma

Other general topics

Abdominal mass

Clinical viva 2
Short cases

Abdominal wall and retroperitoneum

Inguinal hernia — small, large inguinoscrotal, landmarks, sliding, treatment options
Incisional hernia

Breast

Bilateral gynaecomastia

Endocrine

Thyroid/multinodular goitre — Pemberton's sign

Head and neck

Parotid mass-tumours, benign and malignant

Skin and soft tissue

Dupuytren's contracture
Lipoma, sebaceous cyst, BCC, SCC, ganglion

Arterial, venous and lymphatic systems

Leg/ foot ulcers, +/– neuropathy, vascular disease, +/– diabetic foot
Lymphoedema

Other general topics

Median nerve palsy
Ulnar nerve palsy
Abdominal mass (any quadrant) hepatomegaly, splenomegaly, +/– jaundice

Surgical anatomy viva

Abdominal wall and retroperitoneum

Rectus, pyramidalis
Laparoscopic preperitoneal inguinal hernia
Femoral canal/femoral hernia operation anatomy

Breast

Axilla — the anatomy of an axillary dissection: boundaries, contents, arterial branches, brachial plexus

Endocrine

Thyroidectomy anatomy
Recurrent laryngeal nerve/relationships
Parathyroid glands — position

Head and neck

Facial nerve anatomy
Anterior/posterior triangles and contents
Submandibular gland and relations
Thoracic outlet

Upper gastrointestinal and hepatobiliary

Stomach anatomy
Anatomy of a laparoscopic or open cholecystectomy
Pancreas anatomy — embryology, divisum, annular, peripancreatic anatomy
Liver — hepatic resection anatomy

Arterial, venous and lymphatic systems

Superficial venous anatomy
Carotid endarterectomy — internal carotid and external carotid arteries and branches and related nerves
Subclavian artery and branches
Femoral artery
Popliteal artery — medial approach, popliteal fossa image
Aorta and its branches

Other general topics

Median nerve
Ulnar nerve
Femoral triangle — boundaries, floor, contents
Adductor canal

Diaphragm
Retroperitoneal anatomy — ureter (course, blood supply, significance)
CT scan transpyloric plane (L1)
CT scan trans-tubercular plane (L5)
Internal iliac artery branches, lateral pelvic view (hemi pelvis)

Operative surgery viva

Abdominal wall and retroperitoneum

Obstructed femoral hernia/elective femoral hernia operation

Breast

Axillary dissection

Colorectal

Ileostomy closure
Right hemicolectomy, bleeding from hepatic flexure veins, +/– caecal volvulus
Hartmann's procedure
Haemorrhoidectomy

Duodenum and small bowel

Small bowel resection

Endocrine

Total thyroidectomy

Head and neck

Thyroglossal cyst
Submandibular gland excision
Tracheostomy

Trauma

Blunt and/or penetrating injury, trauma laparotomy, damage control, supra coeliac clamp
Trauma splenectomy

Upper gastrointestinal and hepatobiliary

Perforated or bleeding gastric or duodenal ulcer
Common bile duct stones — management, intraoperative cholangiogram

Arterial, venous and lymphatic systems

High ligation long saphenous vein

Other general topics

Consent principles for example laparoscopic cholecystectomy or incisional hernia

Pathophysiology and critical care and clinical reasoning viva

Breast

Breast lumps

Colorectal

Anal sphincter anatomy in conjunction with fistula-in-ano
Pilonidal sinus

Duodenum and small bowel

Small bowel tumours

Endocrine

Thyroid cancer
Multinodular goitre

Sepsis and the critically ill or compromised patient

SIRS
MODS
Peritonitis
Necrotising fasciitis
Mesenteric ischaemia

Surgical oncology

Testicular tumours — classification

Trauma

Trauma case/shock
Tension pneumothorax — chest tube

Upper gastrointestinal and hepatobiliary

Barrett's oesophagus
Oesophageal tumour
Stomach cancer
Cholangitis
Hydatid cyst
Pancreatitis — ICU case scenario, complications, role of ERCP

Arterial, venous and lymphatic systems

DVT, VTE and prophylaxis

Other general topics

Anticoagulation management — warfarin, clopidogrel, aspirin, vitamin K, FFP — in conjunction with any operative emergency, for example bleeding duodenal ulcer, in conjunction with coronary stent, or obstructed femoral hernia patient.

Chapter 1.4

Suggested reading list

What to read? So many books, so little time!

The books, journals and materials listed below provide an indication of the spectrum of resources that are currently used by successful candidates when preparing for the Fellowship Examination in General Surgery. The use of any individual book or resource is clearly a personal decision and is subject to hospital/region/state variation. However, the range, rather than the choice, of specific books appears to be important in determining success in the exam, reflecting the fact that no one book or journal contains enough material to supply the necessary knowledge required in the exam. Accordingly, most candidates end up using an extensive range of books and resources during their preparations.

Some of the books in the following list are useful in more than one section of the examination. Also please note that many books and journals are available online at the RACS website.

Written examinations 1 and 2

ABC of Breast Diseases (ABC Series). Dixon J M. 2006, BMJ Books.
Companion to Specialist Surgical Practice (Series). Various authors. Saunders Limited.
Current Surgical Therapy, 10th edn. Cameron J L. 2010, Churchill Livingstone.
Sabiston Textbook of Surgery, 19th edn. 2012, Saunders.
Schwartz's Principles of Surgery, 9th edn. 2009, McGraw-Hill Professional.
Textbook of Surgery, 3rd edn. Tjandra J. 2006, Wiley-Blackwell.
NZ guidelines provided by the Ministry of Health in NZ, or Australian guidelines provided by NHMRC and NCCN guidelines for melanoma, colorectal and breast cancer.
Compile your own series of power point slides and sets of summary notes.

Clinical vivas

A Guide to Physician Training, 6th edn. Talley N J, O'Connor S. 2009, Churchill Livingstone. (This is a physician's handbook but covers many gastrointestinal conditions and how to deal with cases well.)

Advanced Surgical Recall, 3rd edn. Blackbourne L H. 2007, Lippincott Williams & Wilkins.
Bailey and Love's Short Practice of Surgery, 25th edn. Williams N S. 2008, Hodder Arnold Publishers.
Browse's Introduction to the Symptoms & Signs of Surgical Disease, 4th edn. Browse N L. 2005, Hodder Arnold Publishers.
Clinical Cases & OSCEs in Surgery, 2nd edn. Ramachandran & Gladman. 2011, Churchill Livingstone.
Clinical Cases for Surgery Exams. Lim T, Robless P A, Tan C T K. 2009, World Scientific Publishing Company.
Hamilton Bailey's Physical Signs: Demonstration of Physical Signs in Clinical Surgery, 18th edn. Lumley J S P (ed). 1997, Hodder Arnold Publishers.
Passing the General Surgery Board Exam. Neff M A. 2005, Springer Publishing.
Surgical Short Cases for the MRCS examination. Revised edition. Parchment-Smith C. 2006. Cambridge University Press.

Anatomy viva

Anatomy of General Surgical Operations, 2nd edn. Jamieson G G. 2006, Churchill Livingstone.
Atlas of Human Anatomy, 5th edn. Netter F H. 2010, Saunders.
Colour Atlas of Anatomy, 7th edn. Rohen J W, Lutien-Drecoll E, Yokochi C. 2010, Lippincott Williams & Wilkins.
Instant Anatomy, 4th edn. Whitaker R H, Borley N R. 2010, Wiley-Blackwell.
Last's Anatomy: Regional and Applied, 12th edn. Sinnatamby. C.S. 2011, Churchill Livingstone.
McMinn's Color Atlas of Human Anatomy, 5th edn. Abrahams P H, McMinn R M H, Marks S C, Hutchings R T. 2003, Mosby-Year Book.
Use of prosections in anatomy museums.
Brisbane 2000 Classification system for liver anatomy. Online. Available at: http://www.ahpba.org/index.php?option=com_content&view=article&id=35
or http://www.ihpba.org/mc/page.do?sitePageId=103192

Operative viva

Anatomic Exposure in Vascular Surgery, 2nd edn. Valentine R J, Wind G C. 2003, Lippincott Williams & Wilkins. (operative and anatomy)
Chassin's Operative Strategy in General Surgery, 3rd edn. Scott-Conner C E H. 2002, Springer Publishing. (Gives consideration to surgical pitfalls and how to cope with pathology intra-operatively.)
General Surgical Operations, 5th edn. Kirk R M. 2006, Churchill Livingstone. (Brief, but a good start and covers many procedures.)
Maingot's Abdominal Operations, 11th edn. Zinner M, Ashley S. 2006, McGraw-Hill Professional.
Shackelford's Surgery of the Alimentary Tract, 6th edn. Yeo C J. 2006, Saunders.
Surgical Anatomy and Technique: A Pocket Manual, 3rd edn. Skandalakis L J, Skandalakis J F., Skandalakis P N. 2008, Springer Publishing.

Zollinger's Atlas of Surgical Operations, 9th edn. Zollinger R, Ellison E. 2010, McGraw-Hill Professional.
Your own operation notes that you have collected during the last 5 years of training.

Pathophysiology and critical care and clinical reasoning viva

CCrISP course manual.
DSTC course manual.
EMST/ATLS course manual.
Robin's and Cotran Pathologic Basis of Disease, 8th edn. Kumar V, Abbas A K, Fausto N, Aster J. 2009, Saunders.

General reading

British Journal of Surgery, *Surgical Clinics of North America*, and *Colorectal Disease*
Current Diagnosis and Treatment Surgery, 13th edn. Doherty G. 2009, McGraw-Hill Medical
Last 2 years of relevant articles in the *Australian and New Zealand Journal of Surgery*

Section 2

The written papers

Chapter 2.1

The written examination paper 1 — spot test questions

The secret of getting ahead is getting started. The secret of getting started is breaking your complex overwhelming tasks into small manageable tasks, and then starting on the first one. (Mark Twain, 1835–1910)

The examination format

The first written paper comprises 25 spot test questions, which must be completed within 2 hours, resulting in 4.8 minutes per question. Candidates are allowed into the examination room 15 minutes prior to the commencement of the examination and are given 10 minutes reading time prior to the official start. Candidates receive the 25 spot test questions all in one examination booklet, which is set out with an image on the left-hand side of the page and the questions, with sufficient space to write the answers, on the right-hand side of the page. There are only about 5 to 10 lines in which to write each answer. There is a large bank of images that is continually changed from which the spot test questions are created. The examination booklets cannot be removed from the examination, so the images are not in the public domain. However, there is a tendency for similar questions, and thus similar images, to repeat.

The emphasis of this section of the examination is on factual knowledge and if you know the material you will pass. For each of the 25 questions, the image provides the stimulus or trigger for the ensuing questions. Typically, the questions following each image adhere to the following pattern:

1. What is the diagnosis?
2. What is the differential diagnosis?
3. Which investigations would you perform/are appropriate/are diagnostic in this condition?
4. What is the management?

Exam technique

- A sensible approach is to spend 4 minutes on each question, which will leave you 20 minutes at the end of the examination to check your answers and complete any unanswered questions.

- Irrespective of the order that you choose to answer the questions in, make sure that you answer *all* 25 questions. Remember that a 'good' pass in half the questions will not compensate for a 'fail' in other questions that have been answered inadequately or not at all.
- Once you have read the examination paper you may be happy to answer the questions in order from 1 through to 25. However, many candidates prefer to answer the questions they consider 'easiest' first and tackle 'more difficult' questions last. Regardless of the order, be aware of the time and *do not* write for more than 4 minutes per question!
- Make your answer easy to read and be sure that every word is legible. Examiners can only award marks if they can read the content of your response.
- The written papers are photocopied and sent to the examiners for marking. This means that there will be *no* benefit from using coloured markers or highlighters.

Many of these techniques will be demonstrated in the model answers in Chapter 2.2.

Preparation and practising

Look at the list of common spot test questions in Chapter 1.3 and expand it by discussing with previous exam candidates to establish the topics that they encountered. With this information to hand it is imperative that you practise frequently. Images can easily be found on the internet and in everyday clinical practice and it is a good idea to create 'mock' examinations in your study group to gain experience looking at images and answering questions pertinent to them. It is a good idea to have your tutors check the questions and answers.

There is a limit to what you can write in 4 minutes and thus the examiners are frequently looking for key words/terms/phrases and salient points rather than long verbose responses. It is critical to keep this in mind when writing your responses.

It is helpful to run through the following checklist of interventions that are pertinent for the non-surgical treatment of patients with surgical diseases. It is important to appreciate that not every intervention is indicated in every case, but this list will serve as an *aide-memoire* to prevent you forgetting fundamental components to the answers in the written papers (and vivas).

The ABCDEFG of non-surgical treatment of surgical patients

- **A** Analgesia/antibiotics
- **B** Breathing optimisation (e.g. nebulisers)/bowel preparation
- **C** Catheter/consent
- **D** DVT prophylaxis/drain insertion (NGT)
- **E** Electrolyte correction/emesis prevention
- **F** Fluid resuscitation/ferrous (iron)
- **G** Gastric protection/glucose (nutritional) provision

Chapter 2.2

Common written examination spot test questions: model answers

By identifying the most frequently encountered topics in recent years, we have been able to provide examples of typical images and questions encountered in this section of the examination. In the following pages, we will present images depicting pertinent pathology/abnormalities together with a series of questions and sample answers to help you appreciate the nature and style of questions encountered in this section of the exam.

2.2.1 Scrotal swelling

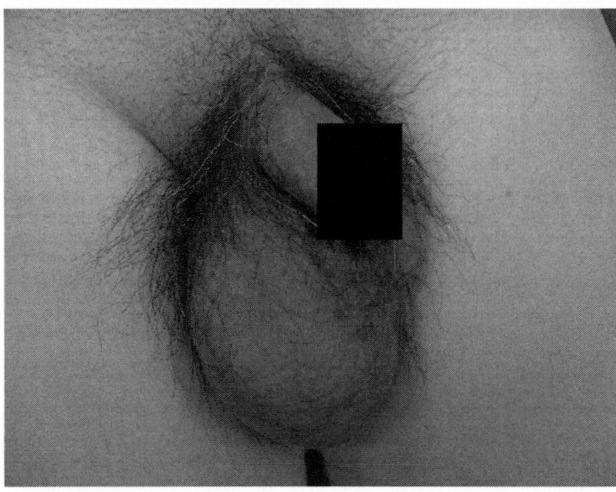

Figure 2.2.1
Right epididymal cyst

Please read in conjunction with 3.5.1, inguinal hernia.

1. What are the causes of this swelling?
   - A swelling arising within the scrotum:
     - epididymal cyst, hydrocoele, spermatocoele, testicular malignancy, infection (epididymal-orchitis/syphilis), varicocoele. If acute — trauma/testicular torsion.
   - Extension of a groin swelling into the scrotum:
     - indirect inguinal hernia, congenital hydrocoele.
2. How do you distinguish between causes?
   - By examination utilising palpation and transillumination to answer the following four questions.
     a. Can I get above it?
        - No = groin swelling.
        - Yes = confined to scrotal structures.
     b. Is it reducible?
        - Yes = hernia.
        - No = scrotal pathology.
     c. Can I palpate the testicle separate from the swelling?
        - Most epididymal cysts are posterior to the testis and most hydrocoeles are anterior.
     d. Do the contents transilluminate?
        - Epididymal cysts, hydrocoeles and (most) spermatocoeles transilluminate.
3. Which investigations would you perform?
   - Scrotal ultrasound (US).
   - May require renal ultrasound and/or CT scan abdomen depending on the results of the scrotal US.
   - If testicular tumour — above plus chest x-ray, α-fetoprotein, β-hCG, LDH.

2.2.2 Breast cancer

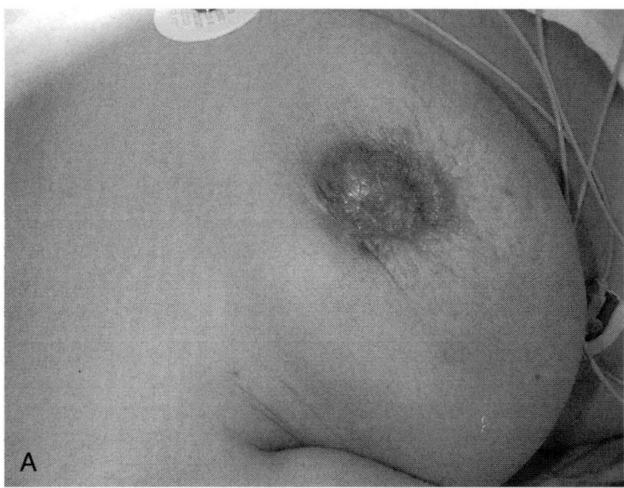

Figure 2.2.2A
Locally advanced central breast cancer (female)

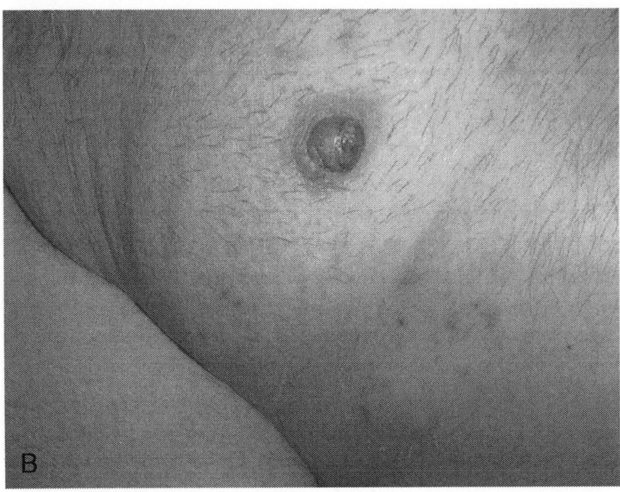

Figure 2.2.2B
Breast cancer (male)

Please read in conjunction with 3.3.1, breast cancer medium case, 4.4.3, axillary dissection, and 4.6.1 synoptic breast pathology reporting.

1. What is the diagnosis in these two images?
   - A: breast cancer in a female patient.
   - B: cancer in a male breast.
2. What are the risk factors for B?
   - Age: male breast cancer typically occurs 15 years later in men than in women.
   - Hyperoestrogenic states: e.g. (i) Klinefelter's syndrome (47XXY), (ii) testicular dysgenesis/cryptorchidism, (iii) obesity, (iv) alcoholism and liver impairment.
   - Chest irradiation: e.g. Hodgkin's disease.
   - Occupational exposures: electromagnetic fields, high temperature.
   - Genetic causes: up to 20% have a first degree relative with breast cancer, and BRCA2 mutations are the most commonly observed alterations in males with breast cancer. Rare: Cowden Syndrome and CHEK2.
3. How would you manage B?
   - Total mastectomy indicated in most men.
   - Post-mastectomy radiotherapy is frequently offered for poor prognostic features such as:
     - large tumour
     - >3 axillary nodes involved
     - high grade disease.
   - Sentinel lymph node biopsy (SLNB) suitable in clinically negative axilla. Clinically or SLNB positive axilla require formal axillary dissection.
   - Male breast cancer is more likely to be at a more advanced stage at presentation than female breast cancer, so overall prognosis is worse, but stage for stage prognosis is the same as for women.
   - Hormone receptor responsive tumours receive Tamoxifen for 5 years with evidence of improved survival.
   - Adjuvant chemotherapy if lymph nodes positive.

2.2.3 Bilateral gynaecomastia

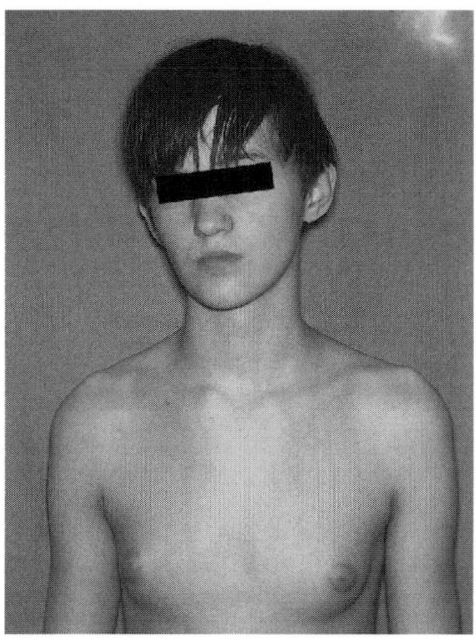

Figure 2.2.3
A teenage boy with Klinefelter syndrome (XXY) and bilateral gynaecomastia (Source: *Before We Are Born*, 8th edn. Moore K L et al. 2011, Saunders: an imprint of Elsevier, Fig 19-7.)

1. What is the diagnosis?
   - Bilateral gynaecomastia, probably physiological, with enlargement of ductal and stromal tissue.
2. What are the causes?
   - Physiological (20%): high serum oestradiol to testosterone ratio, seen in neonates, at puberty and in the elderly.
   - Pharmacological (20%): hormonal supplements (oestrogens), hormone inhibitors (cimetidine, spironolactone), drugs causing hyperprolactinaemia (e.g. phenothiazines, methyldopa, tricyclic antidepressants, metoclopramide), cytotoxic drugs (busulphan, vincristine), recreational drugs (e.g. marijuana). NB: you don't need to list all in the actual exam — any three drugs will do).
   - Pathological (35%):
     - liver disease, commonly alcoholic
     - increased oestrogen production such as hepatoma; testicular, pituitary and adrenal tumours; paraneoplastic syndrome (e.g. bronchial carcinoma)
     - decreased oestrogen clearance such as in cirrhosis, haemochromatosis and Wilson's disease
     - decreased testosterone production such as in Klinefelter's syndrome, mumps, orchitis, bilateral cryptorchidism, or acquired testicular failure secondary to irradiation or hypopituitarism
     - testicular feminisation syndrome.
   - Idiopathic (25%): no other cause found.

3. Which investigations would you perform?
   - Adolescent males do not require investigation. They require reassurance that it is benign and self-limiting and that 75% improve over 2 years.
   - For the rest it depends on history and examination, but will likely include:
     - TFTs, LFTs, α-fetoprotein, β-hCG, prolactin
     - scrotal ultrasound in young men and USS/CT abdomen in older males to assess the liver
     - mammography if appropriate, otherwise breast ultrasound (especially if unilateral and FHx)
     - FNA or core biopsy if a discrete breast mass is palpable.

2.2.4 Paget's disease of the nipple

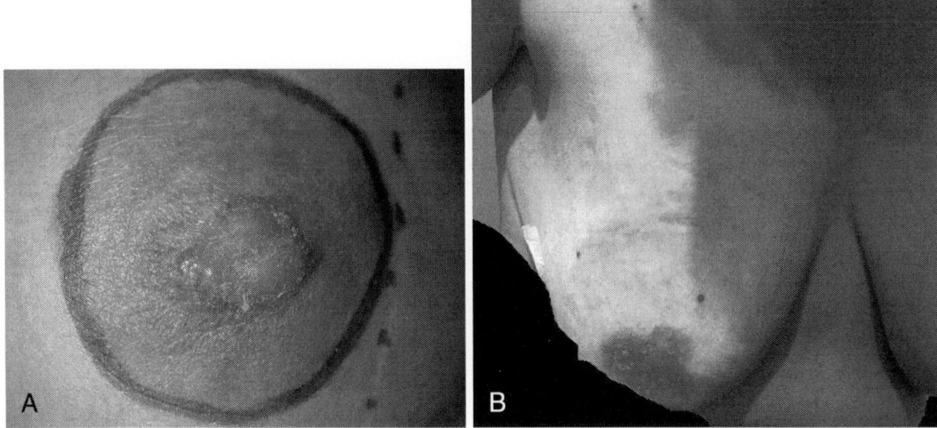

Figure 2.2.4
Paget's disease of the nipple

1. What is the diagnosis?
   - Paget's disease of the nipple.
2. What is the basis of this disease?
   - It is an eczematous change in the skin of the nipple due to Paget's cells (large cells with pale cytoplasm and prominent nucleoli) in the epidermis of the nipple.
   - More than 95% of women with Paget's disease of the nipple have an underlying malignancy (90% invasive, 10% DCIS), although almost half are clinically and mammographically undetectable.
   - Comprises 5% of breast malignancies — most patients are elderly.
3. What is the aetiology?
   Two hypotheses:
   a. The 'in situ transformation' hypothesis suggests Paget's cells arise from transformed malignant keratinocytes (Toker cells) and is thus a type of carcinoma in situ of the skin. This hypothesis is supported by the fact that the Paget's cells and the underlying cancer are often separated by some distance.
   b. The 'epidermotropic' hypothesis suggests ductal cells migrate along the basement membrane of ducts into the nipple epidermis. Immunohistochemical

studies support this hypothesis as there is similar staining of Paget's cells and the underlying carcinoma.

4. How does it present?
   - Symptoms include burning, itching and change in sensation of the nipple and areola.
   - Skin lesion which is raised, irregular and sharply demarcated from surrounding skin. There is often associated erythema and scaling of nipple.
   - Nipple retraction and discharge are uncommon.
5. What is the management of the condition?
   - Confirm diagnosis by core biopsy or wedge biopsy of nipple.
   - Begin with detailed mammographic examination with magnified views of the subareolar region and US of breast and axilla. If no lesion seen in preliminary investigation then MRI of breast.
   - Total mastectomy with sentinel node biopsy: suitable for women with diffuse disease or disease at a distance from nipple.
   - Wide local excision of nipple and underlying ducts is an option when disease localised to subareolar area or nipple areola complex. This is increasingly combined with radiotherapy although evidence is lacking due to rarity of disease.
6. What is the treatment when it occurs with DCIS?
   - Excision of nipple and central ducts if DCIS localised, consider radiotherapy.
   - Mastectomy if extensive underlying DCIS.

2.2.5 Rectal cancer

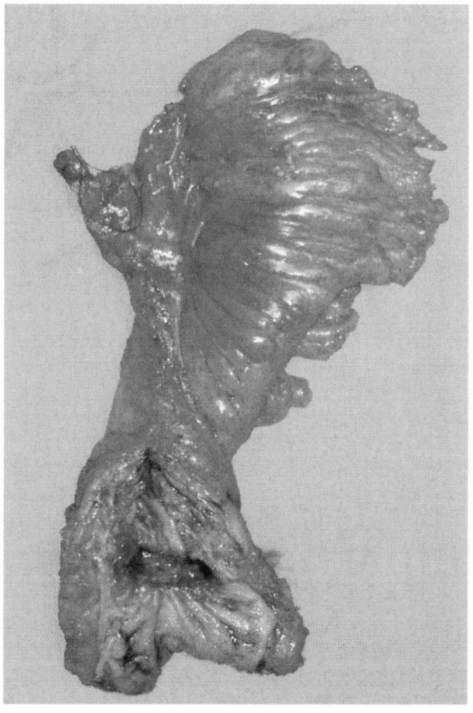

Figure 2.2.5
Low rectal cancer

Please read in conjunction with 3.3.2, rectal cancer medium case.

1. What is the diagnosis?
   - Low rectal cancer.
2. Which patients are more likely to receive this diagnosis?
   - Male > Female (M : F about 55%:45%).
   - Older: >90% of cases occur over 50 years of age. Median age is 68 years.
   - Personal and family history of colorectal cancer.
3. How did this patient most likely present?
   - Asymptomatic:
     - faecal occult blood testing (FOBT)
     - during surveillance colonoscopy.
   - Symptomatic detection:
     - rectal bleeding
     - change in bowel habit (typically to loose stools)
     - tenesmus
     - acute large bowel obstruction (up to one-third of cases).
4. Which histopathological features are associated with a poor prognosis?
   - Tumour factors:
     - tumour penetrating the visceral peritoneum or into an adjacent organ (T4 cancers)
     - obstructed or perforated cancer
     - poorly differentiated histology
     - lymphatic/venous/perineural invasion
     - anterior position of tumour.
   - Presence of lymph node metastases. Positive apical node involvement is even worse.
   - Presence of distant metastases.
   - Cancer at the (circumferential or distal) resection margin.

2.2.6 Clostridium difficile colitis

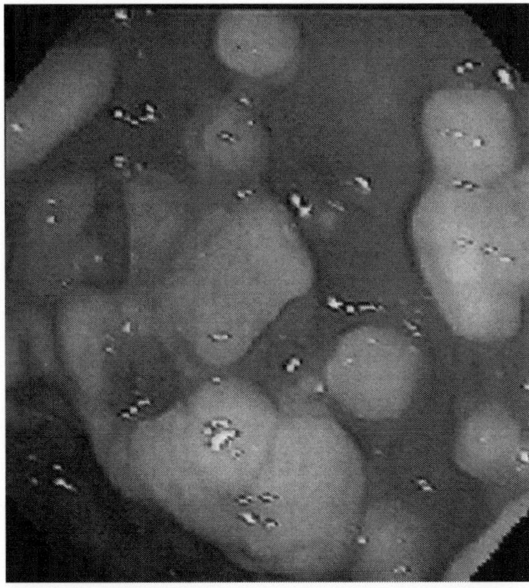

Figure 2.2.6
Pseudomembranous colitis

This patient presented with diarrhoea, abdominal distension and a WCC of 38.2.

1. What is the diagnosis?
   - This is a colonoscopic image of pseudomembranous colitis, with yellow membranes seen on the large bowel wall.
2. What is the cause and pathogenesis of this?
   - It is usually caused by clostridium difficile (C. difficile; spore forming organism, anerobic G+ve).
   - Administration of broad-spectrum antibiotics, especially penicillins, cephalosporins and clindamycin, leads to changes in normal colonic flora with resultant overgrowth of other commensals.
   - Other, rarer organisms: *Salmonella*, *Clostridium*, *Candida*, *Staph aureus*.
   - Proton pump inhibitors have been proposed as a risk factor (*Am J Gastroenterol* 2008; 103:2308–13).
   - C. difficile is resident in the gut of 3% of general population and 10% of patients in hospital.
   - C. difficile produces cytotoxins A (enterotoxin) and B (cytotoxin) which cause inflammation and mucosal damage.
   - Pseudomembranes comprised of bacteria, fibrin, mucus and neutrophils from intercrypt erosions.
   - Oedema and extensive lamina propria neutrophil infiltration.
   - Rectum is spared in one-quarter of cases.
3. What is your initial management?
   - Confirm diagnosis:
     - stool smear
     - C. difficile toxin can be detected in a faecal specimen
     - flexible sigmoidoscopy: elevated, yellow pseudomembranes with mucosal ulceration.
   - Correction of fluid and electrolyte status.
   - Contact isolation.
   - Cease antibiotic administration if possible (stop offending agent).
   - Commence Metronidazole 500 mg po tds for 14 days.
   - Monitor patient for complications (toxic megacolon or perforation).
   - Avoid antiperistaltic agents.
4. Initial management fails to improve the patient's clinical status — what options are now available?
   - Commence vancomycin 125 mg qid if not already receiving it.
   - Adjuncts to normalise colonic flora (probiotics).
   - Consult ID and exclude resistant strain.
   - Cholestyramine may be useful in refractory cases (binds toxin).
   - Up to 20% of patients with fulminant infections will require colectomy.
   - If colectomy required, mortality rate is 35–80%.
   - Recurrence of symptoms after successful treatment occurs in up to 20% of patients, which requires repeated antibiotic treatment. Use vancomycin for recurrences, if severe.

2.2.7 Colitis

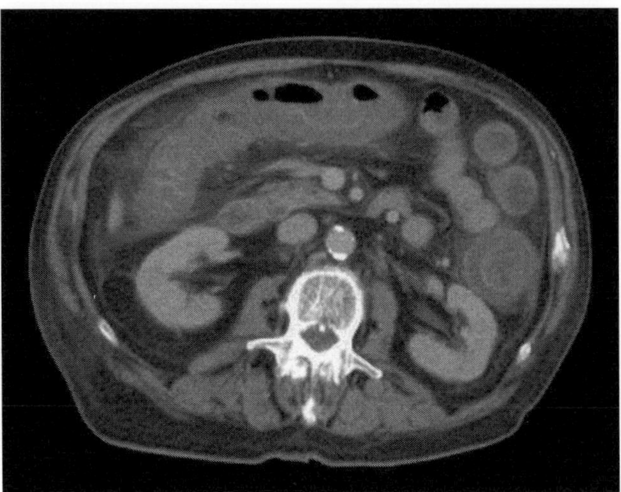

Figure 2.2.7
Colitis CT scan

1. Describe the findings?
   - Axial CT scan image at about L2 level showing thickened large bowel wall consistent with colitis.
2. What are the possible causes and their treatment?
   Infective
   - Bacterial
     - *Campylobacter*: usually self-limiting within a week or can treat with erythromycin 250 mg QID, ciprofloxacin 250–500 mg BD or doxycycline 100 mg BD for 7–10 days.
     - *Clostridium*: C. difficile — see 2.2.6 above.
     - *Escherichia coli*: treatment of toxin-producing *E. coli*: supportive, no antibiotics — may worsen.
     - *Salmonella*: *S. enteritidis* — most require no antibiotic treatment; *S. typhi* ('typhoid fever') — always treat: 3rd generation cephalosporins, but be alert for antibiotic resistance.
     - *Shigella*: usually self-limiting or treat with 3rd generation cephalosporin for 3–5 days.
     - *Vibrio cholerae*: treatment is supportive +/- azithromycin.
   - Viral
     - Rotavirus, Norwalk, CMV (especially in immunocompromised).
     - Usually self-limiting but anti-viral therapy (e.g. famcyclovoir/gancyclovoir) indicated in the immunocompromised.
   - Parasitic
     - Amoebic dysentery: Entamoeba histolytica infection. Treat with metronidazole for 10 days.
     - *Giardia lamblia* (flagellated protozoan). Treat with metronidazole 5 days.
     - *Cryptosporidium* (protozoan). Treatment: nitaxzoxanide.
     - Schistosomiasis (fluke). Treatment: praziquantel.

Non-infective

- Inflammatory bowel disease:
  - ulcerative colitis
  - Crohn's disease
  - indeterminate colitis (≈10%)
  - treat with anti-inflammatory (5ASA/steroids) or anti-TNF agents.
- Ischaemic colitis:
  - SMA/IMA territory of the colon may be affected. Typically, the watershed area of the distal transverse colon/splenic flexure is affected
  - acute infarction usually presents with profound compromise of the patient due to an acute (or acute on chronic) event. Aggressive resuscitation and timely surgical intervention with appropriate resection is indicated. Patient compromise usually makes a primary anastomosis undesirable
  - in the absence of acute infarction, the presentation is less dramatic with pain and/or bleeding PR. Treatment of such cases is usually non-surgical involving appropriate resuscitation and antibiotic administration and serial clinical, laboratory and radiological evaluation to ensure resolution. Occasionally, anticoagulant therapy is indicated.
- Diversion colitis:
  - inflammation of a previously normal segment of colon following formation of a temporary colostomy/ileostomy
  - resolves after stoma reversal
  - administration of short-chain fatty acid enemas may help.

Miscellaneous

- NSAID induced
- Amyloidosis
- Behcet's disease
- Malacoplakia (rare chronic granulomatous disease that can cause colonic strictures and may resemble colitis).
- Collagenous colitis, causes watery diarrhoea.

FURTHER NOTES — MICROBIOLOGY OF ACUTE COLITIS

Bacterial

- Campylobacter (gram -ve rod): usually food-borne. Usually self-limiting within a week, relapses in 20% of untreated patients. If prolonged or severe can treat with erythromycin 250 mg QID, ciprofloxacin 250–500 mg BD or doxycycline 100 mg BD for 7–10 days (enhances elimination but almost no difference to duration of symptoms).
- *Clostridium*: C. difficile — see 2.2.6 above. C. perfringens: enterotoxin from meat/poultry, usually self-limiting, but rarely ('type C' strain) can cause necrotising enteritis.
- *E. coli*: (i) enteroinvasive (serotypes 0124, 0136, 0143): cause necrosis and ulceration; (ii) enteropathogenic (serotypes 044, 0111, 0114, 0125) — unknown mechanism, causes destruction of microvilli; (iii) enterotoxic/enterotoxigenic (serotypes 0115, 0148, 0153) — heat-stable (cholera-like) toxin causes travellers and infant diarrhoea; (iv) enterohaemorrhagic (O157:H7) — has vero toxins which cause haemorrhagic colitis and can be associated with haemolytic uraemic syndrome and thrombocytopenic purpura. Treatment of toxin-producing *E. coli* — supportive, no antibiotics, may worsen.

- *Salmonella. S. enteritidis*: contaminated meat/eggs causes enterocolitis. Most require no antibiotic treatment; S typhi ('typhoid fever'): GI tract mucosa can bleed and/or the gut can perforate (through Peyer's patches), or cause peritonitis (10–20%; rarely require operation). Can get into lymphatics causing lymphadenopathy, splenomegaly, bacteraemia, systemic illness, meningitis. Can infect and colonise the gallbladder for entire life and remain contagious by shedding *S. typhi* in stool. Always treat: cotrimoxazole/amoxicillin, but be alert for antibiotic resistance.
- *Shigella* (gram -ve rod): very contagious person-to-person; direct damage and/or toxin effects. Usually self-limiting or treat with 3rd generation cephalosporin for 3–5 days.
- *Vibrio Cholera*: toxin causes increased cAMP levels in the cell. Treatment is supportive +/− azithromycin.

Viral

- Rotavirus, Norwalk, CMV (especially in immunocompromised).
- Usually self-limiting but anti-viral therapy (e.g. famcyclovoir/gancyclovoir) indicated in the immunocompromised.

Parasitic

- Amoebic dysentery: *Entamoeba histolytica* infection. Treat with metronidazole for 10 days.
- *Giardia lamblia* (flagellated protozoan): cysts survive in water. Treat with metronidazole for 5 days.
- *Cryptosporidium* (protozoan): commonly seen in HIV. Treatment: nitaxzoxanide.
- *Schistosomiasis* (fluke): carried by freshwater snail, especially in Africa/South America. Also can cause glomerulonephritis, CNS lesions, chronic cystitis and TCC bladder. Treatment: praziquantel.

2.2.8 Large bowel obstruction

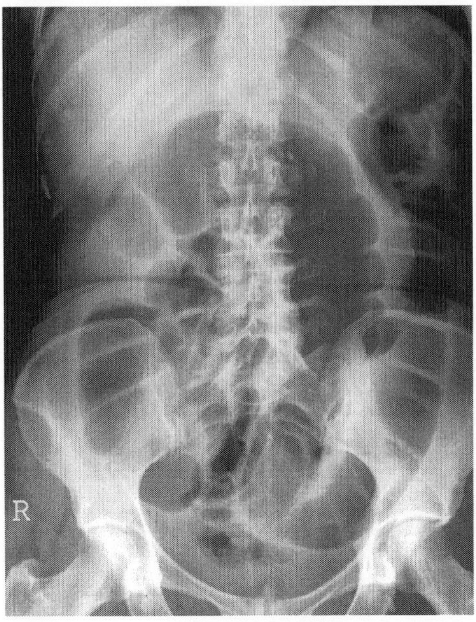

Figure 2.2.8
AXR of large bowel obstruction

1. What does this image demonstrate?
   - Acute large bowel obstruction (LBO). The plane abdominal x-ray shows dilated large bowel, caecum and transverse colon, appearing to stop at splenic flexure with no evidence of gas in the left colon or rectum.
2. What is the differential diagnosis?
   - Mechanical obstruction:
     - neoplasia — malignant but very occasionally a large benign adenomatous lesion
     - inflammatory stricture
     - diverticulitis/stricture
     - volvulus
     - faecal impaction
     - iatrogenic strictures.
   - Pseudo-obstruction.
3. What are the initial investigations and treatment?

   The extent of investigation and urgency of treatment will depend on the clinical context (guided by history and examination, assessing for vital signs, signs of peritonism). If the patient is unwell and has generalised peritonism then an urgent laparotomy without further investigation is indicated.

   About one-third of patients believed to have mechanical LBO on clinical and x-ray findings have no obstruction and one-fifth of patients suspected of having pseudo-obstruction have mechanical LBO. (Computed tomography in the assessment of suspected large bowel obstruction. G.C. Beattie; ANZJS 2007; 77: 160–5)
   - Investigations:
     - AXR: erect and supine
     - rigid/flexible sigmoidoscopy
     - single contrast (Gastrografin) enema:
       - sensitivity 96%, specificity 98% (G C Beattie; ANZJS 2007; 77: 160–5)
       - may be difficult in elderly; failures due to inability to retain the contrast or with very low obstruction.
     - CT scan abdomen pelvis, ideally with rectal contrast:
       - sensitivity 96%; specificity 94% (G C Beattie ANZJS 2007; 77: 160–5)
       - additional targeted CT prone and/or decubitus scanning to shift colonic gas can help with the diagnosis and evaluation
       - colonic mural wall thickening is difficult to interpret on CT scan. Focal mural thickening, resulting in luminal narrowing, with no associated mass or obvious cause is often difficult to clarify, and should lead to further investigation.
   - Treatment:
     - resuscitation ABC
     - intravenous fluids
     - IDC and strict fluid and electrolyte normalisation
     - NGT.
4. What is the definitive management?

   Mechanical obstruction
   - Surgery: Patient in modified Lloyd Davies position. Generous midline incision. If the bowel is tense, decompress it with 16G cannula through the taenia coli.

Exact procedure performed depends on (i) the patient's fitness/physiological status; (ii) disease factors such as position of pathology, condition of proximal colon, presence of complications relating to obstruction (e.g. perforation) etc; (iii) curative or palliative intent. The options include:
  - Hartmann's procedure — resection of primary pathology without anastomosis. Should be preferred in patients with high surgical risk
  - total colectomy with end ileostomy or primary anastomosis, depending on the intra-operative scenario. Restoration of continuity is associated with higher rates of impaired bowel function
  - resection of pathology with manual decompression or intra-operative colonic irrigation and primary anastomosis.
- Self-expanding metallic stents:
  - in the palliative setting, stent placement is associated with similar mortality/morbidity rates and shorter hospital stay
  - when used as a bridge to surgery, stents seem to be associated with a shorter hospital stay and lower mortality and colostomy formation rates.

Sigmoid volvulus
- Flexible/rigid sigmoidoscopy and rectal tube decompression (rigid is associated with more perforation and does not allow such accurate evaluation of mucosal viability).
- Use of Gastrografin/fleet enemas to effect correction of volvulus.
- Percutaneous endoscopic colostomy (like a PEG) to fix the sigmoid colon in frail, unfit patients with recurrent volvulus (Baraza UK BJS 2007; 94: 1415–20).
- Surgery:
  - usually elective after decompression (unless viability in doubt)
  - sigmoid resection +/- total colectomy, if megacolon.

Pseudo-obstruction
- Once a mechanical cause has been confidently excluded the focus is to:
  - aggressively resuscitate to correct fluid/electrolyte disturbances
  - evaluate for signs of ischaemia/perforation
  - treat the underlying conditions (e.g. respiratory or congestive heart failure) and stop any contributing medications (e.g. narcotics, anticholinergics) if possible
  - NG tube if vomiting
  - rectal tube may be therapeutic in some cases
  - colonoscopic decompression (useful in 70–85%); passage of scope to transverse colon is usually enough
  - use of Gastrografin/fleet enemas
  - neostigmine (inhibits destruction of acetylcholine by acetylcholinesterase). With HDU/ICU monitoring. 1–2 mg iv/sc; may repeat in 3 hours if needed. NB: may cause significant bradycardia, so beware in patient with cardiac problems.
  - Surgical options:
    - tube caecostomy/percutaneous caecostomy/lap-assisted caecostomy/subtotal colectomy, usually with end ileostomy.

2.2.9 Rectal prolapse

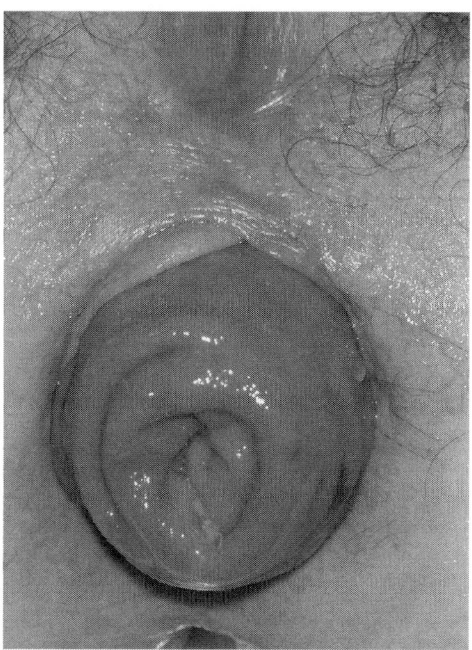

Figure 2.2.9
Rectal prolapse

This 83-year-old woman presented with a lump protruding from her anus.

1. What is the diagnosis?
   - Full-thickness rectal prolapse.
2. Which investigations would you consider/perform?
   - Barium enema/colonoscopy to exclude underlying colorectal organic precipitant.
   - Anorectal physiology, including: (i) endoanal ultrasound to assess structural abnormalities of the anal sphincter; (ii) manometry to assess resting and squeeze anal tone, functional anal canal length; and (iii) electromyography to assess pudendal nerve terminal motor latency.
   - Defaecating proctogram.
   - Routine pre-operative work up: bloods, ECG, CXR.
3. What is the operative management?

   Depends on the patient's fitness. Usually abdominal procedure for fit patient due to lower recurrence rates and perineal procedure for unfit patients. Controversy exists regarding the best procedure. Options include:
   - trans-abdominal (resection) rectopexy: 1–10% recurrence rate; 5–20% morbidity; sutured or mesh rectopexy ± sigmoid resection (may be indicated in patients with history of constipation)
   - perineal proctosigmoidectomy (Altemeier procedure): 5–60% recurrence rate; low morbidity
   - perineal Delormes procedure (rectal mucosectomy and plication of muscle): 5–40% recurrence rate; low morbidity.

2.2.10 Appendiceal mucocoele

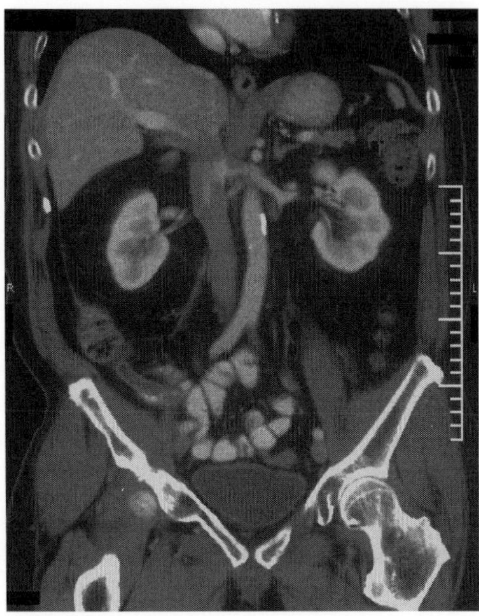

Figure 2.2.10
Mucocoele of the appendix

This is the CT scan of a 62-year-old man who was admitted to hospital with right iliac fossa pain and treated conservatively for an appendiceal abscess with antibiotics 6 weeks previously.

1. Describe the findings of this CT scan.
   - Coronal CT scan image with a 5 × 1 cm diameter dilated tubular structure in the right iliac fossa.
2. What are the possible diagnoses?
   - Mucocoele of the appendix.
   - Acute appendicitis with luminal dilatation.
   - Low grade appendiceal mucinous neoplasm (LAMN).
   - Caecal tumour obstructing the appendix.
3. What is the management?
   - Management always begins with patient assessment, including history and examination.
   - Colonoscopy.
   - Appendicectomy if no caecal pathology and able to transect the appendiceal base safely. Attempt laparoscopic approach initially (if suspect appendiceal mucocoele, open approach is safer to avoid inadvertent perforation and spillage of mucus).
   - Ileocaecal resection if caecal or base of appendix pathology.

2.2.11 Fistula in ano

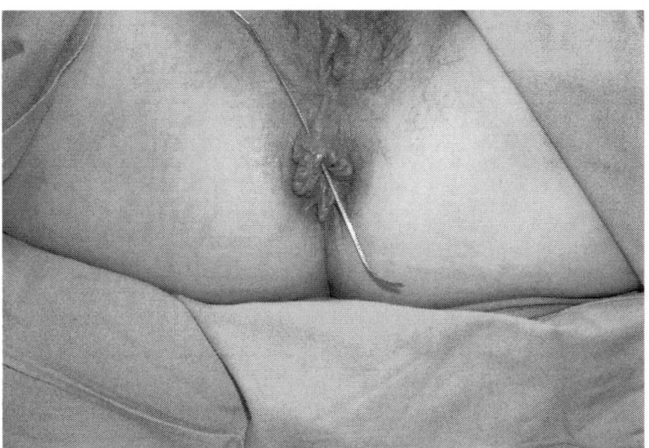

Figure 2.2.11
Fistula in ano with probe in situ

Please read in conjunction with 4.6.5, fistula in ano.

1. What is the diagnosis?
   - Fistula in ano in the right anterior position (assuming patient in lithotomy position), with a Lockhardt-Mummery probe in situ. Appears to be a low fistula, either intersphinteric or low trans-sphincteric.
2. What are the likely causes?
   - Primary (cryptoglandular) vs secondary (inflammatory e.g. Crohn's disease, malignancy, radiation, foreign body).
   - Cryptoglandular theory most likely (blocked anal gland that subsequently becomes infected). Tracking/resolution of sepsis results in fistula formation.
   - Usually no predisposing factors, but more common in patients with diabetes, immunocompromised, previous perianal abscess/fistula, perianal Crohn's disease, male and smoker.
3. What do you tell the patient prior to surgery?
   - Explain aetiology and likely natural course without intervention.
   - Explain operative risks: trauma to anal sphincter (flatus/faecal incontinence, temporary/permanent), bleeding, recurrence (30–50%), wound healing complications. Possibility of insertion of a seton and need for staged approach with additional procedures.
   - Other: expected time off work, expected time in hospital.
4. What is the operative management?
   - EUA rectum and anus.
   - Assess sphincter and fistula anatomy to determine whether intersphincteric, low trans-sphincteric or high trans-sphincteric.
   - If intersphincteric/low trans-sphincteric with good anal canal length proximally, suitable for excision (fistulectomy) or, more commonly, laying open (fistulotomy) ± marsupialisation of tract after fistulotomy. Be cautious of fistulotomy in an anterior fistula in a female no matter how much sphincter is involved.

- Insertion of seton and subsequent reassessment if:
  - fistula is high trans-sphincteric
  - short anal canal length
  - previous history of anal sphincter injury/dysfunction.

2.2.12 Fissure-in-ano

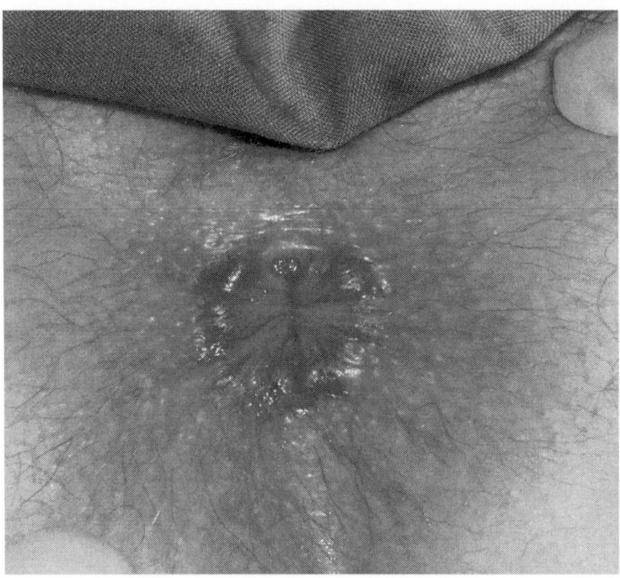

Figure 2.2.12
Anterior anal fissure

1. What is the diagnosis?
   - Chronic anal fissure.
2. What is the initial management?
   - History and examination.
   - Exclude underlying pathological causes and identify any evacuatory dysfunction.
   - Acute fissures: non-operative approach using application of topical local anaesthetic agents and increasing dietary fibre and fluid intake.
   - Decrease internal anal sphincter tone using topical application of glyceryl trinitrate (rectogesic) or diltiazem ointment.
3. What operative intervention would you proceed with if initial treatment fails?
   - Colonoscopy/EUA — confirm diagnosis, exclude other disease such as inflammatory bowel disease and malignancy.
   - Botox injection into the internal anal sphincter.
   - Lateral sphincterotomy — 98% cure, 1% risk of incontinence. Not in inflammatory bowel disease. Care in post-partum woman where sphincter damage suspected. Can be repeated on the contralateral side if fails.
   - Advancement flap: consider if all above fail, or if significant sphincter defect exists (higher risk of incontinence).

2.2.13 Anal squamous cell carcinoma

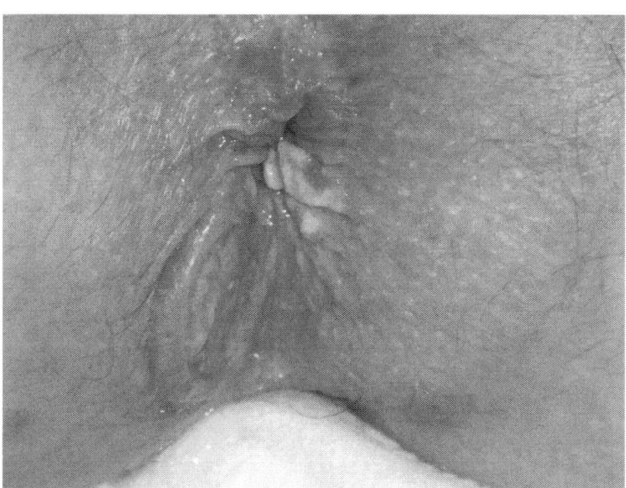

Figure 2.2.13
Anal squamous cell carcinoma

1. Describe the findings (patient is in lithotomy position)
   There is a 4–5 cm diameter, right posterior perianal ulcer that is extending into the anal canal. The edges are raised and everted.
2. What is the diagnosis?
   - Squamous cell carcinoma (SCC). There appears to be an anal canal SCC extending out onto the perianal skin.
3. What is the differential diagnosis?
   - Other epidermoid carcinoma of the anal canal: basaloid (cloacogenic) or muco-epidermoid. Benign causes may include infections (including STDs) and inflammation.
4. What are possible predisposing factors?
   - Chronic benign perianal conditions: fistulae, leukoplakia, radiation changes.
   - Viral infection (human papilloma virus): perianal warts, AIN.
   - Immunosuppression: HIV, IFN renal transplant patients.
5. What is the management?
   - History and examination (check for evidence of groin lymph nodes).
   - Investigation:
     - confirm diagnosis: EUA+ (punch) biopsy
     - stage the cancer: CT/MRI ± PET scan.
   - Treatment determined in a multidisciplinary setting:
     - chemoradiation (Nigro 1974) first line of treatment with 5-FU, mitomycin C and radiation.
     - +/− salvage abdomino-perineal excision of rectum and anus if radiation fails or for recurrence.

2.2.14 Small bowel obstruction

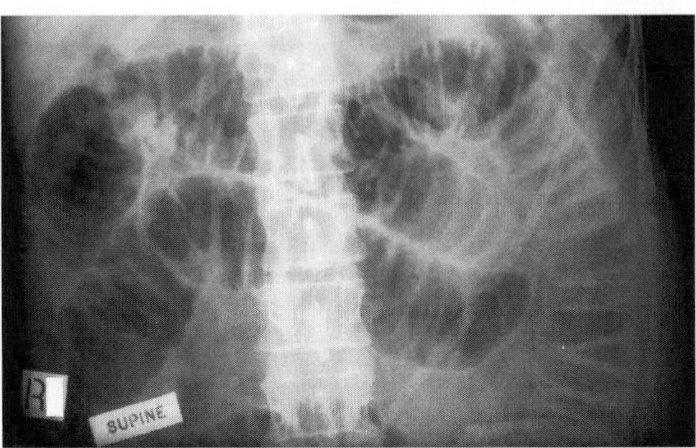

Figure 2.2.14
AXR of small bowel obstruction

This 63-year-old male patient presented with vomiting, central abdominal pain and distension.

1. What are the possible diagnoses?
   Small bowel obstruction (SBO) from:
   - adhesions from previous surgery (60%)
   - neoplasms: intrinsic or extrinsic (20%)
   - hernias (10%):
     - external; for example, inguinal, incisional, para stomal
     - internal — post-surgical; for example, mesenteric defect, after Roux-en-Y gastric bypass, under a stomal loop
     - congenital; for example, paraduodenal fossa, ileocaecal recess, Foramen of Winslow.
   - Inflammatory; for example, Crohn's disease. Also extrinsic inflammation; for example, acute appendicitis or appendix mass, or pancreatitis.
   - Miscellaneous causes:
     - congenital bands
     - cystic fibrosis
     - volvulus
     - intussusception ± tumour
     - gallstone ileus
     - post-radiotherapy stricture
     - vascular — haematoma (e.g. from anticoagulants), post-ischaemic stricture
     - ingested foreign bodies.
2. How would you investigate this patient?
   - Bloods: FBC (especially WCC) and EUC for renal dysfunction/electrolyte disturbances).
   - ABG: acid-base balance looking for lactic acidosis (from strangulation).
   - X-rays: looking for dilated bowel loops, air-fluid levels, 'string of beads' sign, thumb-printing or bowel wall thickening and paucity of large bowel gas.
   - CT abdomen/pelvis or contrast study: helpful when looking for volvulus (swirl in mesentery) if plain films are non-diagnostic, if there is disparity between clinical and radiological findings, or if malignancy is suspected.

3. How would you manage this patient?
Reminder: Use the ABCDEFG of non-surgical treatment of surgical patients (see Chapter 2.1 — preparing and practising).
   - Assess the patient for signs of peritonism, previous abdominal scars, hernia:
     - aggressive correction of fluid and electrolytes
     - insert a NGT and IDC, and +/- nutritional support
     - thromboprophylaxis.
   - Indications for immediate or early surgery:
     - peritonitis on examination
     - suspicion of strangulation (fever, raised WCC, tachycardia, metabolic acidosis, continuing pain).
   - Nearly all SBO in a virgin abdomen require surgical intervention.
   - Patients with partial SBO, who do not resolve within 48 hours should also be considered for surgery.
   - Aim to avoid surgery in Crohn's disease, disseminated carcinomatous and the post-operative period (6 weeks to 6 months), if possible.
   - Adhesional SBO without acute findings can be treated conservatively in about 90% of cases.
   - Patients who do not resolve with conservative treatment should undergo a water-soluble contrast (Gastrografin) study or proceed to surgery. A water-soluble contrast study activates movement of water into small bowel lumen and can decrease small bowel oedema and enhance smooth muscle contractility; its use can be diagnostic and therapeutic.

FURTHER NOTES — SMALL BOWEL OBSTRUCTION

- A longer trial of non-operative management may be considered if diffuse metastatic disease is likely. Rather than resection, a small bowel bypass may be a quicker, safer alternative if end stage disease is present. This may shorten operative time and dissection and may decrease the risk of enterotomy.
- The use of hyaluronic acid-carboxymethyl cellulose (seprafilm) membrane decreases the incidence and extent of adhesions, but there is no evidence of decreased SBO post-operatively. There may be an increased risk of anastomotic leak if wrapped around anastomoses.
- After surgery for adhesion-related SBO, the probability of recurrent SBO is 20–30%.

2.2.15 Meckel's diverticulum

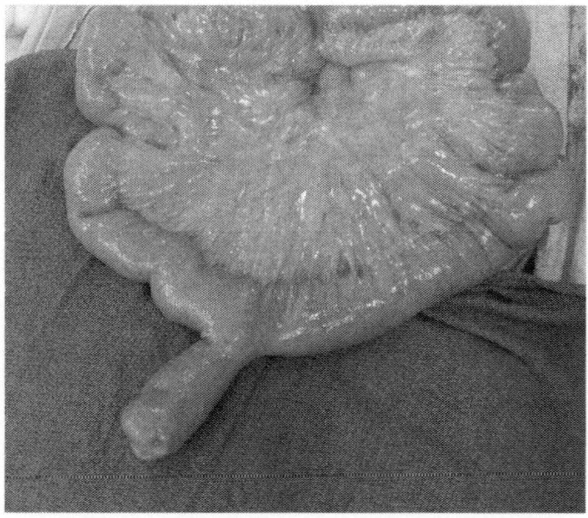

Figure 2.2.15
Meckel's diverticulum

This 44-year-old male presented with intermittent abdominal pain, and a CT scan report of a small bowel intussusception.

1. What is the diagnosis?
   - Meckel's diverticulum.

   Additional information:
   - named after Johann Friedrick Meckel, the Younger, B1781–D1833
   - it is true diverticulum with all bowel wall layers and its own artery, and is a persistence of the vitello-intestinal tract, which usually obliterates in the 5th to 7th week of gestation
   - the rule of **2**s:
     - most common congenital GI tract malformation, occurring in **2**% of the population
     - usually occurs within **2** feet of the ileocaecal junction
     - **2** inches long
     - commonly contains **2** types of epithelial tissue (stomach/pancreas).
2. How may this patient present?
   - With complications:
     - haemorrhage (20–30%): more common in children, due to bleeding from heterotopic gastric mucosa
     - small bowel obstruction (20–25%) due to intussusception or adhesive band
     - inflammation/diverticulitis (10–20%)
     - umbilical anomalies (<10%)
     - neoplasia (1–2%)
     - ulceration
     - perforation.
   - Incidental finding at laparotomy or on imaging.
3. How is it commonly diagnosed?
   - Technetium-99m pertechnetate scan, enhanced by pentagastrin before the scan. Relies on contrast concentrating in gastric and heterotopic gastric mucosa.
   - Coincidental or intentional discovery at laparoscopy/laparotomy.
4. What do you do if you encounter this at laparotomy?
   - If symptomatic: small bowel resection. Simpler to perform a limited small bowel resection along with diverticulum than a diverticulectomy which may narrow the bowel lumen. Also may leave mucosa adjacent to diverticulum if only resect diverticulum which can cause problems later.
   - If asymptomatic or incidental finding — controversial:
     - no resection is favoured where morbidity risk is high
     - resection is favoured where there is a high risk of later becoming symptomatic:
       - males <45 years old; diverticulum >2 cm length; presence of a fibrous band and presence of ectopic tissue in the diverticulum (can't be determined by palpation)
     - evidence against resection:
       - a systematic review reports a significantly higher post-operative morbidity for resection than leaving in situ, with resection being necessary in 758 patients to save one life (Zani A et al. Ann Surg 2008; 247:276–81)
       - 20% complication rate in asymptomatic resection group vs 13% in symptomatic resection group in retrospective 'Mayo study' by Park J J et al Ann Surg 1994; 241:529–33
       - lifetime rate of symptoms or complications estimated at 4% (>50% in children under 10 years).

2.2.16 Gastrointestinal stromal tumour

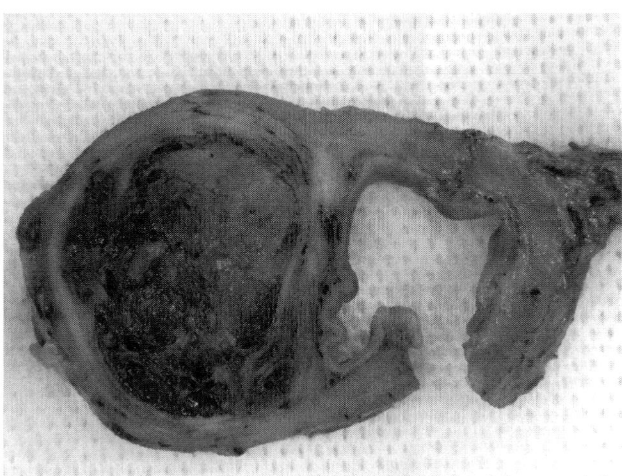

Figure 2.2.16
Gastric gastrointestinal stromal tumour

This image shows a tumour attached to the stomach on the greater curvature.

1. What is the diagnosis?
   - Gastrointestinal stromal tumour (GIST), which arises from the interstitial cells of Cajal.
2. What is the differential diagnosis?
   - Atypical adenocarcinoma.
   - MALT lymphoma.
   - Other lymphoma.
   - Leiomyoma.
   - Leiomyosarcoma.
3. How do you confirm the diagnosis?
   - c-kit (or CD 117) positive (>95%) and CD34 positive (70%) immunohistochemical staining. Negative staining for desmin and S100.
4. What is the operative treatment and principles it is based on?
   - Surgery usually indicated for GISTs with (i) no evidence of metastases and (ii) that are resectable in patients fit for surgery, since:
     - all GISTs have malignant potential that is dependent on size and mitotic rate
     - must differentiate GIST from other tumours such as adenocarcinoma that need different surgical management.
   - Surgical options: depend on size, site and biopsy:
     - local resection if R0 resection with negative margin is possible and intact pseudocapsule
     - distal gastrectomy and Roux-en-Y reconstruction
     - total gastrectomy — no lymphadenectomy routinely required, as lymph node metastases are rare in GISTs.
5. What other treatment options are there?
   - Chemotherapy has no role in primary GIST treatment.

- Tyrosine kinase inhibitor (TKI) therapy:
  - imatinibmesylate (Glivec) is used for non-resectable, metastatic and recurrent GISTs
  - sunitinib malate (Sutent) is used for metastatic or non-resectable GISTs that have failed imatinibmesylate treatment.

2.2.17 Parathyroid adenoma

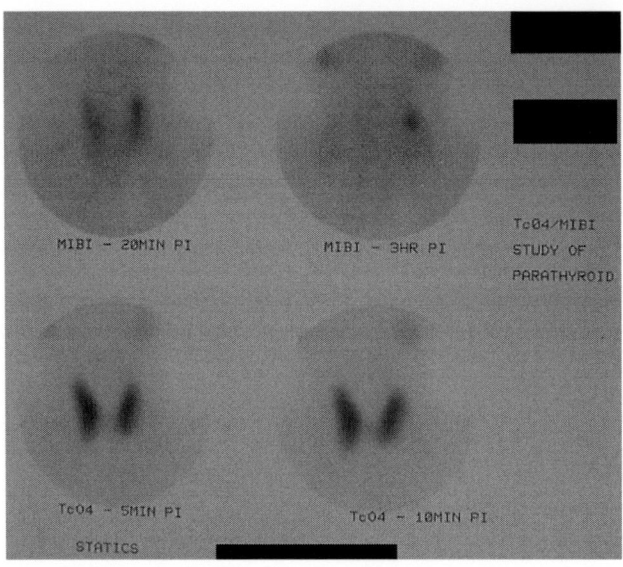

Figure 2.2.17
Sestamibi scan of left superior parathyroid adenoma

Please read in conjunction with 2.4.8, primary hyperparathyroidism.

1. What is this test and what is the diagnosis?
   - Test: sestamibi or MIBI parathyroid scan; that is, Technetium (Tc99m)-sestamibi.
   - Diagnosis: left-sided parathyroid adenoma.

   Extra note: sestamibi or MIBI parathyroid scan (i.e. Technetium(Tc99m)-sestamibi) is absorbed more quickly by hyperfunctioning parathyroid gland than by normal parathyroid. This is a functional study and does not give exact anatomical localisation.
2. What other investigations would you perform?
   - Investigations are focused on confirming the diagnosis and ruling out secondary causes of hyperparathyroidism.
     - Bloods: PTH, calcium, albumin, phosphate, ALP, EUC, Vit D.
     - 24-hour urine calcium and calcium/creatinine clearance ratio.
     - Bone mineral density assessment.
     - Ultrasound scan of the neck.
     - ± CT scan neck.
     - ± MRI neck.
3. What is the operative management?
   - Minimally invasive parathyroidectomy, guided by sestamibi results and intra-operatively by ultrasound.

2.2.18 Pancreatic cystic lesion

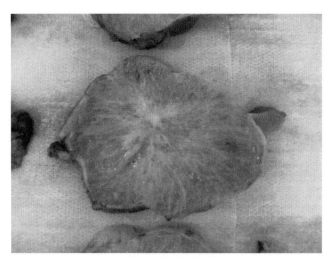

Figure 2.2.18
Pancreas serous cystadenoma

1. This lesion was removed during a Whipple's procedure. Which organ is it likely to be in?
   - Pancreas.
2. What is the likely pathology?
   - Pancreatic cystic neoplasm (10–15% of cystic pancreatic collections):
     - mucinous cystadenoma and cystadenocarcinoma (MCNs)
     - serous cystadenoma
     - intraductal papillary mucinous neoplasm (IPMN)
     - papillary cystic neoplasm
     - acinar cell cystadenocarcinoma
     - choriocarcinoma
     - teratoma
     - islet cell tumours.
3. What investigations would you perform?
   - CT scan abdomen:
     - serous tumours have central calcification, 'sunburst' pattern and small microcysts (like grapes); mucinous tumours have peripheral calcification and macrocysts.
   - Endoscopic ultrasound (EUS).
   - EUS-fine needle aspiration (EUS-FNA):
     - cytopathology to differentiate mucinous and serous tumours
     - biochemistry — CEA high in mucinous tumours, glycogen high in serous tumours.
   - MRI.
4. What is the management?
   - Management is complex and will depend on patient (symptoms and fitness) and lesion (risk of malignancy) factors.
   - Following investigation, non-malignant *serous tumours* can be observed. Surgery is required for serous tumours if they are symptomatic or if it is not possible to differentiate between serous and mucinous tumour.

- MCNs and IPMN are premalignant.
- *Mucinous tumours* require resection if cysts are >3 cm diameter, or symptomatic; for example, pain or pancreatitis.
- Resection recommended if raised CEA on EUS-FNA, or EUS reveals papillary projections or septation.

2.2.19 Submandibular duct stone

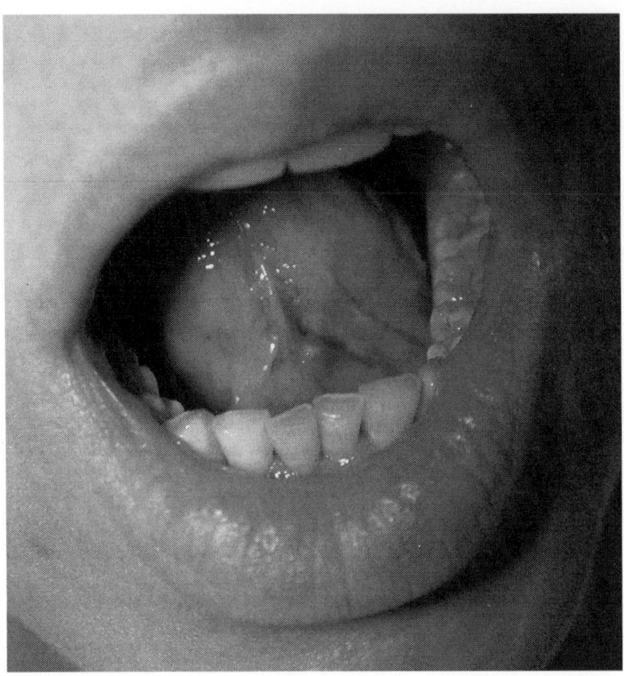

Figure 2.2.19
Left submandibular calculus

1. Describe the findings?
   - This is the open mouth image with tongue lifted to the top of the mouth. There is a swelling of the frenulum with a small part of a calculus visible just to the left of the frenulum.
2. What is the diagnosis?
   - Calculus in the distal left submandibular duct (Wharton's duct) also known as sialolithiasis.
   - Sialolithiasis occurs 80–90% in the submandibular glands or ducts, 5–10% in the parotid glands or ducts, and 0–5% in the sublingual and minor salivary glands.
3. What is the operative management?
   - The stone in this case is quite large, about 1 cm long and is located at the distal end of the duct. It requires trans-oral incision over the distal duct, removal of the stone, and marsupialisation of the duct.

- Prior to incision over the duct, a suture may be placed proximal to the stone, encircling the duct, to prevent the stone passing proximally into the duct while it is being manipulated.
- General operative principals are:
  - distal duct stones, for stones that are palpable or bimanually palpable:
    - duct dilatation and stone removal
    - incision and dissection ± marsupialisation of the duct
    - duct excision from the papilla until the stone is visible followed by hilar marsupialisation
    - small stones <3 mm diameter may be removed using sialoendoscopy and wire baskets
  - proximal duct stones/hilar or intraparenchymal stones:
    - transoral removal may be successful as described above
    - ESWL or endoscopic laser lithotripsy can be performed for stones in the gland
    - gland excision (sialoadenectomy), if the above procedures have failed or are not indicated.

2.2.20 Malignant melanoma

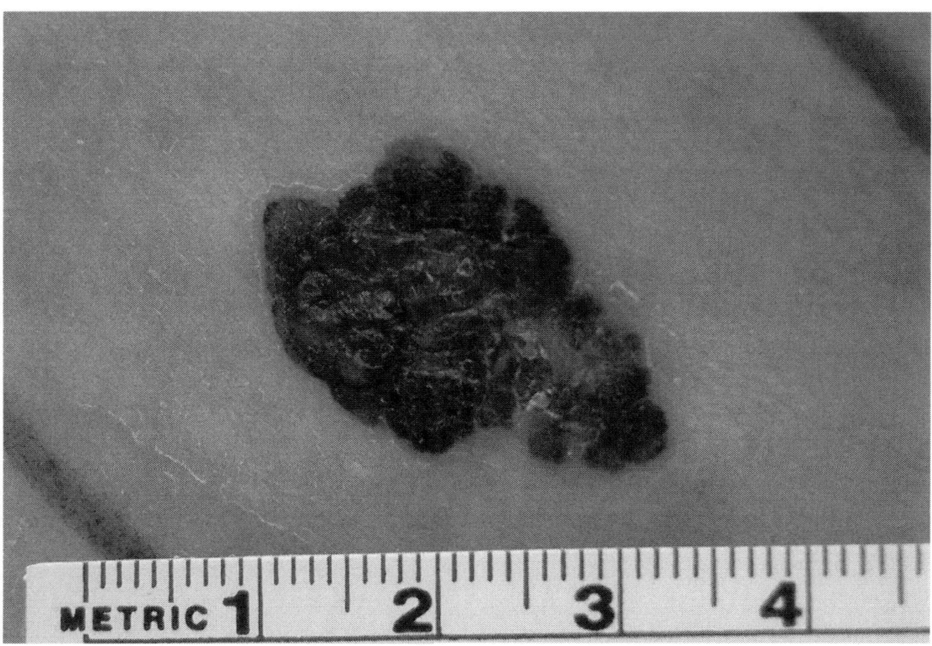

Figure 2.2.20
Malignant melanoma

Please read in conjunction with 3.3.9, malignant melanoma medium case.

1. What is the diagnosis?
   - Superficial spreading malignant melanoma.

2. What are the principles of management?
   - Patient assessment: for risk factors and evidence of metastasis.
   - Confirm diagnosis:
     - small lesions — excision biopsy
     - large lesions — punch (incision) biopsy to assess depth of melanoma prior to definitive excision as per below.
   - Treatment of primary melanoma:
     - wide excision margins (NCCN guidelines):
       - melanoma in situ (Tis): 5 mm margin
       - <1 mm (T1): 1 cm margin
       - 1–2 mm (T2): 1–2 cm margin
       - >2 mm (T3,4): 2 cm margin
     - sentinel lymph node (SLN) biopsy; indications for SLN biopsy:
       - Breslow >1 mm
       - patients with melanomas 0.75–1.2 mm with primary tumour demonstrating ulceration, Clark level IV or V or high mitotic rate should have discussion of SLNB (12% risk of metastases)
       - lymphatic mapping aims to identify the first lymph node. Patent blue dye intra-operatively. Retrieval of lymph node intra-operatively.
   - Treatment of metastatic melanoma:
     - regional lymph node metastases:
       - lymph node dissection
       - +/– adjuvant therapy
     - systemic metastases:
       - resection of isolated metastasis (up to three)
       - radiotherapy
       - chemotherapy
       - immunotherapy.
3. What are the prognostic factors?
   - Most important is clinical stage (TNM).
   - Patient factors:
     - age (risk of death greater >60 yo)
     - gender (men greater risk of death).
   - Primary tumour:
     - Breslow thickness (mm) (Clark level in thin melanomas)
     - ulceration
     - mitotic rate.
   - Nodes:
     - microscopic versus macroscopic
     - number involved.
   - Metastases:
     - number of sites
     - visceral
     - serum LDH
     - poor performance status.

2.2.21 Basal cell carcinoma

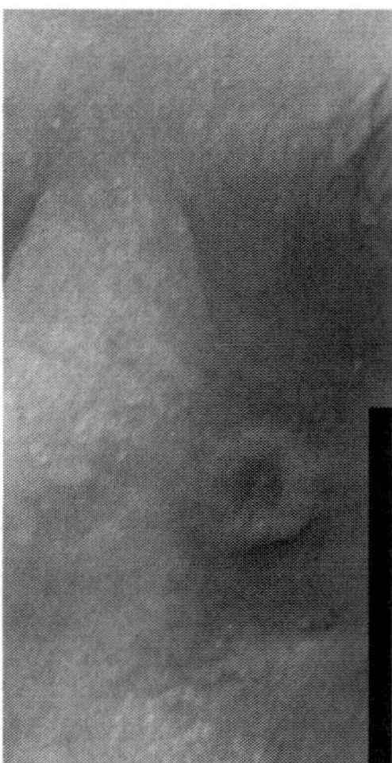

Figure 2.2.21
Basal cell carcinoma

1. What is the diagnosis?
   - Basal cell carcinoma (BCC).
2. What is the management?
   - Excision with histologically confirmed negative margins, both deep and wide.
     - In this case I would excise with a 2 mm margin.
     - Due to the site in this case a wider excision margin is not suitable.
     - Ideally most BCCs can be excised with a 2–3 mm margin and an adequate microscopic margin is 0.5 mm.
     - A 4 mm margin in a tumour with a diameter <6 mm and a >6 mm margin in a tumour with a diameter >6 mm has a control rate of 95% at 5 years.
     - In case of incomplete excision, re-excision to achieve clear margins should be considered.
   - Maintain normal function and achieve a good cosmetic result. This lesion may require a local flap to close the defect.
   - BCCs rarely metastasise and are usually cured by complete excision.
   - Radiation has a role in unfit patients not suitable for surgery, or where surgical excision would be disfiguring.
3. What is the follow-up?
   - There are no specific recommendations supported by evidence. However, I recommend 6–12 monthly review to identify new lesions or recurrent lesions and identify metastatic disease.
   - About 44% will develop another BCC within 3 years of a BCC excision.
   - Local recurrence is <2%.
   - Regional recurrence is very rare.

2.2.22 Squamous cell carcinoma

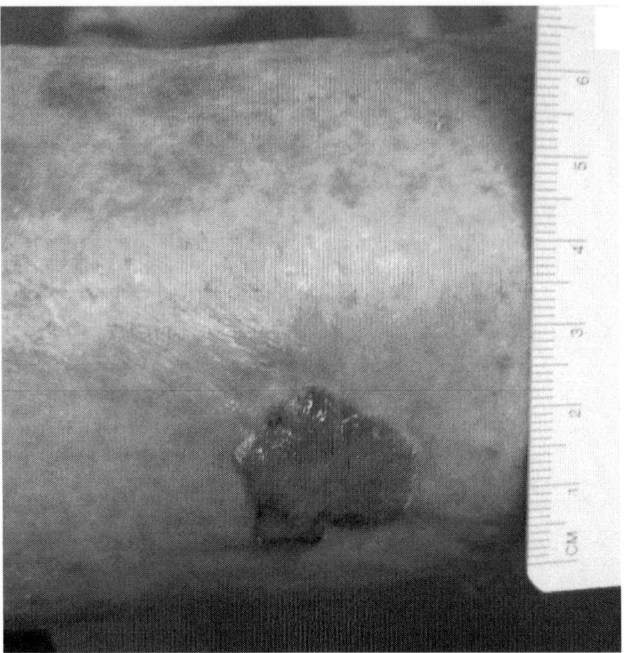

Figure 2.2.22
Squamous cell carcinoma

1. What is the diagnosis?
   - Squamous cell carcinoma of the limb, measuring approximately 2 cm in diameter.
2. What is the management?
   - Complete excision with 5 mm margins and histologically confirmed negative margins, both deep and wide.
     - Elliptical incision with length to width ratio for the ellipse of 3–4 : 1.
     - The majority of SCCs <2 cm in diameter can be excised with a margin of at least 4 mm resulting in good long-term control.
   - Risk of lymph node metastases is small (<1%), but occur more often in lesions:
     - >2 cm in diameter
     - that are poorly differentiated
     - >4 mm thick
     - that are recurrent
     - on the ears and lips
     - with peri-neural invasion.
   - Lymph node metastases are usually excised.
   - Role of radiotherapy:
     - indicated in primary SCC in unfit patients not suitable for surgery, or where surgical excision would be disfiguring, or in cases of positive margin following excision where further excision is not considered appropriate or would be disfiguring

    - following lymphadenectomy in patients at high risk of recurrence
    - in palliative inoperable cases.
- In-transit metastases; uncommon, when occur—wide excision and adjuvant radiotherapy.

2.2.23 Lymphoscintogram

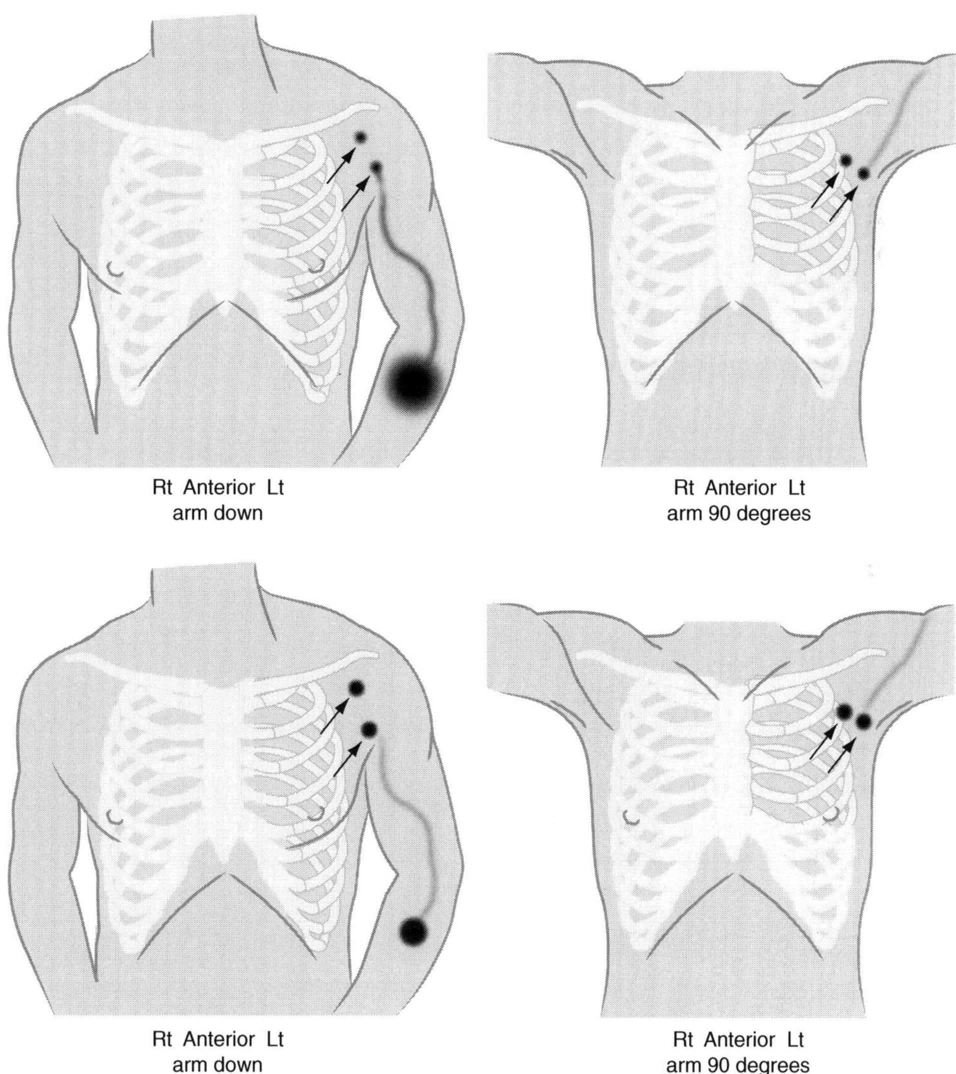

Figure 2.2.23
Lymphoscintogram

The two upper images were achieved 10 minutes after injection and the bottom two images 1 hour later.

1. What are these images of?
    - A lymphoscintogram.

2. What do they show and why was this test performed?
   - Two sentinel lymph nodes are seen in the left axilla. The initial injection site is in the left forearm.
   - This case is most likely of a left forearm malignant melanoma that has already been excised. The sentinel lymph node biopsy (SLNB) was indicated on the basis of the histology of the excised melanoma.
3. What is the test's purpose and how is it performed?
   - A lymphoscintogram is performed to identify a sentinel or sentinel lymph nodes(s), which are thought to be the first lymphatic basin that tumour will metastasise or drain to.
   - A few hours before the SLNB, a filtered sulphur colloid tagged with Tc-99m is injected next to the primary lesion site, and scintigraphic imaging is performed at 10 and 60 minutes.
   - In the operating theatre, lymphatic mapping to identify the first lymph node is achieved by injecting patent blue dye intra-operatively near the primary lesion excision site, where the radionuclide was injected.
   - Using a gamma probe intra-operatively to identify the sentinel lymph node(s) position, a small skin incision(s) is accurately placed, followed by dissection, identification and retrieval of the node(s), using the blue dye colour of the node and the gamma probe as guidance.

2.2.24 Pelvic fracture

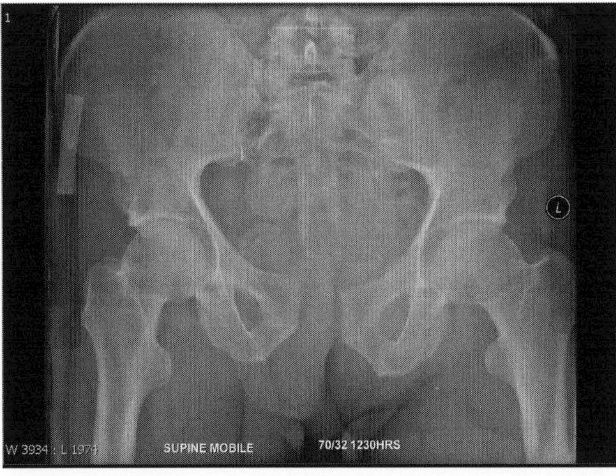

Figure 2.2.24
Pelvic fracture x-ray

1. Describe the findings of the x-ray and give the diagnosis.
   - Pelvic fracture with widening of the right sacroiliac joint (approx 1 cm) and diastasis (approx 2 cm) of the pubic symphysis.
2. What is the initial management?
   - EMST/ATLS principles: ABCDE.
   - IV fluid/PRC resuscitation with restoration of circulating volume is crucial.
   - C-spine XR and CXR to complete the trauma panel.
   - External stabilisation of fracture: use a sheet or some other device to bind pelvis.

3. The patient becomes hypotensive. What is the cause of the bleeding in this patient?
   - Consider other sites of bleeding:
     - external; for example, femur fracture, scalp laceration
     - internal:
       - abdomen (e.g. spleen, liver, mesentery)
       - chest
       - retroperitoneum
   - Bleeding directly from the pelvic fracture:
     - life threatening haemorrhage rarely due to pelvic arterial injury
     - a focused assessment with sonography for trauma (FAST) can be useful to determine whether bleeding is due to other associated intra-abdominal trauma injury, which will mandate exploratory laparotomy (and entry of peritoneal cavity) as well as extraperitoneal packing of the pelvis
     - exploratory laparotomy (and entry of peritoneal cavity) as well as extraperitoneal packing of the pelvis may be necessary to establish the extent of the trauma/injuries
     - more common due to retroperitoneal venous plexus bleeding or cancellous bone bleeding.
4. What treatment is available to deal with bleeding associated with this?
   - Bleeding due to the pelvic fracture:
     - angiographic embolisation (when available) if patient condition/stability allows
     - extraperitoneal circumferential packing of the pelvis
     - formal external fixation of the pelvic fracture
     - in an unstable patient exploratory laparotomy to identify and treat sources of haemorrhage. Placement of external stabilisation device and then angiography if indicated.

2.2.25 Splenic trauma

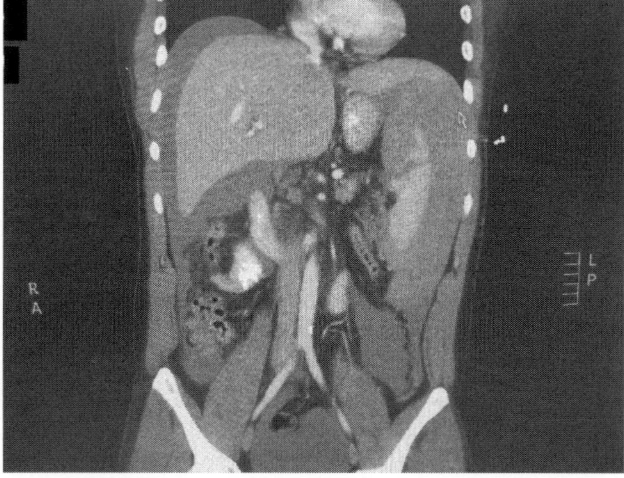

Figure 2.2.25
CT scan splenic trauma grade IV

Please read in conjunction with 4.4.15, trauma splenectomy.

1. What does this CT image show?
   - Splenic injury organ injury scale grade (OIS) IV (i.e. OIS4) with free blood in the peritoneal cavity.
2. What is your initial management?
   - EMST/ATLS Principles: ABCDE.
   - IV fluid/PRC resuscitation with restoration of circulating volume is crucial.
   - A focused assessment with sonography for trauma (FAST) may be useful, if available.
   - If haemodynamically unstable and requiring large fluid volumes, immediate operative management required.
   - If haemodynamically stable, CT scan to assess abdomen: For splenic injury define the OIS and assess for contrast extravasation:
     - OIS1 = (subcapsular <10% surface, capsular tear <1 cm)
     - OIS2 = (subcapsular 10–50% surface, <5 cm diameter, capsular tear 1–3 cm)
     - OIS3 = (subcapsular >50% surface, >5 cm diameter, capsular >3 cm depth or trabecular vessels)
     - OIS4 = (laceration to segmental or hilar vessels with >25% devascularisation)
     - OIS5 = (completely shattered or hilar vascular injury that devascularises spleen).
   - Successful non-operative management has been reported in 68% of splenic injuries, with failure rates of approximately 4%, 9%, 20%, 44% and 83% for OIS1 to OIS5, respectively.
   - Splenic artery embolisation may improve the rate of splenic preservation and avoid splenectomy.
   - Patients with OIS4 and 5 and contrast extravasation usually require operative intervention.
3. What is the operative management if the patient becomes haemodynamically unstable?
   - Laparotomy and assessment of the splenic injury with simultaneous resuscitation.
     - Operative management usually involves splenctomy but splenic preservation should be considered when possible, particularly in young patients.
4. What complications can occur after operative management?
   - Following preservation:
     - delayed haemorrhage
     - pseudoaneurysm formation
     - infection.
   - Post-splenectomy:
     - overwhelming post-splenectomy infection (OPSI):
       - higher susceptibility to encapsulated organisms; for example, S. pneumonia, H. influenza, N. meningitis, and other infectious diseases such as malaria
     - thrombocytosis and risk of thrombosis
     - damage to adjoining organ; for example, tail of pancreas.

2.2.26 Seatbelt injury

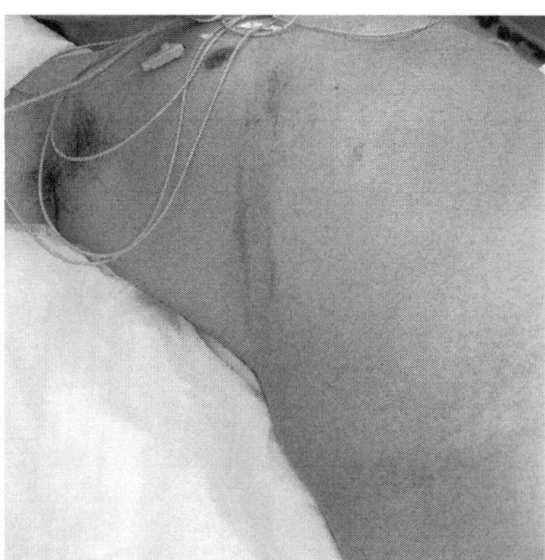

Figure 2.2.26
Seatbelt injury

1. Describe the findings?
   - Image of a man lying supine with right arm out. There is a seatbelt injury mark, commencing at the medial edge of left clavicle that extends across the lower right chest and upper right abdomen and into the right flank. Ecchymosis present from left supraclavicular fossa downwards with some skin abrasion along the line of the injury.
2. What are the potential injuries?
   - General injuries directly due to high velocity blunt trauma/deceleration injury:
     - airway
     - head and neck
     - thorax: lung, cardiac, great vessels, ribs
     - abdomen/pelvis
     - upper and lower limbs.
   - Direct blunt injury to any organ underlying the seatbelt injury or damaged secondarily to compressive force:
     - left clavicle: thoracic outlet, potential subclavian vessel or left first rib injury, left apex of lung
     - mediastinum: heart, oesophagus, trachea, great vessels
     - right chest: chest wall, ribs, lung, diaphragm, major veins (azygous, SVC)
     - right upper quadrant: liver, gallbladder, duodenum, pancreas, IVC
     - right flank: kidney, ascending colon.

2.2.27 Barium swallow: oesophageal cancer and achalasia

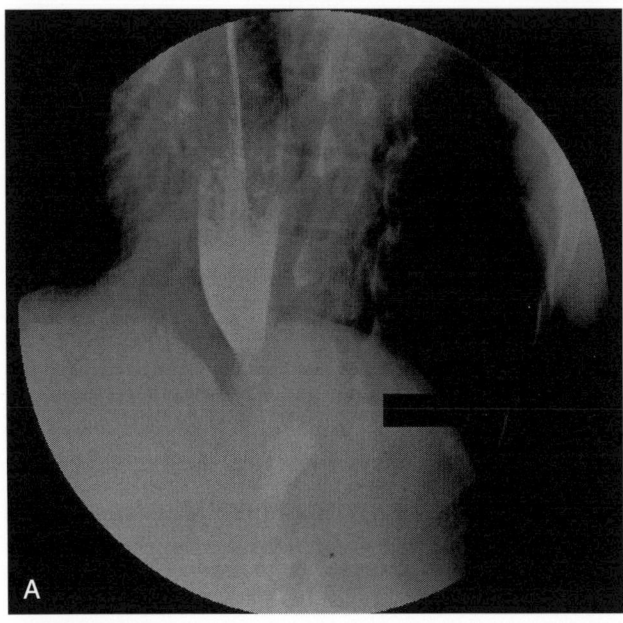

Figure 2.2.27A
Barium swallow of achalasia

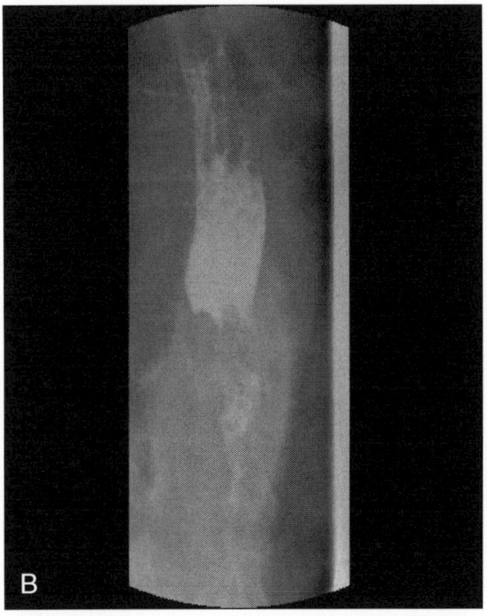

Figure 2.2.27B
Barium swallow of oesophageal cancer

1. What is the diagnosis in these two images?
   - A: Achalasia.
   - B: Carcinoma of the distal oesophagus.
2. How might these patients present?
   - Achalasia: halitosis, regurgitation of undigested contents, dysphagia, odynophagia, retrosternal chest pain, in the elderly recurrent respiratory infections.
   - Carcinoma of the distal oesophagus: dysphagia to solids initially, then to liquids, weight loss, prior symptoms of GORD.
3. What is the pathogenesis?
   - Achalasia: a progressive degeneration of the myenteric plexus of Auerbach. In South America could be due to Chagas disease from *Trypanosoma cruzi*.
   - Carcinoma of the distal oesophagus:
     - SCC — higher rates seen in tobacco smokers and high alcohol intake, higher rates following caustic injury, digestion of smoked foods, and in patients with achalasia
     - Adenocarcinoma — may be due to Barrett's oesophagus, GORD, higher rates in smokers and obesity.
4. What are the treatment options?
   - Achalasia: depends on the age and fitness.
     - Medical: calcium antagonists, not very effective.
     - Endoscopic:
       - botox injection, but needs to be repeated; multiple injections associated with scarring and fibrosis, and decreasing ability to subsequently perform a dilatation or a Heller's myotomy
       - balloon dilatation under direct vision
       - both botox and balloon dilatation is usually reserved for older patients not fit to undergo a Heller's myotomy.
     - Surgical:
       - Heller's myotomy, laparoscopic or open
       - 5–6 cm myotomy from GOJ proximally, and 2–3 cm distally from the GOJ, with a gastroscope to guide the myotomy
       - if myotomy is done properly, 100% of patients will suffer reflux, and so should add a fundoplication, usually a 180 degree anterior wrap.
   - Carcinoma of the distal oesophagus: depends on patient and disease factors, usually a combination of radiation, chemotherapy and/or surgery.
     - SCC — usually treated with definitive chemoradiation.
       - Surgery only if recurrent disease, fit and potentially curable.
     - Adenocarcinoma — neo-adjuvant chemoradiation, then reassess.
       - Surgery (Ivor-Lewis cardio-oesophagectomy) if fit and potentially curable.

2.2.28 Gastric ulcer

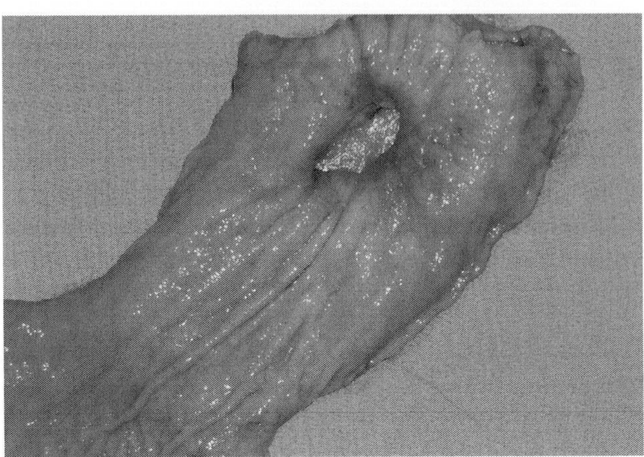

Figure 2.2.28
Perforated gastric ulcer

1. What is the diagnosis?
   - A 3 × 2 cm perforated ulcer in the posterior wall of the upper part of the body of stomach. Gastrectomy specimen.
2. What is the differential diagnosis?
   - Gastric cancer.
   - Gastric lymphoma.
   - Gastric GIST.
3. What is the treatment?
   - Usually surgical:
     - close the defect if possible with an omental patch
     - biopsy the edge of the ulcer in case of malignancy:
       - if gastric cancer usually already disseminated
       - if gastric lymphoma treatment usually medical
       - therefore no benefit usually from immediate gastrectomy and best if can close defect and patch perforated gastric ulcers.
     - if cannot close the defect — distal gastrectomy and reconstruction most likely gastro-jejunostomy Roux-en-Y.

2.2.29 Choledochal cyst

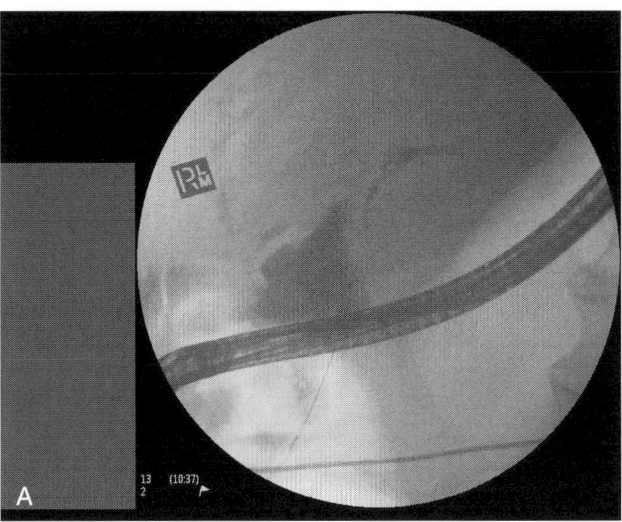

Figure 2.2.29A
ERCP Choledochal cyst

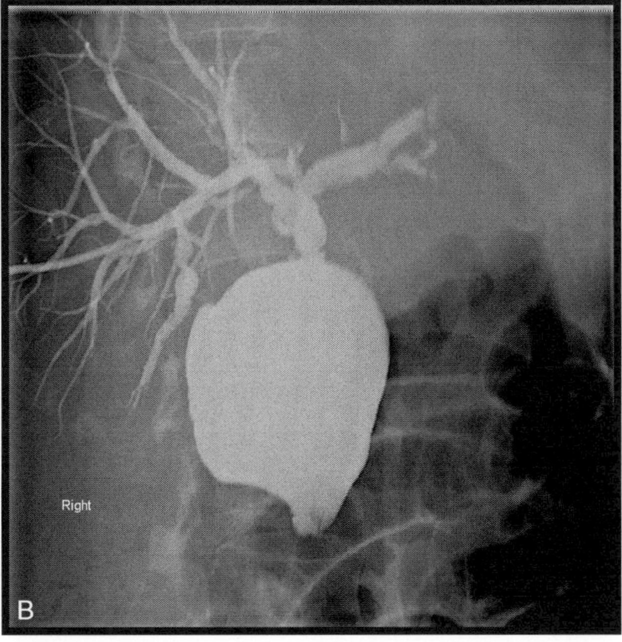

Figure 2.2.29B
PTC Choledochal cyst

1. Describe the findings.
   - A is an ERCP image and B is a percutaneous transhepatic cholangiogram image. Both images show a choledochal cyst.
2. What causes this?
   - An abnormality at the pancreaticobiliary duct junction. Normally separate ducts.
   - Common channel theory is that there is a common pancreatic and biliary duct, and then only controlled by common channel sphincter, with increased reflux of pancreatic juice into bile duct resulting in cystic dilatation and increased ductal pressure, and abnormal sphincter of Oddi function.
3. What is the treatment?
   - Depends of the type of choledochal cyst.
   - High rate of malignancy, so all need to be treated in fit patients.
   - Todani classification (1977) according to site and shape.
     - Type 1: fusiform or saccular extra-hepatic, 50–80%. Requires complete or near-complete excision with Roux-en-Y hepaticojejunostomy and cholecystectomy.
     - Type 2: isolated protrusion or diverticular outpouching of the CBD, <1%. Requires cholecystectomy, simple cyst excision, and common bile duct reconstruction over a T-tube.
     - Type 3: choledochocele with cyst located at most distal part of the CBD in the intra-duodenal portion of the CBD, 10%. If no evidence of malignancy, ERCP and sphincterotomy, or sphincteroplasty. If malignant requires pancreaticoduodenectomy.
     - Type 4: intra- and extra-hepatic ducts. 4a multiple intra- and extra-hepatic, 4b multiple extra-hepatic. 30–40%. If cirrhosis and portal hypertension: need liver transplant. If unilateral require hepatic and CBD resection and hepaticojejunostomy.
     - Type 5: multiple intra-hepatic with hepatic fibrosis (Caroli's disease); 10%. If diffuse (bilobar) requires transplant. If unilobar hepatic resection and hepaticojejunostomy.

2.2.30 Pancreatic pseudocyst

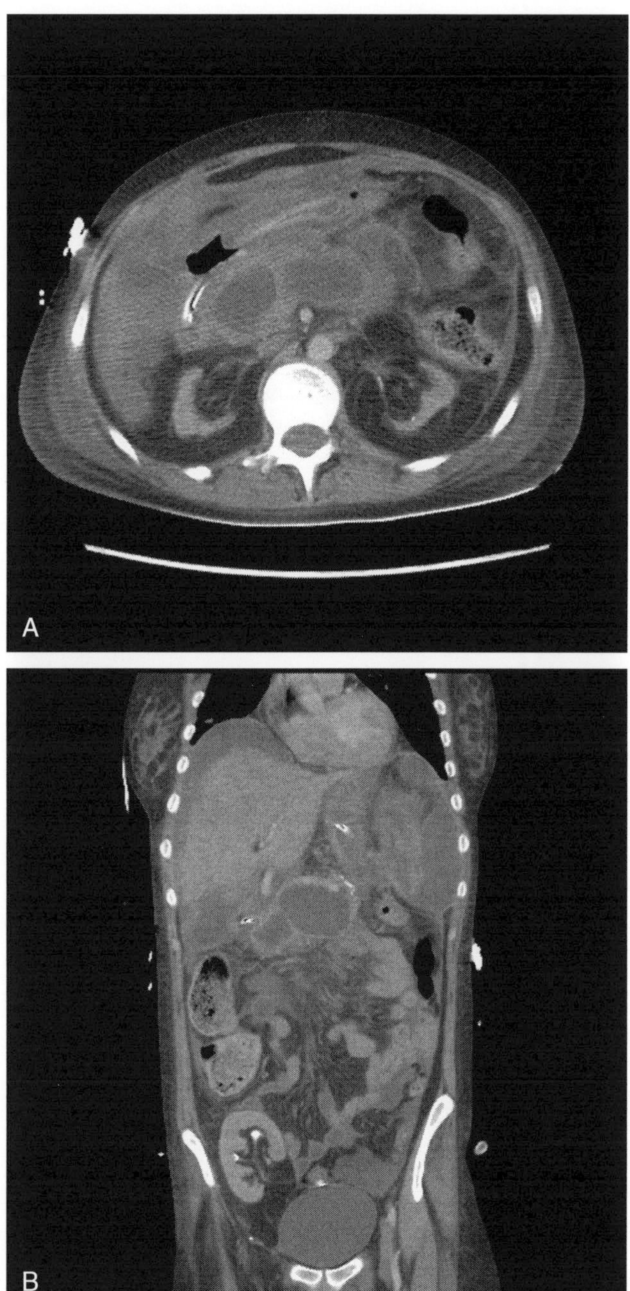

Figure 2.2.30
CT scan pancreatic pseudocyst

Please read in conjunction with 4.6.11, systemic inflammatory response syndrome SIRS, 4.6.12, multi-organ dysfunction syndrome, and 4.6.21, pancreatitis.

This is the CT scan of a 47-year-old man 6 weeks post-pancreatitis.

1. What is the diagnosis?
   - Pancreatic pseudocyst. Also very low right pelvic kidney, maybe renal transplant.
2. What are the complications of pancreatitis?
   - Local, adjacent organs, vascular and to rest of abdomen:
     - pancreas — haemorrhagic or necrotising pancreatitis 25–35%, may become secondarily infected
     - pseudocyst formation
     - infected pseudocyst
     - sequelae of a ruptured pseudocyst- pancreatic ascites
     - vascular complications — pseudoaneurysm of any arteries around pancreas; for example, splenic artery or small arteries around pancreas (e.g. superior pancreaticoduodenal)
     - portal vein thrombosis, splenic vein thrombosis, superior mesenteric vein thrombosis
     - abscess which may track through abdomen, down the paracolic gutters, or present as a iliopsoas abscess
     - bile duct or duodenal obstruction from oedema of the head of pancreas
     - paralytic ileus.
   - Systemic:
     - SIRS
     - MODS.
3. What options are there for drainage procedures?
   - Endoscopic: transpapillary stent or transmural drainage usually through the posterior wall of stomach.
   - External: usually for critically ill patients. CT guided retroperitoneal approach percutaneous drainage.
   - Operative (laparoscopic or open):
     - depends on where the pseudocyst is and where best drainage may occur. Cystogastrostomy, cystoduodenostomy or Roux-en-Y cystojejunostomy are options
     - if pseudocyst is in the tail of pancreas may perform a distal pancreatectomy with or without splenectomy.

2.2.31 Diabetic foot

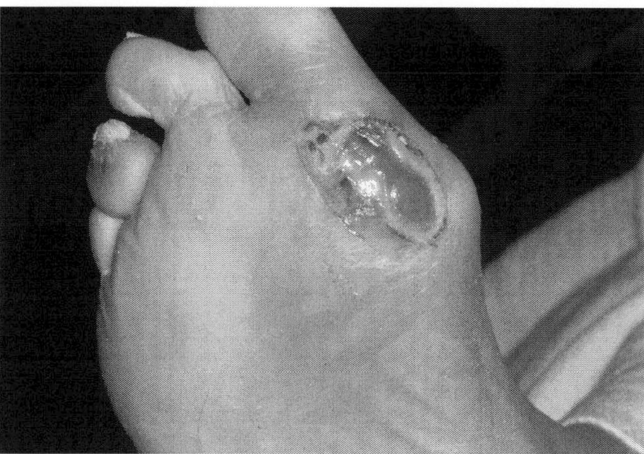

Figure 2.2.31
Diabetic foot ulcer

1. What is the diagnosis and describe the findings?
   - The image shows the typical location of a neuropathic diabetic foot ulcer over a pressure point (in this case, the first MTP joint).
   - There is also a smaller ulcer on the plantar aspect of the third toe.
   - It also shows changes in the foot architecture with subluxation of the first MTP joint.
   - Other features of note are the dry, flaky skin associated with autonomic neuropathy and the callous formation around the ulcer.
2. What is the differential diagnosis?
   - Ischaemic foot ulcer (may be neuropathic and ischaemic).
   - Osteomyelitis.
   - Septic arthritis of the 1st MTP joint (note that the first 3 points in this list may all be present together).
   - Foreign body.
3. How would you investigate this patient?
   - ABPI (note: may be falsely elevated in diabetes due to calcified vessels).
   - MC&S swab of ulcer.
   - Bloods:
     - FBC, EUC, Coags, HbA1c.
   - Plain x-ray of the foot looking for:
     - osteomyelitis
     - foreign body
     - gas in the tissue.
   - Duplex ultrasound.
   - Digital subtraction angiography if there is evidence of impaired blood supply on the less invasive tests.
     - Care with abnormal renal function (elevated) creatinine and implications of the use of nephrotoxic contrast agents.
   - Consider CT or MRI if you suspect deeper infection or foreign body, but would only suggest this if pushed by the examiner.

4. How would you manage this patient?
   Goals:
   - address sepsis
   - optimise blood supply to promote healing and offload pressure
   - optimisation of diabetes management/other risk factors
   - MDT approach (podiatrist, endocrinologist, vascular surgeon).
   - Management of the sepsis:
     - appropriate antibiotic therapy; i.e., broad spectrum to cover polymicrobial infection including anaerobes
     - debridement if necessary:
       - preferably after confirmation/restoration of adequate blood supply
       - may require debridement prior to restoration of blood supply if life-threatening sepsis.
       - debridement back to healthy, bleeding tissue. Often in diabetes the visible ulcer is only the tip of the iceberg (important for consenting the patient)
     - more rarely, plastics may need to be involved for free flaps, rotations flaps, SSG.
   - Management of the blood supply:
     - percutaneous transluminal angioplasty (PTA) +/– stenting of large vessel inflow
     - open surgical bypass +/– endarterectomy.
   - Optimisation of diabetes management/other risk factors:
     - endocrinological input for diabetes management, education, and eye/kidney/foot follow-up
     - anti-platelet agent (aspirin) and statin for plaque stability regardless of cholesterol level
     - consideration of ACE inhibitors if microalbuminuria.

2.2.32 Ischaemic leg

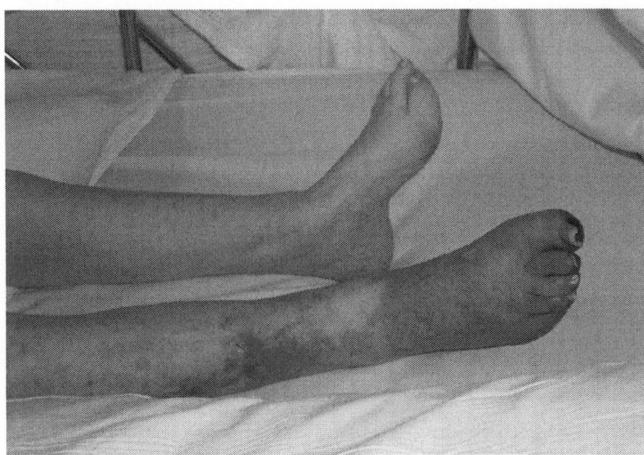

Figure 2.2.32
Ischaemic leg

Please read in conjunction with 3.5.8, peripheral occlusive arterial disease short case.

1. What is the diagnosis?
   - Acutely ischaemic lower right leg and foot.
2. What is the potential aetiology?
   Embolic:
   - cardiac source (AF, endocarditis)
   - from aneurysm in aorta or ipsilateral leg vessel
   - atherosclerotic plaque in aorta or ipsilateral leg vessel.

   Thrombosis:
   - atherosclerosis — acute thrombosis/plaque event in context of chronic peripheral occlusive arterial disease
   - bypass graft occlusion
   - thrombotic conditions.

   Rarer causes:
   - large vessel arteritis:
     - Takayasu's
     - Buerger's disease
     - giant cell
     - polyarteritis nodosa
   - small vessel disease:
     - diabetes
     - Raynaud's disease
     - connective tissue disorders
       - scleroderma
       - rheumatoid arthritis
       - SLE.
   - Miscellaneous:
     - vessel dissection
     - trauma/external compression
     - compartment syndrome
     - frost-bite
     - cold agglutinins (seen in Hep C)
     - myeloproliferative disorders
     - drug-related (vasoconstrictors e.g. noradrenaline in ICU)
     - sepsis, such as pneumococcus, meningococcus.
3. How would you investigate?
   - Basic investigations/pre-operative work-up:
     - urinalysis — glucose, microspot for proteinuria
     - bloods:
       - FBC (Hb, WCC)
       - EUC (renal function)
       - fasting BSL, HbA1C and glucose tolerance tests as required
       - coagulation studies and thrombophilia screens may be indicated in a small number of patient with family history
       - total cholesterol/TG/LDL/HDL
       - vasculitic screen
     - ECG (pre-operative)
     - CXR (pre-operative).
   - Definitive investigation — may be completed *after* intervention:
     - echocardiography (exclude emboli)

- duplex imaging
- radiological investigation:
  - diagnostic digital subtraction angiogram
  - CT angiography (if proximal disease is suspected)
  - MR angiography.

4. How would you manage this patient?
   - Assess patient for risk factors and cause (is patient in AF?), determine if acute embolic phenomena or acute on chronic ischaemia (based on previous history of peripheral occlusive arterial disease/claudication).
   - Determine severity of ischaemia using the Rutherford Classification (see Table 2.2.32), which is based on capillary return, audible arterial and venous pulse, sensory loss and muscle weakness.
   - Immediate treatment:
     - resuscitation with fluids and oxygen
     - pain control
     - antibiotics, keep foot dependent, avoid extremes of temperature
     - intravenous heparin (5000 IU) followed by an infusion.
   - Definitive treatment (revascularisation) will depend on Rutherford classification:
     - irreversible acute ischaemia (unsalvageable — class III) with complete neurological deficit, tense muscles, absent capillary return and no Doppler signal:
       - palliation
       - amputation.
     - Critical acute ischaemia (*threatened* leg — class IIb) with partial neurological deficit and no audible Doppler signal or if thrombolysis is contraindicated in patients with subcritical ischaemia:
       - immediate surgical exploration of the femoral artery with balloon catheter embolectomy ± on table arteriography.
     - Subcritical acute ischaemia (*viable* leg — class I/IIa) with no neurological deficit and an audible Doppler signal:
       - arteriography
       - probable embolus — aspiration or embolectomy
       - probable thrombus — thrombolysis.

Table 2.2.32 Rutherford classification of acute limb ischaemia

	CLINICAL FINDINGS			DOPPLER		PROGNOSIS
Class	**Capillary return**	**Sensory loss**	**Motor weakness**	**Arterial signals**	**Venous signals**	
I. Viable	Intact	None	None	Audible	Audible	Not immediately threatened
IIa. Marginal threat	Intact/ slow	Minimal sensory loss	None	Often not audible	Audible	Salvageable if prompt treatment (there is time for angiography)
IIb. Immediate threat	Slow/ absent	Rest pain with sensory loss	Mild to moderate	Inaudible	Audible	Salvageable with immediate treatment (no time for angiography)
III. Irreversible	Absent	Severe anaesthesia	Paralysis with muscle rigor	Inaudible	Inaudible	Not salvageable, permanent nerve/muscle damage needs amputation

2.2.33 Psoas abscess

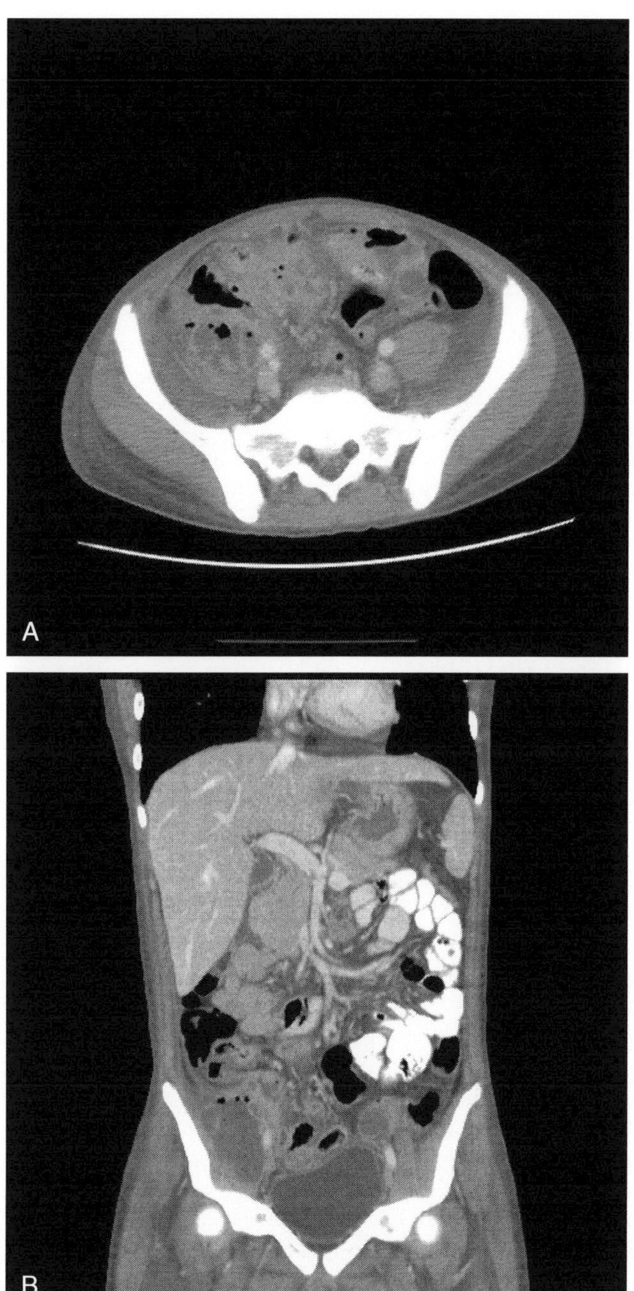

Figure 2.2.33
CT scan of bilateral psoas abscesses

1. What is the diagnosis?
   - Right-sided psoas (or iliopsoas muscle compartment) abscess, and what appears to be a smaller left-sided psoas abscess.
2. What are the possible causes?
   - Primary abscess (20–40%). Infection occurs via haematogenous spread from distant source. Pathogens include *Staph. aureus*, *Escherichia coli* and *streptococcus*. Occurs more often in:
     - diabetes
     - HIV/AIDS
     - IVDU
     - alcohol abuse
     - renal failure
     - haematological disease such as haemophilia or cancer
     - immunosuppression
     - malnutrition.
   - Secondary abscess (60–80%): infection spread from adjacent structures, commonly *Escherichia coli* and bacteroides, while M. tuberculosis is the most common cause in developing countries in which tuberculosis is still common.
     - Potential origins:
       - vertebral bodies — osteomyelitis, tuberculosis of the spine (Pott's disease)
       - large bowel — appendix (appendicitis), caecum or ascending colon (cancer) on right and sigmoid colon on left (Diverticulitis)
       - small bowel — terminal ileum (Crohn's disease)
       - urinary tract — kidney/renal pelvis (pyelonephritis), ureter (urinary tract infection)
       - psoas muscle — haematoma, spontaneous or iatrogenic (e.g. femoral nerve block catheter)
       - abdominal aorta — mycotic aneurysm
       - pancreas — pancreatitis
       - hip joint — infected total hip prosthesis, septic arthritis
       - iliac lymph nodes.
3. What is the management?
   - Appropriate IV antibiotics.
   - Drainage, mostly CT-guided percutaneous drainage and culture of fluid to guide the antibiotic cover.
   - Abscess may require surgical drainage/debridement if failed percutaneous drainage or multiloculated abscess.
     - Open drainage approaches via an extraperitoneal approach:
       - flank for upper retroperitoneal and around the kidney
       - iliac fossa muscle splitting for lower retroperitoneal
       - abscess may extend to the thigh and require drainage there.
   - Identify the cause of the abscess if secondary abscess.
   - Treatment of the underlying pathology if present.

Chapter 2.3

The written examination paper 2 — short answer questions

The common denominator of success, the secret of success of every man who has ever been successful, lies in the fact that he formed the habit of doing things that failures don't like to do. (Albert E N Gray, 1940)

The examination format

The second written paper comprises eight short answer questions, which must be completed within 2 hours, (i.e. 15 minutes per question). Candidates are allowed into the examination room 15 minutes prior to the commencement of the examination and are given 10 minutes reading time prior to the official start. Candidates receive answer booklets consisting of 35 pages which are blank on one side and lined on the other. Answers are only to be written on the lined sides of the answer booklets. Candidates can ask for more booklets if required.

Exam technique

- Once you have read the examination paper, you may be happy to answer the questions in order from one through to eight. However, many candidates prefer to answer the questions they consider 'easiest' first and tackle 'more difficult' questions last. Whilst this is an excellent strategy to build confidence, it requires exceptional discipline to ensure that you do *not* write for more than 15 minutes!
- Whichever order you chose to answer the questions in, make sure that you answer *all* eight questions. Remember that a 'good' pass in one or two questions may not necessarily make up for a 'fail' in other questions that have not been answered adequately or at all.

- Ensure that you do not write for more than 15 minutes on any one question. Be aware of the time and pace yourself. It is useful to position a watch clearly on the desk in front of you so that you are mindful of the time while writing. This sounds so obvious but it is easy to lose track of time during the exam, particularly when you are in full-flow writing on a topic that you know well!
- Most trainees can write approximately four pages in 15 minutes, so aim to achieve the same.
- You must be confident knowing how many pages you can write and exactly how much detail you can incorporate within the allotted time. You will be surprised how few points you can make. Only through repeated practise can you expect to know this information.
- Make your answer easy to read and be sure that every word is legible. Examiners can only award marks if they can read the content of your response.
- Generally, the response is most efficiently organised in point format, using tables, diagrams or flow charts. Avoid writing an essay since the majority of the words written are redundant in terms of scoring.
- Direct the examiner to keywords by underlining or using upper case to emphasise important points or phrases of particular significance.
- Phrases which imply deeper understanding to the examiner but require very few words are useful as they are likely to receive disproportionately more recognition than the time required writing them down (e.g. 'damage control').
- The written papers are photocopied and sent to the examiners for marking. This means that there will be *no* benefit from using coloured markers or highlighters.
- Consider writing a plan before launching into the written response. This can be included on the first answer page. A plan helps provide a schema for your answer and enables you to identify and list the 'suburbs, streets and houses' (as detailed in Chapter 1.2). It will also ensure that you have your thoughts, ideas and responses ordered in a logical fashion and thus may paradoxically save you time in the long run; it will help keep you to time while answering your question.
- Be certain to structure your answer to facilitate presentation of the facts to the examiner to ensure that you pick up all available marks. Refer back to Chapter 1.2 for further information relating to this point.
- It is quite reasonable to use 'dot points' when writing answers, so that you can cover the main areas in a short period of time. The use of simple diagrams and/or charts to elaborate your answer can also be useful.

HINT

We strongly recommend breaking the question down into its constituent components and highlighting each of these in your plan/answer. This will ensure that, under the pressure of the exam, you answer every part of the question without omission and thus secure maximum marks available. It will also make sure that you don't run out of time before addressing every section of the question. It is advisable to write your answer using the components of the question as subheadings. This will direct the examiner to the important points within your answer and improve your chances of picking up all the available marks on offer.

The following is an example of a past question that will be considered in Chapter 2.4.7.

Question: a 40-year-old woman is referred to your office with thyrotoxicosis. What are the common causes of thyrotoxicosis and what is the role of surgery in each? How would you prepare a thyrotoxic patient for surgery?

Accordingly the components of the question to be highlighted in the plan are:

1. common causes of thyrotoxicosis
2. what is the role of surgery in each
3. how do you prepare a thyrotoxic patient for surgery.

When writing the answer, these same subheadings should be used. Many of the above techniques will be demonstrated in the model answers in the Chapter 2.4.

Preparation and practising

Although each of the above points seems very obvious, our experience from marking 'mock answers' is that candidates very frequently forget to pay attention to this advice. Indeed, we have observed that candidates tend to despise practising short answer questions and tend to prefer attending tutorials or rehearsing the *viva voce* examinations. However, you cannot possibly expect to pass this section of the examination if you have not repeatedly practised answering the questions in 15 minutes without needing to refer to any textbooks or notes. It is also worth practising writing eight answers in 2 hours to simulate the exam and to discover how challenging it is on your hand and your brain! You must force yourself to practise this section of the exam and include adequate time to do so in your study plan. Finally, don't forget to ask colleagues, mentors and supervisors to critique and mark your answers.

Chapter 2.4

Common written examination short answer questions

2.4.1 Genetics of colorectal cancer syndromes

Question: discuss the genetics of hereditary colorectal cancer syndromes.

Answer

Plan or overview

- Syndromes — account for 5% of all colorectal cancers, the remainder are sporadic:
  - HNPCC/Lynch Syndrome
  - FAP
  - Familial juvenile polyposis
  - MUTYH-associated polyposis (MAP).

1. HNPCC (hereditary non-polyposis colorectal CA)/Lynch syndrome

DEFINITION

- The most common form of hereditary CRC.
- Four cardinal features:
  1. earlier average age (40–45 yrs) at onset of CA than in general population
  2. presence of associated cancers within the pedigree
  3. improved survival when compared stage for stage to sporadic cases
  4. presence of a germ-line mutation in affected family members.

INCIDENCE

- Account for 2–3% of CRC.
- Onset in 40s (compared to 60s for general population).

CLASSIFICATION

1. Lynch I = FHx of CRC.
2. Lynch II = FHx of CRC and other extra-colonic manifestations:
   - Muir-Torre Syndrome (= subtype of HNPCC/Lynch II):
     - skin tumours (sebaceous neoplasms) and GIT and GU adenoCAs
     - 12% risk of breast CA.

GENETICS

- Autosomal dominant.
- Germ-line mutation: genetic defect of mismatch repair genes on chromosome 2p:
  - MLH1, MSH2, MSH6, PMS1 and PMS2
  - NB MLH1 and MSH2 account for 90%.
- The defects occur in the setting of microsatellite instability.

PATHOLOGY

- Typical histology associated with microsatellite instability:
  - presence of tumour infiltrating lymphocytes, Crohn's-like lymphocytic reaction
  - mucinous/signet ring differentiation, or
  - medullary growth pattern.

HINT

Pathology can be remembered as LAMPS:

i) **l**ymphocytes/**l**ymphoid aggregates
ii) **a**ssociated extracolonic cancers (endometrium, stomach, ovary, urothelium, small bowel)
iii) **m**ucinous/**m**etachronous tumours
iv) **p**oorly differentiated/**p**roximal colon tumours
v) **s**ignet ring/**s**ynchronous tumours.

- Mutations in chromosome 2p or 3p in 90% — mismatch repair (MMR) protein genes (MLH1, MSH2, MSH6, PMS1, PMS2, etc) → accumulation of unrepaired replication errors detectable in tumour (RER+).
- Loss of nuclear expression of MMR protein can be detected by immunohistochem.
- When a MMR gene mutation is inherited, the loss/silencing (through methylation) of the second copy of the gene results in total loss of the mismatch capacity associated with that gene → accumulation of error.

2. FAP (familial adenomatous polyposis)

DEFINITION

A rare familial disease associated with development of CRC before age 40 in nearly all untreated patients.

INCIDENCE

Accounts for 0.5% of CRC.

CLASSIFICATION

- Attenuated form of FAP ('weaker'): <100 adenomas, uneven distribution in colon, later age of onset (risk rises sharply after age 40 and is >50%), usually R colon; often have rectal sparing.
- FAP with extracolonic manifestations:
  - Gardener's/Gardner's syndrome = a variant of FAP distinguished by the presence of prominent extra intestinal lesions, such as desmoid tumours, osteomas (of mandible or skull), sebaceous cysts and thyroid CA
  - Turcot's syndrome: polyposis and childhood cerebellar medulloblastoma.

AETIOLOGY

- Autosomal dominant (AD) mutations of the tumour suppressor APC gene (Chr 5q) are responsible for FAP:
  - >300 mutations have been described
  - lead to a loss of β-catenin regulation → β-catenin accumulation → activated transcription factor Tcf-4
  - somatic APC mutations have been discovered in the majority of sporadic desmoids
  - AD inheritance, but incomplete penetrance.

PATHOLOGY

- Attenuated FAP: variant associated with mutations at the 3' or 5' end of the APC genes.
- Patients with APC 3' mutations → 65% risk of developing desmoids post-operatively (BJS 2007; 94:1009–13).

3. Familial juvenile polyposis syndrome

- Harmartomatous polyps
- ↑risk of:
  - CRC (lifetime risk 9–25%)
  - gastric CA
  - duodenal CA
  - pancreatic CA.
- Screening: colonoscopy 1–2 yrly from age 15.

4. MUTYH-associated polyposis(MAP)

- MAP is suspected in an individual who has:
  - colonic adenoma count between one and ten before age 40 years
  - colonic adenoma and/or hyperplastic polyp count between ten and a few hundred
  - colonic polyposis (i.e., >100 colonic polyps) in the absence of a germline APC mutation
  - colorectal cancer (CRC) with the somatic KRAS mutation c.34G>T in codon 12
  - family history of colon cancer (with or without polyps) consistent with autosomal recessive inheritance.
- The diagnosis of MAP is confirmed by the presence of biallelic MUTYH mutations [Al Tassan et al 2002, Sieber et al 2003].

2.4.2 Autonomic innervation of the pelvis

Question: discuss the hypogastric nerve plexuses highlighting the sites of possible surgical injury. Emphasise the consequences of injury that you would include in your discussion when obtaining informed consent from a patient.

Answer

Plan

Superior hypogastic plexus (predominately Sympathetic Nervous System [SNS] Fibers) → hypogastric nerves → connect to inferior hypogastric plexus.

Inferior hypogastric plexus x 2 = pelvic plexus. Formed from expansion of S2-4 anterior rami (Parasympathetic Nervous System [PNS] fibres join) and receives sympathetic fibres from hypogastric nerves.

Sites of injury:

- IMA ligation
- sigmoid mobilisation
- rectal mobilisation:
  - mesorectal plane
  - anterior rectal mobilisation.

Consent:

- erectile dysfunction
- urinary retention
- ejaculatory failure and retrograde ejaculation
- inadvertent injury vs intentional sacrifice.

Anatomy

- *Superior hypogastic plexus* is a singular, midline structure close to the origin of IMA. It arises from convergence of preganglionic *SNS fibres* from the sympathetic trunk.
  - Lies deep to the parietal peritoneum in front of the left *common iliac vein*.
- It breaks up to give rise to right and left *hypogastric nerves (singular or bundle)*:
  - descend on the posterolateral pelvic wall just underneath the parietal endopelvic fascia of the rectum
  - the hypogastric nerves run down into the pelvis to join the pelvic plexus.
- The parasympathetic supply to the pelvis arises from the S2-4. The pelvic splanchnic nerves (*nervi erigentes*) continue as visible condensations, expanding to form the right and left *inferior hypogastric plexuses*, which are collectively known as the *pelvic plexus*.
  - The right and left *inferior hypogastric plexuses* are flat plexuses lying beneath the parietal layer of endopelvic fascia lateral to mid rectum.
- Fibres from pelvic plexus project forward and medially to the pelvic viscera (bladder, rectum, seminal vesicles, erectile tissue of corpus cavernosa, uterus and vagina).

Sites of injury during surgery and consequences

- Ligation of IMA: the pre-aortic sympathetic fibres may be damaged.
- Mobilisation of the sigmoid mesocolon: the superior hypogastric plexus at risk:
  - damage to SNS structures → ejaculatory failure or retrograde ejaculation.
- Posterior rectal mobilisation if the mesorectal plane is not respected: the inferior hypogastric plexus and pelvic splanchnic nerves at risk.
- Anterior rectum dissection from the seminal vesicles: terminal branches of the pelvic plexus at risk:
  - damage to the pelvic plexus, or mixed PNS and SNS → erectile impotence, urinary retention or both.

Informed consent

The patient needs to be made aware that these structures may be damaged inadvertently or scarified intentionally in an attempt to achieve *R0* resection, potentially leading to the symptoms described above.

2.4.3 Management of large bowel obstruction/role of colonic stents

Question: outline the management of large bowel obstruction. Include differential diagnoses and discuss the role of colonic stents.

Answer

Causes of LBO

Causes of LBO can be divided into:
- pseudo-obstruction vs mechanical obstruction
- mechanical obstruction
  - intraluminal
    - faecal impaction
    - foreign body
  - mural
    - diverticular stricture
    - carcinoma (colonic or rectal)
    - IBD stricture
    - ischaemic stricture
  - extramural
    - volvulus: sigmoid or caecal
    - tumour extrinsic to bowel eg. ovarian or endometrial CA in the pelvis.

Management

Resuscitation — CCrISP principles:
- correct hypovolaemia due to any vomiting and 'third' space losses.

Assessment:

- History:
  - characteristic symptoms (CAVE) — constipation; abdominal pain; vomiting; enlarged abdomen
  - presence of pain, ask about characteristics of peritonitis
  - recent change in bowel habit, PR bleeding, and weight loss preceding presentation
  - personal or family history of colorectal cancer
  - previous presentations with diverticulitis/IBD/colitis
  - previous colonoscopy
  - medications: contribute to constipation and volvulus
  - social circumstance and level of function: volvulus typically occurs in elderly/nursing home residents.
- Examination:
  - presence of peritonitis raises level of urgency to investigate and intervene
  - RIF peritonism = suspect caecal perforation (Laplace's law)
  - perform a digital rectal examination/rigid sigmoidoscopy.

Investigation:

- bloods: ↑WCC suspicion of complications; anaemia
- erect CXR: if pneumoperitoneum present then needs urgent laparotomy
- erect and supine AXR: if appearance consistent with sigmoid volvulus then try to decompress with rigid/flexible sigmoidoscopy and rectal tube
- CT abdo/pelvis if stable and large bowel obstruction confirmed on AXR
- gastrografin enema useful to distinguish pseudo-obstruction and mechanical obstruction. May also reduce sigmoid volvulus. Also provides useful 'roadmap' if stenting considered.

Intervention:

- depends on findings of investigation
- if malignant cause or stricture identified — plan for surgery
  - urgency determined by clinical signs and patient's condition
  - if malignant lesion then consider stenting vs resection (see below)
- if sigmoid volvulus unable to be decompressed 'on-ward' then will need Gastrografin enema or colonoscopic (CO2) decompression
  - if unsuccessful then may resection if patient fit for surgery
  - if caecal volvulus then may need ileocolic resection
- if extrinsic compression and not suitable for stent then may need stoma to decompress colon
- if faecal impaction and not perforation, needs disimpaction and regular enemas.

Role for stents

- May be used for malignant obstruction of the colon.
- Role in:
  - palliation of stage IV disease: case series suggest safe and effective in this setting

- 'bridge' to surgery i.e. temporising measure to allow elective resection (one-stage)
- patient 'unfit' for surgery.
- Stents are deployed endoscopically and avoid need for laparotomy and stoma formation in malignant large bowel obstruction.
- Risks:
  - inability to stent
  - bowel perforation
  - stent migration
  - stent occlusion
  - pain/tenesmus if stent low in rectum.
- Minimal evidence for use in benign causes of obstruction.

2.4.4 Colonoscopic surveillance and complications

Question: write short notes on the recommendations of the use of colonoscopy in surveillance of patients with common colorectal diseases (e.g. cancer, IBD) and briefly outline the main complications of colonoscopy and management.

Answer

Surveillance guidelines

ADENOMA SURVEILLANCE: NHMRC 2012 GUIDELINES

- High risk: colonoscopy @ 3 yrs → if –ve then subsequent @ 3–5 yrs:
  - adenoma ≥10 mm
  - ≥3 adenomas
  - villous/tubulovillous lesions and/or high grade dysplasia
  - adenomas + FHx of CRC.
- Low risk: colonoscopy at 5 yrs +/– consider discontinuing surveillance if normal:
  - adenomas with none of high-risk features above and no FHx of CRC.
- Other:
  - 3 months — excision of malignant adenoma or incompletely excised large adenoma
  - within 1 yr — incomplete/inadequate exam.

FHX OF CRC (NZ GUIDELINES GROUP)

- low risk: → no scope; report symptoms
  - only ONE 1st or 2nd degree rel >55 yrs only.
- medium risk:
  - ONE 1st or 2nd degree rel <55 yrs with CRC
  - or TWO 1st/2nd degree rels same side.

  } → 5 yrly from age 50 (or 10 yrs ealier than Dx of relative)
- high risk:
  - if THREE + 1st/2nd degree rels same side with CRC.

  } → suspect HNPCC/FAP & refer to genetics

FAMILIAL SYNDROMES: (NZ GUIDELINES GROUP)

- FAP:
  - 1–2 yrly from age 12–15 yrs then 3 yrly from age 35 if all normal
    - and gastroscopy from age 30–35
  - NB offer prophylactic colectomy in late teens.
- HNPCC:
  - 2 yrly from age 25 (or 5 yrs earlier than relatives developed CA)
  - NB endometrial surveillance too.

IBD SURVEILLANCE: NHMRC 2012 GUIDELINES

- UC pts with colonic involvement beyond sigmoid colon and pts with Crohn's disease involving > one-third of the colon NO later than 8 years after disease onset.
  - If primary sclerosing cholangitis detected BEFORE this time — immediate colonoscopy.
  - Strong PHx or FHx should commence surveillance sooner.
- Annual surveillance recommended if 1 or more of the following present:
  - active disease
  - primary sclerosing cholangitis
  - family history of colorectal cancer in first degree relative < 50 years old
  - colonic stricture, patients with multiple inflammatory polyps or shortened colon
  - previous dysplasia.
- Three yearly colonoscopy is recommended for patients with:
  - inactive ulcerative colitis extending proximal to the sigmoid colon without any of the above risk factors
  - patients with Crohn's colitis affecting more than one third of the colon without any of the above risk factors
  - IBD patients with a family history of colorectal cancer in a first degree relative > 50 years old.
- Five yearly colonoscopy recommended for patients in whom two previous colonoscopies were macroscopically and histologically normal.
  - NB if high grade dysplasia found in UC — pt should be referred for colectomy.
  - NB if low grade dysplasia found in UC — interval of colonoscopic surveillance should be shortened to yearly or colectomy considered in healthy patients.
  - Consider chromoendoscopy.

CRC SURVEILLANCE: NHMRC 2012 GUIDELINES

- Three to six months after resection if no/incomplete colonoscopy pre-operatively.
- 1 year after resection of a sporadic cancer (assuming no other post-operatively colonoscopy).
  - If +ve adenoma — 3 yrly.
  - If –ve adenoma — 5 yrly.
- For rectal CA: also 6 monthly sigmoidoscopy for 2 yrs.

Colonoscopy complications and management

- Complications related to bowel prep.
- Complications related to sedation/anaesthetic.
- Complications related to procedure:
  - perforation (1/2000), risk higher if polypectomy performed
  - bleeding (approx. 1%).

Management of such complications is dependent on the clinical signs and symptoms of the patient as well as their haemodynamic stability.

PERFORATION

Clinically well patient, no signs of sepsis, mild abdominal pain can be treated non-operatively with intravenous antibiotics, analgesia, nil by mouth, IV fluids and serial imaging (CT with oral and IV contrast). Surgical management will depend on site of perforation, size of defect, underlying pathology, degree of contamination and patient factors.

Clinically unwell patient, signs of sepsis, peritonism and free air on x-ray require operative management.

BLEEDING

Clinically well patient, haemodynamically stable — treated non-operatively, daily Hb checks, correct any coagulopathy, nil by mouth.

Haemodynamic compromise but stable — resus ABC, early ICU involvement, transfuse with PRCs, administer other blood products if required, CTA +/– angiography with embolisation of bleeding vessel, surgery if signs of ongoing haemodynamic instability or failure of angiography + embolisation. Occasionally, endoscopy with a plan to clip or diathermise the bleeding site.

2.4.5 Enterocutaneous fistula

Question: a 43-year-old man presents to a peripheral metropolitan hospital with small bowel obstruction. He has a history of appendicectomy as a child and three subsequent laparotomies for small bowel obstruction. After conservative treatment fails, he undergoes a further laparotomy. The operation is prolonged and difficult and two enterotomies were sustained and repaired primarily without resection during the adhesiolysis. Six days after surgery, enteric fluid is noticed leaking from the wound. The patient is transferred to your institution without evidence of peritonitis but is still not able to tolerate enteral nutrition. Outline your management of this problem.

Answer

Plan

Principles of management summarised by acronym SNAP:

S — **s**epsis control and **s**kin care

N — **n**utrition

A — define **a**natomy
P — **p**lan surgery

Fistula volume: high vs low:

- High: >500 ml/day. Indicative of: proximal origin, major underlying abnormality, likelihood of sepsis, skin breakdown, electrolyte and nutritional disturbances. Most require resection under optimal conditions.

Treat **sepsis** using broad spectrum ABx and possibly antifungal treatment if required. Screen and isolate if resistant infection — VRE and ESBL common. Infectious disease advice about ABx.

- Drain abscess — 80% amenable to radiological drainage.
- Surgical drainage only in patients with uncontrolled leakage of enteric contents into the peritoneal cavity or radiological drainage is not possible.
- Resection of leaking segment (with proximal and distal exteriorisation; anastomosis is rarely safe); formation of a proximal diverting loop stoma or conversion to a laparostomy.
- Early surgery to control sepsis should not be confused with early definitive surgery. *Early attempts at definitive surgery appear to increase mortality.*

Skin care: stomal therapy nurse. Protect skin from excoriation using stoma appliance, barrier cream.

Nutrition — no evidence that suspending enteral nutrition will increase rate of closure or ultimate outcome of fistula. However, until anatomy defined and need for surgery clear, reducing output may be beneficial in management. Place NG tube and use continuous low wall suction to reduce gastric contents. Start octreotide 25 mcg/tds SC daily and proton-pump inhibitors (e.g. pantoprazole 40 mg BD) to reduce output (and acidity). Initiate TPN. Resuscitation may be necessary in early stages.

- Calories: 35–40 kcal/kg/day(d).
- Volume: 30 ml/kg/day.
- Electrolytes: Na 1.5 mmol/kg/d; K 1 mmol/kg/d; Cl 1.3 mmol/kg/d; Mg 0.2 mmol/kg/d; PO_4 1 mmol/kg/d.
- Trace elements: Zinc, manganese, Fe — given as multivitamin preparation.
- Essential fatty acids: 15 g each of arachidonic acid and linoleic acid/day.
- Ratio: 50% carb; 30% lipid and 20% protein.
- Adjust each requirement according to bloods and extent of illness.

Enteral nutrition can be re-established even when fistula has not closed provided volume is controlled, electrolyte imbalances are addressed, sepsis is controlled and adequate drainage of any collections is achieved.

Define **anatomy** once sepsis and nutrition controlled — use CT scan and/or gastrografin follow-through. Issues:

- high or low in small bowel?
- distal obstruction
- ongoing disease (radiological evidence of Crohn's disease etc.)
- length of fistula tract.

Plan definitive surgery:

- if a fistula persists > 6 weeks after control of sepsis and adequate nutrition, spontaneous closure is unlikely, especially when output > 500 ml
- definitive surgery is planned for 3–6 months after injury to allow adhesions to settle
- mobilisation, fistulating bowel ends resected
- anastomosis should be goal
- cover anastomosis with omentum
- inspect for inadvertent enterotomy
- other options include bypass or conversion to an internal fistula (for duodenal fistula).

2.4.6 Solitary thyroid nodules

Question: discuss the aetiology and management of solitary thyroid nodules.

Answer

Definition: a thyroid nodule is a discrete lesion within the thyroid gland that is palpably and/or ultrasonographically distinct from the surrounding thyroid parenchyma.

Aetiology

Subdivided dependent upon whether the patient has thyrotoxicosis or not.

Thyrotoxic:

- Graves'
- multinodular goitre
- toxic adenoma — in the setting of a solitary nodule, toxic adenoma will be demonstrated on I^{131} scan and is the most likely diagnosis in thyrotoxic patients.

Euthyroid:

- degenerative cysts
- nodular thyroiditis
- neoplastic lesions
  - follicular adenoma
  - primary thyroid cancer
    - papillary, follicular, medullary, anaplastic, and other
  - secondary metastases.

Management

ASSESSMENT

Aims to:

- differentiate whether the nodule is in a thyrotoxic or euthyroid patient
- stratify risk for thyroid cancer.

HISTORY

- Symptoms of thyrotoxicosis (heat intolerance, palpitations, tremor etc.).
- Involvement of adjacent structures — notice voice change.
- Mechanical symptoms (stridor, dyspnoea, dysphagia).
- Associated symptoms of familial syndromes: phaeochromocytoma (hypertension, sweats), hypercalcaemia (stones, bones, groans, psychic moans).
- PHx: history of radiation — increases index of suspicion.
- FHx: familial thyroid cancer syndromes — medullary thyroid cancer, MEN 2a, MEN 2b and Cowden's syndrome (PTEN).

EXAMINATION

Neck:

- nodule characterisation: fixed, texture, size, solitary
- lymph nodes — lateral nodes: level 2 to 5
- change of voice.

Eyes:

- lid retraction, thyroid stare, ophthalmoplegia etc.

General:

- thyrotoxicosis — tremor, tachycardia, sweating etc.

Surgical planning:

- can I get above it, can I get below it
- retrosternal/retroclavicular.

INVESTIGATION

Bloods:

- TSH: initial evaluation of a patient with a thyroid nodule — Recommendation C (American Thyroid Guidelines).

Imaging — USS/CT:

- USS excellent at differentiating solid from cystic lesions.
- Generally, only nodules larger than 1 cm should be evaluated, because they have the potential to be clinically significant cancers. Occasionally, there may be nodules smaller than 1 cm that require evaluation, because of suspicious ultrasound findings, a history of head and neck irradiation, or a positive family history of thyroid cancer.

Pathology:

- Ultimately, fine needle aspiration cytology (FNAC) will differentiate between causes for the nodule.
- The potential codes for a euthyroid patient can be subdivided into insufficient, indeterminate, suspicious, benign, malignant.

Nuclear medicine scans:

- ^{123}I scan ONLY useful for patient with thyrotoxicosis (TSH <0.01).
- UNHELPFUL in euthyroid patients as poor sensitivity/specificity for diagnosis of cancer.

Ancillary tests:

- Suspicion medullary thyroid cancer — calcitonin, CEA, calcium, PTH, urinary and plasma catecholamines. MIBG (if high urinary catecholamines), genetic counselling: RET proto-oncogene testing.
- Papillary thyroid cancer: thyroglobulin: helpful in adjuvant assessment.

TREATMENT

Thyrotoxic patients:

- ^{123}I: >3 cm — surgery
- ^{123}I: <3 cm — radioactive ^{131}I

Euthyroid — guided by initial cytology result:

- cystic lesions — surgery if:
  - >4 cm diameter
  - blood-stained aspirate
  - recurrence after 2/3 aspirations
- benign FNAC — indications for surgery
  - mechanical symptoms
  - increasing size lesion
- indeterminate FNAC
  - often reported as 'suspicious,' 'follicular lesion' or 'follicular neoplasm'
  - found in 15–30% of FNAC specimens
  - assessment of capsular invasion is the most accurate determinant for differentiating adenoma from follicular carcinoma
  - initial management would be hemithyroidectomy
  - completion thyroidectomy without nodal dissection is recommended in patients with a finding of carcinoma on pathology.
- malignant FNAC:
  - differentiated thyroid cancer
    - **p**apillar**Y** = **p**aed = occurs in 20s; **Y** = yellow = lymph spread
    - micropapillary (<1 cm), intrathyroidal, and extrathyroidal
    - **f**ollicula**R** = **f**orties/fifties; **R** = red = blood spread
    - total thyroidectomy and ipsilateral central neck dissection
    - ^{131}I adjuvant treatment: for patients with high risk features (AGES [age, grade, extent, size] or AMES [age, metastasis, extent, size]) or close margins and central nodal involvement. Also allows for post-operative surveillance with thyroglobulin
  - medullary thyroid cancer:
    - treatment is determined based on stage of cancer
    - total thyroidectomy and bilateral central neck dissection if incidental finding/impalpable
    - total thyroidectomy, bilateral central neck dissection and ipsilateral lateral neck dissection (level 2–5) if palpable (risk lateral node involvement ~15%)
    - exclude concomitant phaeochromocytoma.

2.4.7 Thyrotoxicosis

Question: a 40-year-old woman is referred to your office with thyrotoxicosis. What are the common causes of thyrotoxicosis and what is the role of surgery in each? How would you prepare a thyrotoxic patient for surgery?

Answer

Common causes

- Autoimmune (Graves') (80%).
- Toxic multinodular goitre (Plummer's) (15%).
- Solitary toxic nodule 3%.
- other 2%.

Indications for surgery

Manage jointly with endocrinologist the 6 Ms:

- **m**alignancy (or suspicion)
- **m**edical therapy failure
- **m**echanical compression
- **m**enacing consequencesof radioactive iodine (pregnancy, allergy, severe eye disease)
- **m**ediastinal extension (unable to monitor changes clinical)
- **m**arred beauty (young/patients with large goitres).

Role of surgery

- Autoimmune – Graves' disease:
  - failure of thioamide drug treatment
  - RAI contra-indicated: pregnancy, allergy, severe eye disease
  - patient preference
  - the common procedures are total thyroidectomy and lifelong T4 or subtotal thyroidectomy. The latter has a greater chance of recurrence of thyrotoxicosis but the former necessitates life-long T4 treatment.
- For thyrotoxicosis due to De Quervain's thyroiditis, post-partum or that associated with Hashimoto's — the disease is transitory and surgery is not indicated.
- For large multi-nodular goitre or in the presence of compressive symptoms or suspicious nodules:
  - surgery is the procedure of first choice
  - ^{131}I less effective and also does not address the risk of malignancy (3%).
- For *small* (<3 cm) solitary toxic nodule either ^{131}I or hemithyroidectomy are acceptable treatments. The risk of malignancy is <1% if there is a solitary functioning nodule and the efficacy of both treatments is equal. Larger toxic nodules (>3 cm) should be treated surgically (hemithyroidectomy).

Preparation for surgery

- Check TSH, T_3 and T_4 to confirm, toxicosis. Anti-thyroid antibodies.
- US scan to check for suspicious nodules, neck masses or nodes with FNAC of suspicious nodules. CT if suspicion of retrosternal extension.
- Ophthalmology review if Graves' eye disease present.
- Render patient euthyroid using carbimazole 20 mg TDS initially and titrating to T_4 and serum TSH in conjunction with endocrinologist.
- Autonomic symptoms can be controlled with propranolol.
- ^{123}I scan to determine the appropriate procedure (total thyroidectomy or subtotal for Graves' disease, total for multinodular goitre or hemithyroidectomy for solitary nodule).
- Pre-operative flexible laryngoscopy to document RLN function.

Surgery depends on cause of toxicosis:

- Graves': total thyroidectomy plus lifelong T4 or subtotal. Depends on patient preference after full discussion of risks and benefits
- solitary toxic nodule: hemithyroidectomy (but also see 2.4.6)
- multinodular goitre: total thyroidectomy
- transient thyroiditis (low uptake on ^{123}I scan): no surgery.

2.4.8 Primary hyperparathyroidism

Question: discuss the aetiology and management of primary hyperparathyroidism.

Answer

Definition: hyperfunction of the parathyroid glands, with raised parathyroid secretion; 'recurrent' if recurs after ≥ 6 mths of normocalcaemia in a cured case.

Aetiology

- Parathyroid adenoma (80–90%).
- May be multiple (3%).
- Hyperplasia (10%):
  - primary: involves all of the parathyroid glands
  - secondary; for example, in secondary and tertiary hyperparathyroidism:
    - chief cell hyperplasia
    - water-clear cell (Wasser-Heller) hyperplasia.
- Parathyroid Carcinoma: rare — <1% of primary HPT.
- Parathyroid cysts (v rare! McKay ANZJS 2007; 77: 297–304).

Management

CLINICAL ASSESSMENT

- Asymptomatic or 'stones, bones, abdominal groans, psychic moans and fatigue overtones'.

- GI:
  - peptic ulcer disease
  - constipation
  - pancreatitis
  - anorexia/nausea/vomiting.
- CVS:
  - bradycardia
  - arrhythmias
  - heart block.
- Renal:
  - nephrolithiasis, nephrocalcinosis
  - polyuria and polydypsia (↑Ca impairs sodium and water reabsorption)
  - renal failure.
- Musculoskeletal:
  - osteopoenia, osteoporosis, osteitis fibrosa cystica → fractures
  - muscle weakness
  - ataxia.
- Neuropsychiatric:
  - anxiety
  - headaches
  - confusion
  - depression
  - coma.

INVESTIGATIONS

- Urine:
  - ↑Ca — excludes benign familial hypercalciuria
  - 24-hr urine Ca +/− Ca/creat clearance ratio.
- Bloods:
  - ↑corrected Ca
  - ↑PTH
  - ↓ Serum phosphate (tubular reabsoption of phosphate ↓) or normal
  - ALP may be raised
  - check renal function
  - Cl : P ratio >33 suggests PHP.
- Imaging and pre-operative localisation — localises lesion and to ensure lesion is solitary:
  - ultrasound → 95–97% accuracy (BJS 2007; 94:42–7)
  - CT — difficulty localising adenomas in the lower neck. Not useful in isolation
  - MRI (T2 weighted) — sensitivity 75%
  - ^{99}Tc-labelled sestamibi scanning (?dual isotope subtraction scintigraphy) +
    - sestamibi scan alone: sensitivity 63–100%, good at predicting the side, but not quadrant, of adenoma
    - NB sestamibi scanning in recurrent hyperparathyroidism or if planning a targeted/minimally invasive operation.

- Pre-operative localisation important if:
  - planning minimally invasive approach
  - for persistent hyperparathyroidism (i.e. following recent excision)
  - for recurrent hyperparathyroidism
  - generally U/S and sestamibi will suffice.
- Intra-operative tools for parathyroid localisation:
  - quick parathyroid hormone assay (QPTH) — 50% ↓ (from highest pre-operative level), 10–15 minutes after adenoma removal
  - frozen section (commonest intra-operative assessment)
  - intra-operative ultrasound
  - hand-held gamma probe
  - venous sampling (rarely used).

Treatment

ACUTE MX OF ↑CA

Medical management:

- observation may be appropriate in pts with mild and asymptomatic primary hyperparathyroidism
- IV rehydration (N. Saline 200–500 mls/hr to generate UO >100 mls/hr)
- loop diuretics
- bisphosphonates
- calcitonin
- oestrogen therapy in postmenopausal women — to ↑ bone density.

Surgery:

- approach dependent on localisation
- minimally invasive approach preferred if lesions localised
- bilateral neck exploration is challenged by pre-operative/intra-operative techniques to localise
- unilateral approach through an incision <2.5 cm
- excision of enlarged glands with preservation of 'normal' glands
- use of QPTH studies in difficult cases.

2.4.9 Phaeochromocytoma

Question: discuss the aetiology, clinical features, investigations, and treatment of phaeochromocytoma.

Answer

Definition: catecholamine-secreting tumour arising from chromaffin cells of the adrenal medulla.

Aetiology

- Adrenal (90%).
- Extra-adrenal (10%) — arise from paraganglia (e.g. organ of Zuckerkandl).
- Sporadic.

- Familial (≥ 10%) — should be considered in pts <40 yo:
  - MEN-2
  - von Hippel-Lindau disease
  - Carney's syndrome
  - NF-1.

HINT

Pathology: rule of 10s*
10% bilateral
10% extra-adrenal (aka functional paraganglionomas)
10% malignant (usually spread haematogenously but lymph spread is possible)
10% hereditary (likely closer to 30% due to occult germline mutations)
10% of cases are clinically silent

*Note: this has been challenged recently (Tischler AS. Arch Pathol Lab Med 2008; 132: 1272-84.

Clinical features

NB: adrenal phaeo secrete mainly epinephrine; extra-adrenal sides secrete NE Clinical.

- CVS:
  - hypertension — chronic or paroxysmal episodes
  - palpitations
  - chest pain/SOB
  - complications (e.g. MI) or CVA may occur.
- General:
  - sweating
  - anxiety
  - tremor
  - headaches.
- GI:
  - abdo pain
  - nausea.

Paroxysmal secretion/symptoms can be brought on by stress, exercise, trauma, etc.

Investigations

- Urine:
  - 24 hr urinary catecholamines (dopamine, adrenalin and noradrenalin)
  - 24 hr urinary metanephrines
  - 24 hr urinary cats + mets combined = *best specificity*; sensitivity 90–98%; specificity 96–99%
  - vanillylmandelic acid +/– urinary dopamine and — its metabolite — methoxytyramine.
- Bloods:
  - plasma catecholamine levels — unhelpful for diagnosis as levels fluctuate in many physiologic and pathologic states

- plasma free-metanephrines — excellent sensitivity so if negative essentially rules out phaeo but specificity only 85–89% so approx 15% false +ve
- chromogranin A — ↑ in 80% of patients with phaeo.

- Imaging:
  - CT: appearance variable as may have varying degeneration necrosis/calcification/cystic or lipid degeneration
  - I-131 MIBG scintigraphy scan (or MIBG/MRI scan): useful for extramedullaryphaeo and recurrence — for localisation
  - MIBG = metaiodobenzylguanidine = a structural analogue of norepinephrine not taken up by normal adrenal medullary tissue. Whole body imaging 24 and 72 hrs after administration of MIBG → 80–90% sensitivity and 90–100% specificity for detection of phaeochromocytoma
  - +/– ^{111}In nucleotide.
- Additional:
  - PET? (F-18-FDG) — cannot distinguish between phaeo and adrenal metastases
  - MRI: T1 = low signal intensity; T2 = high signal intensity. Enhancement ++ with contrast (Gadolinium).

Treatment

Medical:

- pre-operative: α blockade +/– β blockade (only after α blockade) for ≥10/7 pre-operative:
  - α-blockers: phenoxybenzamine or doxazocin (shorter acting) then β-blockers (propranolol), if still tachycardic
  - β-blockers should only be instituted after adequate α-blockade and hydration, in order to avoid effects of unopposed α-stimulation (i.e. hypertensive crisis and CHF)
- IV hydration:
  - repletion required when initiating anti-hypertensives pre-operative
  - post-operative to prevent hypotension (from loss of vasoconstriction after tumour removal)
- Mg also given, especially intra-operative.

Surgery:

- usually laparoscopic adrenalectomy if tumour <6 cm
- if bilateral (eg in hereditary cases): (BJS Sept 2008; 95)
  - bilateral adrenalectomy (disadvantage = life-long steroid replacement)
  - subtotal cortical-sparing adrenalectomy in benign disease +/– pts with MEN2, VHL and SDHD germ-line mutations (because risk of malignancy is low <5%) (ANZJS 2009 79:371–7) *but* drawback is risk of recurrent tumours in remnant (some medullary tissue inevitably left behind with spared cortex)
  - if unresectable → debulk +/– radiotherapy and α-blockade.

2.4.10 Anterior and posterior neck triangles

Question: describe the anatomy of the neck relating it to lymph node dissection for head and neck squamous cell carcinoma.

Answer

The neck is divided into two main triangles by the sternocleidomastoid muscle (SCM).

1. Anterior triangle

- Borders:
  - anterior border SCM
  - mandible (lower border)
  - midline.

2. Posterior triangle

- Borders:
  - posteriorly border SCM
  - middle third of clavicle
  - anterior border trapezius muscle.

The roof of both triangles is the investing layer of deep cervical fascia. The floor is formed by the prevertebral fascia.

The lymph nodes of the neck are divided into levels I to VII.

The nodes of the jugular vein (levels II to IV) are not contained in either the anterior or posterior triangle and are mostly *behind* SCM.

In a level I-IV neck dissection the posterior border of the dissection is the posterior border of SCM which is approached deep to the muscle (from anterior to posterior and identified by the cervical plexus branches as they curve laterally around the posterior border of SCM.

Lymph node levels

(See Figure 2.4.10.)

- I — submental + submandibular.
- II — base of skull to level of hyoid.
- III — between level of hyoid and level of cricoid cartilage.
- IV — level of cricoid to clavicle.
- V — posterior triangle.
- VI — hyoid→ supra-sternal notch, between carotids.
- VII — retromanubrial/sternal→ inominate.

Note level III→IV is from the posterior border SCM→ lateral sternohyoid.

Neck dissection

Comprehensive (levels I to V in head and neck squamous cell carcinoma [SCC]):

- radical — includes SCM, jugular vein, accessory nerve
- modified radical — preserves one or more of the above.

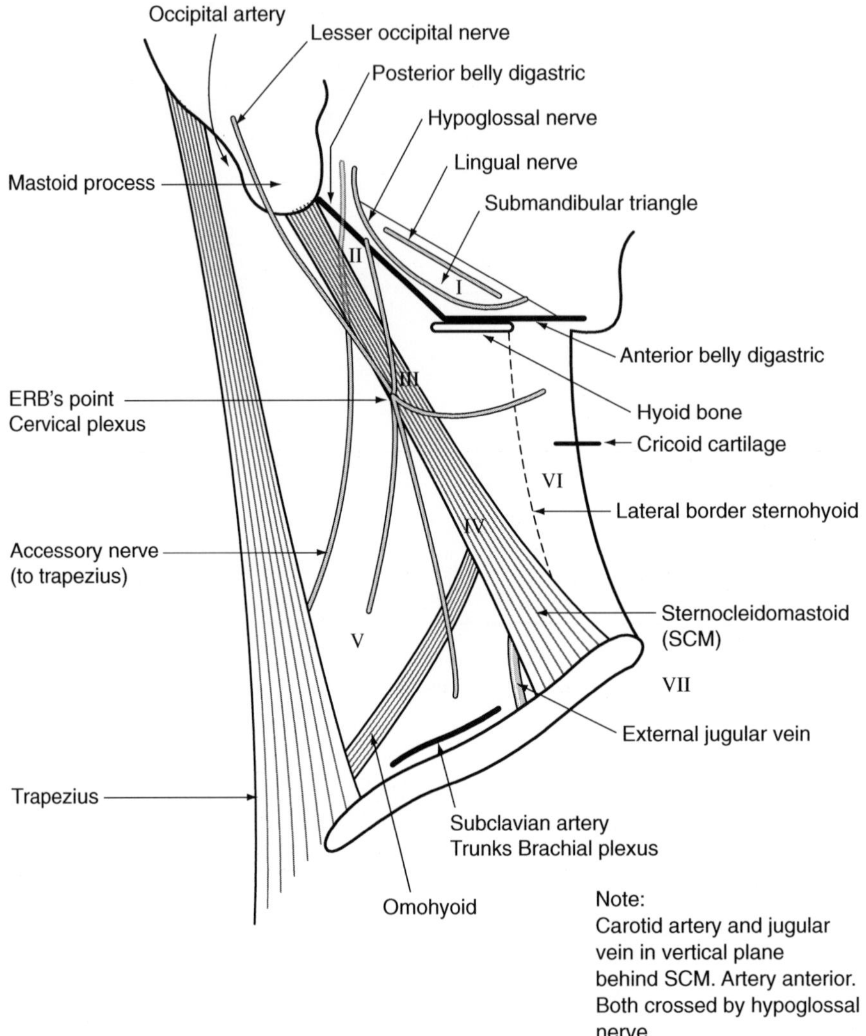

Legend:
View of right side of neck showing relevant LYMPH NODE levels

- I – submental + submandibular
- II – base of skull to level of hyoid
- III – between level of hyoid and level of cricoid cartilage
- IV – level of cricoid to clavicle
- V – posterior triangle
- VI – hyoid → supra-sternal notch, between carotids
- VII – retromanubrial/sternal → inominate

Note level III → IV is from the posterior border SCM → lateral sternohyoid

Figure 2.4.10
View of right side of neck showing relevant lymph node levels

Selective:

- depends on primary tumour site
- usually in the clinically and radiologically negative neck
- usually the draining node group and adjacent groups (e.g. level I, II and III for floor of mouth SCC).

Patterns of drainage by primary site

- Anterior floor of mouth, anterior two-thirds of tongue, lip, cheek mucosa→ level I.
- Nasopharynx→ level II, III, IV, parotid nodes.
- Oral cavity/pharynx→ level III, IV, V (often bilateral).
- Cutaneous primary→ sentinel node biopsy assists in predicting drainage.
- Note: enlarged supraclavicular nodes — thyroid, pirifom sinus, cervical oesophagus, or could be from a primary below clavicle (gastric, oesophageal).

2.4.11 Laparostomy

Question: describe in detail the role of laparostomy in abdominal surgery. Include the pathophysiological basis, indications and their causes, management and closure techniques.

Answer

Plan

- Definition: the peritoneal cavity is opened anteriorly and deliberately left open.
- Physiology: abdominal perfusion pressure (APP) = MAP — IAP.
- APP <50 or IAP >20 poor outcome → laparostomy.
- Indications: ACS, sepsis, damage control.
- Management: short term – long term: if early closure not possible.

PATHOPHYSIOLOGY

- Abdominal cavity distensible (unlike skull).
- However, a limit is reached where compliance (P/V) drops dramatically.
- Beyond this small ↑ in volume of contents (oedema fluid, gas, blood) results in rapid ↑ in intra-abdominal pressure (IAP) — similar to Monroe-Kelly doctrine.
- Abdominal perfusion pressure (APP): APP = MAP — IAP.
- When APP is <50–60 mmHg, perfusion ↓ and ischaemia to solid organs and viscera results in organ dysfunction. Then a strong association with poor outcome.

INDICATIONS AND CAUSES

- Abdominal compartment syndrome (ACS): IAP raised by blood (retroperitoneal haematoma), oedema fluid (pancreatitis, massive resuscitation, SIRS), gas (ileus or bowel obstruction).
- For intractable intra-abdominal sepsis (analogous to draining an abscess) — fistulation or pancreatic necrosis.

- Abdominal wall dehiscence: unsafe to re-close abdomen usually because of increase IAP/sepsis.
- Facilitate re-look in 'damage control surgery' after trauma/control of bleeding and contamination.

MANAGEMENT (SHORT-TERM)

- General: ICU, control sepsis, prevention of organ failure, control evisceration and prevent complications (entero-cutaneous or entero-atmospheric fistula) usually with temporary abdominal closure (TAC). Attempt early closure if safe.
- TAC: control evisceration, exudate and prevent fistula formation. ↓damage to fascia from multiple re-closure. Help ↓ retraction of muscle. Probability of early closure highest for trauma; lowest for sepsis/fistula.
  - VAC dressing: plastic on bowel, sponge on plastic, second layer of plastic and apply suction (~120 mmHg). Opsite sandwich.
  - Bogota bag: bag from irrigation fluid sutured to wound edge.
  - Absorbable mesh sutured to fascia.
  - Absorbable mesh and VAC.
- ACS: identify at risk patients (ICU setting). Bladder monitoring of IAP.
  - If IAP >12 but <20 mmHg: sedation, pain control, repositioning, restrict fluid boluses, decompress GIT (NG, rectal tube, trophic enteral nutrition only)
  - If IAP >20 mmHg *without* organ dysfunction: paralysis, drain (abscesses, paracentesis, decompressive colonoscopy), haemofiltration or dialysis.
  - If IAP >20 mmHg *with* organ dysfunction: laparosotomy.
- Sepsis — washout, multiple drains. Continuous peritoneal lavage (e.g. after pancreatic necrosectomy). Regular return to theatre for re-look. Dressings often without TAC. Allow abdomen to granulate. Skin graft.
- Abdominal fascial failure managed by controlling infection, improving nutrition and allowing abdomen to granulate. Skin graft.

CLOSURE TECHNIQUES

- Primary fascial closure: best option if feasible.
- Planned hernia approach: used when fascia will not come together, risk of recurrent ACS, fistula (especially entero-atmospheric). Skin graft to serosa of bowel. Reconstruction delayed some months. Re-laparotomy when viscera herniate. Adhesiolysis, resect/internalise fistula.
- Early-delayed closure once sepsis and ACS risk reduced: absorbable mesh-assisted gradual fascial closure, component separation or non-absorbable mesh closure (if no infection and enough skin to cover prosthesis).
  - Giant ventral hernia repair then required using component separation, rectus sheath transposition, mesh, staged surgery to regain 'right of domain' or pedicled microvascular flaps (TRAM, tensor fascia lata).

2.4.12 Malignant melanoma

Question: you are referred a 54-year-old man who has had a suspicious skin lesion removed from his right posterior calf by his local doctor.

Pathology demonstrates a superficial spreading melanoma, Breslow thickness of 2.5 mm, no ulceration, mitoses 4/mm, closest lateral margin 3 mm. Discuss further management of his melanoma with respect to:

- **further management of his excision site**
- **further management of his regional lymph node basin**
- **important features on pathology of the primary lesion.**

Answer

- A detailed history including:
  - medical comorbidities
  - risk factors for melanoma (e.g. family history, sun exposure, skin type).
- Detailed examination of whole body for:
  - other suspicious skin lesions
  - evidence of sun damage
  - examination of the right leg to assess for any clinical groin or popliteal lymphadenopathy suggestive of LN metastases, presence of satellite nodules or in transit metastases
  - assess wound for healing/infection.

Management of excision site

- Needs wide excision to prevent local recurrence.
- Meta-analysis of RCTs comparing adequate margins demonstrates no difference in 2 cm compared to 3 or 5 cm margins.
- Current guidelines recommend margins of:
  - pT1: melanoma <1.0 mm: margin 1 cm
  - pT2: melanoma 1.0–2.0 mm: margin 1–2 cm
  - pT3: melanoma 2.0–4.0 mm: margin 1–2 cm
  - pT4: melanoma >4.0 mm: margin 2 cm.
- This man should have a re-excision of his melanoma site down to deep fascia with 2 cm margins.
- Closure of wound needs to be considered:
  - may be too large for primary closure
  - options for closure include split skin graft or a local flap (such as keystone flap)
  - consent needs to include risks of infection, bleeding, graft necrosis, injury to adjacent structures e.g. sural nerve, SSV.

Management of regional lymph node basin

- Further management depends on whether or not there is evidence of clinical metastasis.
- If lymphadenopathy then groin ultrasound with FNA is indicated. If metastatic melanoma is demonstrated on FNA then a groin dissection is indicated for local control. Groin dissection may be subinguinal or ilioinguinal depending on bulk of disease. A positive FNA result confers Stage III disease and patient

should be staged with CT brain and PET-CT to assess for distant metastasis prior to any surgery as their presence may change management.

- If no lymphadenopathy/proven LN metastases then SLN biopsy is indicated for all melanoma with Breslow thickness >1 mm. Risk of LN metastases increases with increasing Breslow thickness such that:
  - <1 mm — risk <5%
  - 1–4 mm — risk 8–30%
  - >4 mm — risk >30%.
- LN mets are a poor prognostic feature and impact on survival. MSLT-1 demonstrates significant survival advantage in treatment arm where completion lymph node dissection was performed for positive SLN compared with arm where patients had a therapeutic lymph node dissection performed for subsequent clinical lymph node metastases (70% vs 55% 5 year survival)
- Risks of SLN biopsy included in consent — infection, bleeding, injury to major structures in groin (<1%), lymphoedema (<1%), anaphylaxis to blue dye injection (1/1000)

Important pathological features of primary

Three most important features that confer increased risk of LN metastasis and are used for T staging of melanoma:

1. Breslow thickness
2. presence of ulceration
3. presence of mitoses.

Other features of primary with less established significance:

- Clarks level (impact greatest in thin melanomas <1 mm, decreasing evidence for importance in thicker melanomas when compared with Breslow thickness. Clark IV in thin melanoma 0.75 — 1 mm is an indication to consider SLN biopsy)
- lymphovascular invasion
- tumour infiltrating lymphocytes
- neurotropism.

2.4.13 Renal transplantation: short- and long-term complications

Question: when obtaining informed consent from a potential recipient of a kidney transplant, describe the possible complications, their causes and the potential outcomes.

Answer

Plan

- Immediate vs early vs late.
- Vascular, urological, immunological, infectious and neoplastic.
- Complication → Cause → Treatment → Outcome.
- Alternative or no treatment options.

COMPLICATIONS

Immediate:

- bleeding:
  - re-operation
- vessel thrombosis due to kinking or intimal dissection:
  - re-operation
- hyperacute rejection due to pre-formed complement-fixing Ab. Failure of cross-match. Intra-renal thrombosis:
  - requires nephrectomy.

Early:

- infection in wound, lung, UTI
  - Abx and/or drainage
- bleeding with haematoma
  - possible evacuation
- lymphocoele with vascular or ureteric compression. If same Cr concentration as serum then lymphocoele
  - if small observe; if large drain via a peritoneal window
- urine leak — from bladder, ureteric anastomosis or calyx
  - small leaks — nephrostomy
  - large leaks — exploration
- anastomotic obstruction of ureter
  - stenting
- general risk: MI, pneumonia, DVT/PE, death
- delayed graft function — dialysis in first week — rejection, vascular and ureteric complications.

Late:

- vascular:
  - renal artery stenosis or stenosis at anastomosis (can present with HTN)
    - in anastomotic stricture, PTA is less successful than surgery
  - false aneurysm: anastomotic or mycotic aneurysm
    - Abx and removal of graft
- ureteric:
  - stricture at anastomosis: ischaemic +/– polyoma virus infection
    - stent, endoscopic stricturoplasty, re-implantation (Boari flap)
  - VUR
- immunosuppression complications:
  - infection — increased risk of viral (CMV, EBV, HSV, Varicella, BK virus), bacterial (TB, Listeria, nocardia), fungal (Candida, aspergillus, cryptococcus), protozoal (PCP).
    - prophylaxis for CMV using ganciclovir, PCP using co-trimoxazole, fluconazole for candida, TB prophylaxis for patients with history or PPD conversion. BK virus infection (causes tubulitis) requires reduction in immunosuppression
  - infection-related malignancy — ↑ risk of SCC skin (SCC; BCC ratio 2:1 — usually 1:5), Kaposi sarcoma (HHV8). Anal carcinoma due to HPV.

Post-transplant lymphoproliferative disorder ranging from polyclonal proliferations (reduced immunosuppression) to monoclonal NHL B cell lymphoma (EBV)

- metabolic — diabetes, HTN, vascular disease all more common with immunosuppression

- graft failure:
  - may be due to acute rejection (treat by increasing immunosuppression)
  - may be due to chronic allograft nephropathy — combination of chronic rejection, damage due to immunosuppression
  - return of renal disease (esp. FSGS).

ALTERNATIVE

- No renal replacement therapy: death if severe renal failure.
- Remain on dialysis: risk of death increased due to complications from dialysis access and vascular disease.
- Pre-dialysis Tx better than post-dialysis Tx.

2.4.14 Blunt abdominal injury

Question: a 25-year-old man has been severely injured in a motor vehicle accident where he was ejected from the vehicle. He is on transit to the hospital, his blood pressure is unstable and he has a painful and tender abdomen. Discuss management principles.

Answer

Plan

- General approach — trauma team.
- Primary survey — ABCs; treatment in primary survey of tension pneumothorax, tamponade, refractory ⇓BP, cardiac arrest.
- Secondary survey — if appropriate.
- Operative approach — laparotomy, thoracotomy, diaphragmatic injury, damage control.
- Definitive management — ICU, tertiary survey, definitive plan.

PRINCIPLES OF MANAGEMENT

- This patient is an acute trauma patient and should be managed according to the EMST guidelines.
- The patient is shocked and a cause needs to be established and corrected to prevent loss of life.
- Life-threatening injuries should be sought and excluded/addressed in the primary survey. Injuries requiring *immediate* correction can be remembered by the acronym (ATOMIC):
  - **a**irway obstruction
  - **t**ension pneumothorax
  - **o**pen pneumothorax

  - **m**assive haemothorax
  - **i**ncomplete (flail) chest
  - **c**ardiac tamponade.
- If cardiogenic shock has been excluded in the primary survey, his unstable blood pressure is likely to be due to haemorrhagic shock, particularly in view of the abdominal signs which suggest a likely intra-abdominal source of haemorrhage, such as:
  - solid organ injury (liver, spleen, kidney)
  - hollow organ injury (bowel)
  - major vascular injury
  - mesenteric vascular injury
  - pelvic fracture.
- The priority is to establish and maintain haemodynamic normality.
- *Definitive* haemorrhage control may only be possible at laparotomy.
- Ideally, primary and secondary surveys and key investigations are completed prior to definitive management.
- However, if haemodynamic normality can *not* be established during resuscitation, then transfer for laparotomy to achieve haemorrhage control will be required BEFORE completing the remainder of the trauma assessment.
- The patient's clinical (haemodynamic) status will dictate the appropriateness of diagnostic investigations (FAST/CT scan etc.).

PRE-ARRIVAL

- Assemble trauma team in the resuscitation trauma bay and plan for the arrival of the patient.
- Trauma team should discuss the specifics of the 'BAT' call from the ambulance crew and set out a preliminary management plan.
- All equipment should be made ready — e.g. fluid warmers, portable x-ray, IV and central lines/intubation equipment/chest drains/IDC set up and O- blood should be readily available in the emergency department.
- On arrival of the trauma patient, a primary survey should be performed (ABCDE).

PRIMARY SURVEY

Airway with C-spine control:

- three-point fixation (hard-collar, sand bags and a spinal board) should be applied
- assess airway patency
- respiratory distress (stridor, wheeze, cyanosis) should prompt urgent assessment to exclude airway compromise from facial fractures, bleeding into the airway, inhalation burns, etc.
- airway management protocol from suction/chin lift and jaw thrust to oropharyngeal airway to rapid airway stabilisation by ETT intubation
- intubation if appropriate (GCS <8, combative)
- if not possible and emergency airway required — cricothyroidotomy should be performed until a definitive airway with tracheostomy is established.

Breathing:

- the patient's respiratory rate, breath sounds and oxygen saturations should be assessed
- if stable the patient should be placed on 100% O2 via facemask. Measure SaO_2
- if compromised a tension pneumothorax/haemopneumothorax should be excluded or definitively treated by insertion of a chest drain.

Circulation:

- assess colour, diaphoresis, temperature, and mental status for signs of shock
- haemorrhage control with external compression of obvious bleeding
- the pulse should be assessed for rate, rhythm, volume, character, radial-radial symmetry, and radio-femoral delay
- the blood pressure should be taken
- at the same time IV access should be established with at least two large bore IV lines (14G preferably) and blood sent for FBC, EUC, amylase, coagulation screen, pregnancy test in a female and group and cross match for 4 units packed red cells
- 2–3 L of crystalloids (Hartmann's solution) should be given and the patient's response assessed — i.e. good response, transient responder, non-responder etc. — this is determined by feeling the pulse volume, pulse rate, systolic pressure, mental status, oxygenation
- during resuscitation, if the patient is a transient or non-responder, transfusion of 4 units of O –ve packed red cells (or cross-matched blood if available) is required.

Disability:

- determine the level of consciousness using the AVPU (alert, responds to vocal or painful stimuli, unresponsive) scales; GCS reserved for secondary survey
- assess pupils for size, equality and reaction.

Exposure/environmental control:

- completely expose the patient whilst keeping the patient warm:
  - be aware lethal triad: hypothermia/acidosis/coagulaopathy.

SECONDARY SURVEY

- May not be completed *before surgery* if the patient is sufficiently shocked and unstable.
- Systematic skull-to-toe examination.
- Thorough examination of all body systems.
- Particular attention to abdomen and perineum in this case.
- Tubes/fingers in all orifices: an IDC should be inserted if no evidence of urethral injury (high riding prostate/ blood at the urethral meatus), consider NGT.
- The patient should be log-rolled and all orifices examined

C-spine, CXR and pelvic x-ray:

- if stable then x-rays in resus bay
- to assess for bony injury, missed or subtle pneumothorax/ haemothorax, mediastinal great vessel injury and a pelvic fracture.

FAST scan +/− DPL/CT scan:

- should only be performed if the patient is haemodynamically normal
- assess for intraperitoneal blood. Ultrasound assessment of Morrison's pouch (hepato-renal recess), spleno-renal recess, pelvis, and pericardium should be performed; FAST should be performed again within 30 minutes if negative
- DPL can be useful if the patient clinically and radiologiclly has a pelvic fracture and there is uncertainty whether the bleeding is from the pelvis or intra-abdominal source
- a negative DPL may change the decision from laparotomy to angiography +/− embolisation if pelvic bleeding (arterial) is suspected.

DEFINITIVE MANAGEMENT — LAPAROTOMY

- If haemodynamically unstable, laparotomy is indicated if the primary survey excludes other causes of shock relating to the cardiorespiratory systems.
- Ideally this decision should be made within minutes of arrival in the emergency department after assessment and initiation of resuscitative measures.
- Liaise with the operating theatre staff to initiate 'the massive transfusion protocol' and schedule an immediate laparotomy for control of intra-abdominal haemorrhage.
- Prepare cell savers, large-bore suckers, numerous packs and vascular instruments, haemostatic agents (surgical/flowseal, etc.).
- At laparotomy, make an incision from the xiphisternum to the pubic symphysis and perform 4-quadrant packing.
- Use assistants to retract the abdominal wall with retractors.
- Assess each quadrant carefully by removing packs and methodically assessing all organs and vascular structures to find the source of bleeding, beginning with quadrant LEAST likely to be source of haemorrhage.
- In blunt abdominal trauma, the most common sites of injury would be solid organ injury (liver, spleen and kidneys).
- Initially, bleeding should be controlled by 'packing'.
- Definitive control of haemorrhage may require complete or partial (anatomical or extra-anatomical) removal of the offending organ.
- 'Damage control' laparotomy to allow correction of the components of the lethal triad may be appropriate.
- Return to theatre in 24 hrs or sooner if necessary for definitive treatment.
- This patient should be managed post-operatively in an ICU setting.

Post-operative management:

- transfer to *ICU* for monitoring
- the secondary survey is completed (if not already) or a tertiary survey performed to identify other missed injuries
- a definitive management plan should be formulated with ICU team
- DVT and stress ulcer prophylaxis.

2.4.15 Burns

Question: a 28-year-old man presents to the emergency department having sustained a significant thermal injury to his torso and both upper limbs, although the details of the events leading to the injury are unclear. Outline your immediate management of this patient in the ED. What issues are important in the definitive management of his burns?

Answer

Plan

Resuscitation and limit 'delayed injury' and assessment of burn/management of burn shock:

- ABCDE — assess risk to airway and lungs!
- analgesia
- cool the wound
- extent of burn — 'rule of 9s'
- depth of burn
- fluid replacement strategies.

Important issues in definitive management of burn wound:

- local management of burn wound
- burns unit
- managing complications:
  - infection
  - nutrition
  - scars.

Immediate management in ED

RESUSCITATION AND LIMIT 'DELAYED INJURY'

- ABCDEF: patients may have also sustained low/high velocity trauma so demand full resuscitation using ATLS/EMST protocols:
  - particular attention to assess risk to airway and lungs!
  - burned airway creates swelling and complete occlusion if not proactive — look for loss of hair/perioral/nasal deposits/nasopharyngeal blisters/ deep burns around mouth/neck
  - early elective intubation *preferable* before signs (stridor/respiratory difficulties)
  - Rx inhalation injury aggressively (physio/Nebs/humified O_2)
  - objective is achieving approp IV access to facilitate fluid resuscitation and prevention of burn shock (see below)
- Analgesia is crucial in partial-thickness injury (see below).
- Cool the wound:
  - aim to achieve 15°C for minimum 10 mins
  - reduces delayed microvascular damage
  - effective up to 1 hour after injury.

ASSESSMENT OF BURN/MANAGEMENT OF BURN SHOCK

- Extent of burn:
  - estimation of total body surface area (TBSA) affected
  - initially 'rule of 9s' then Lund and Browder chart
  - bigger the burn and/or older the pt = worse prognosis.
- Depth of burn:
  - partial thickness (spares some epidermis and/or dermis)
  - full thickness — complete destruction of epithelium and dermis — can only prevent healing by scarring by grafting
  - differentiation not easy:
    - partial — red, blistered, moist, very sensitive
    - full — parched and pale (like marble), absence of sensation.
- Fluid replacement strategies:
  - must maintain intravascular volume
  - IV resus mandatory for burn >10% TBSA in child or >15% in adult; consider CVP/more sophisticated monitoring if TBSA > 30%
  - oral fluid consumption should incorporate added sodium
  - resus volume is constant in proportion to TBSA burned
  - choice fluid: Hartmann's solution is commonest — hypertonic saline, human albumin solution or FFP alternatives
  - simplest formula — Parkland:
    - TBSA x weight (kg) x 4 = volume (mls)
    - Half given in first 8 hours, second half next 16 hrs
  - Monitor adequacy of resus using:
    - urine output (0.5–1.0 ml/kg/hr) — if low increase IVI by 50%
    - PR, BP, CVP.

IMPORTANT ISSUES IN DEFINITIVE MANAGEMENT OF BURN WOUND

- Burns unit:
  - airway/inhalation injury
  - burn likely to require IV fluid resus/surgery
  - burns to hands/face/perineum
  - extremes of age.
- Local management of burn wound:
  - tetanus
  - antibacterial topical treatment (sulphadiazine cream/silver nitrate solution)
  - simple dressings
  - > 10% TBSA/circumferential — consider escharotomy.
- Managing complications:
  - infection
  - nutrition
  - scars.

2.4.16 Gastro-oesophageal reflux disease

Question: discuss the investigations, treatment and indications for surgery of gastro-oesophageal reflux disease.

Answer

- Gastro-oesophageal reflux disease (GORD) is a common condition affecting between 10–40% of the population in western countries.
- Patients commonly present with acid regurgitation, heartburn, waterbrash, and dysphagia. They can also present atypically with respiratory or cardiovascular symptoms and be investigated for pathology in these systems.

Investigation of GORD

- The objectives of investigating patients for GORD are:
  - confirm the diagnosis of GORD
  - define the anatomy of the oesophagus
  - exclude a motility disorder.
- With consideration of:
  - endoscopy
  - manometry
  - 24 hr pH monitoring.

CONFIRM DIAGNOSIS OF GORD

- Patients who have had a transient or sustained improvement of symptoms on a PPI strongly suggest GORD.
- Further investigation for GORD should be performed, especially in patients who have not responded to medical treatment. These investigations are:
- Endoscopy and biopsy:
  - mandatory prerequisite
  - objective evidence of reflux (e.g. oesophagitis, ulceration, stricturing or bleeding) can be documented
  - strictures can be dilated
  - position of squamo-columnar junction can be assessed
  - presence/size of hiatus hernia can be assessed
  - biopsy of mucosal abnormalities (Barrett's).
- Oesophageal pH monitoring:
  - routine vs selective assessment
  - a good test to confirm acid regurgitation and reflux but not the gold standard as not sufficiently accurate
  - useful in cases where endoscopy is NEGATIVE
  - can clarify whether symptoms are associated with reflux events.

DEFINE THE ANATOMY

The next step is to define the anatomy of the oesophagus to exclude:
- hiatus hernia
- 'short oesophagus' caused by Barrett's/cancer/achalasia.

This can be assessed at endoscopy or by barium swallow.

EXCLUDE A MOTILITY DISORDER

- Oesophageal manometry useful in excluding a primary motility disorder, such as achalasia.
- Ability to document adequacy of peristalsis (patients with weak peristalsis can get worsening dysphagia post-operatively).

Treatment of GORD

MEDICAL TREATMENT

- Simple measures:
  - antacids
  - avoidance of precipitating factors
  - weight loss
  - smoking cessation.
- H_2 receptor antagonists:
  - can be effective in mild to moderate reflux disease
  - diminished effectiveness with time.
- Proton-pump inhibitors:
  - most effective therapy and can achieve healing
  - long-term use can be associated with atrophic gastritis and parietal cell hyperplasia.
- Prokinetics:
  - Cisapride only demonstrable effective agent but withdrawn due to cardiac toxicity (arrhythmias).

Indications for surgery

- Patient preference (i.e. does not wish to be on medication long-term).
- Medical treatment no longer effective.
- Regurgitation is the main symptom.
- Hiatus hernia is present.
- Complicated GORD (Barrett's oesphagus/bleeding/stricture/ulceration).

The aim of surgery is to:
- create a competent lower oesophageal sphincter by fundoplication
- reduce a hiatus hernia if present
- return the gastro-oesophageal junction back into the abdomen
- tighten the hiatus
- protect the vagus nerves.

The operation of choice by majority of surgeons is a laparoscopic fundoplication. The fundoplication (wrap) can either be a complete (Nissen) or partial (Tuopet). Partial wraps are more suitable for patients with weak peristalsis.

2.4.17 Obesity/bariatric surgery

Question: what are the indications, management and complications of surgery for obesity?

Answer

Introduction

- Incidence of obesity in Australia is approximately 24% of the population with 2.5% being morbidly obese.
- Obesity is the second leading cause of preventable death in the USA with 300,000 deaths annually.

Indications for bariatric surgery for morbid obesity

- BMI of 40 kg/m^2 or greater.
- BMI 35 to 40 kg/m^2 with significant obesity-related comorbidities (hypertension, diabetes).
- Unsuccessful attempt at weight loss by non-operative means.
- Clearance by dietician and mental health professional.
- No medical contraindications to surgery.

Management of morbidly obese patient

- Weight-loss surgery is not designed to achieve a cosmetic result but rather to reverse obesity related disease and improve overall health and quality of life.
- Patients need to be aware that although most operations are reversible, weight-loss surgery should be viewed as a lifelong commitment to behavioural and dietary modification and medical supervision.
- These patients should be evaluated by a multidisciplinary team consisting of:
  - surgeon
  - dietitian
  - psychiatrist
  - anaesthetist
  - medical specialist as indicated (cardiologist/respiratory/endocrinologist/renal).

ASSESSMENT

- History and physical examination:
  - symptoms and signs of HTN, diabetes, obstructive sleep apnoea, asthma, cardiac disease, renal disease, musculoskeletal problems, non-alcoholic steatohepatitis (NASH)
  - refer to appropriate specialist for evaluation and optimisation.
- Bloods:
  - FBC, EUC, Coag, G + H, LFT's, ABG, Glucose.
- Imaging:
  - x-rays: CXR, US-Liver and GB to assess for fatty liver complications/gall stones.

- Special tests:
  - ECHO/ stress test (nuclear)/ gastroscopy if GORD.
- Control diabetes pre-operatively to reduce morbidity.
- If high risk for DVT/ PE — Greenfield filter as the most common cause of mortality is VTE.
- If NASH, Optifast diet for 8 weeks pre-operatively to reduce the size of the liver.

Peri-operative Mx:

- bariatric table and instruments
- Abx on induction and continue 24 hrs post-operative
- thromboprophylaxis: low MW heparin/TEDS/leg compressors
- intra-operative TOE if cardiomyopathy
- remove GB if stones/planning malabsorption procedure.

Post-operative Mx:

- early ambulation 6–8 hrs post-operative
- air mattress to prevent pressure sore
- DVT prophylaxis and continue for 2/52 post-operative
- Abx for 24 hrs
- control blood sugars
- respiratory physiotherapy +/– CPAP/Nebulisers/ICU — hypoxia can be disastrous
- control HTN.

Complications of bariatric surgery

- Overall 30-day mortality is <1%.
- Mortality rates are higher in men than in women and for those aged 65 and older.
- Both in-hospital and 30-day mortality are decreased when bariatric surgery is performed by surgeons and hospitals that perform more than 100 procedures a year.
- Failure to lose weight 10–15% due to failure to change behavioural pattern
- The most common causes of early re-hospitalisation are nausea, vomiting, and dehydration, abdominal pain, and wound problems.
- The most common causes of early mortality are pulmonary emboli and complications related to leaks.
- Roux-en-Y gastric bypass complications are diverse and include:
  - gastric remnant distension, stomal stenosis, marginal ulcer formation, cholelithiasis, ventral hernias, internal hernias, hypoglycaemia, dumping, metabolic and nutritional derangements and weight regain
  - some complications are seen during the early post-operative periods while others may present weeks to months following the surgery.
- Laparoscopic adjustable gastric banding complications include:
  - acute stomal obstruction, band erosion, band slippage leading to gastric prolapse, port malfunction, oesophageal dilatation, oesophagitis, and infection.

- Laparoscopic sleeve gastrectomy complications include:
  - bleeding, narrowing or stenosis of the stoma and leaks.
- Vertical banded gastroplasty complications include:
  - staple line disruption, stomal stenosis, band erosion, reflux, nausea/vomiting, marginal ulcers, and weight regain.
- Biliopancreatic diversion complications include:
  - significant protein calorie malnutrition, anaemia, metabolic bone disease and deficiencies of fat-soluble vitamins A,D, E, K and vitamin B12 due to lack of IF.

2.4.18 Upper GI haemorrhage

Question: a 50-year-old man presents with haematemesis and melaena. A duodenal ulcer was diagnosed on an endoscopy performed at another hospital 1 month ago. He has a HR 110, BP 90/40. He is on pantoprazole as his only medication. Outline your management.

Answer

- Management involves:
  - aggressive resuscitation/initial management
  - assessment of severity
  - definitive management.
- This patient has evidence of haemorrhagic shock and represents a surgical emergency.
- Mortality is 10%. It is highest in the elderly and those with comorbidities. Paradoxically, surgical intervention must not be delayed in such patients.
- Causes include: peptic ulcer (35–50%), gastroduodenal erosions (8–15%), oesophagitis (5–15%), varices (5–15%), Mallory Weiss tears (15%) and CA (1%).

Initial management — aggressive resuscitation

Airway:

- ensure airway protected — blood in stomach is a potent stimulant of emesis — risk of aspiration with vomiting of gastric contents
- in setting of significant haemetemasis, protect airway with early intubation.

Breathing/oxygenation:

- generous supplementary O_2 via facemask to ensure maximal O_2 saturations — important to protect elderly/comorbid patients from consequences of myocardial/cerebral ischaemia.

Circulation:

- 2 x large bore cannula
- commence 2L warmed Hartmann's
- bloods for FBC, coagulation, X match 6 units, EUC and LFTs

- insert IDC to allow hourly urine output monitoring
- consider use of NGT
- commence IV PPI infusion
- ICU/HDU.

Assessment of severity

- Severity is assessed using scoring systems (e.g. Rockall), which incorporate:
  - age
  - haemodynamic status
  - comorbidity
  - endoscopic findings.
- High-risk patients are those with:
  - increasing age
  - comorbidity
  - tachycardia/hypotension
  - endoscopic stigmata of haemorrhage (clot/bleeding vessel).
- History to assess risk factors — anticoagulation, liver disease, ethanol, steroids, NSAIDs.

Definitive management

- Endoscopy should be undertaken in all patients and may enable haemostasis.
- If re-bleeding occurs, one further attempt at endoscopic haemostasis is acceptable.
- High dose PPI infusion reduces re-bleed rates but not mortality.
- Surgical intervention indicated for:
  - unable to identify source of bleeding due to large amount of blood/clot
  - unable to control bleeding endoscopically
  - ongoing bleeding, significant re-bleed after initial endoscopy (repeat endoscopy and attempt endoscopic haemostasis first).

ENDOSCOPIC MANAGEMENT

- Identify bleeding point, exclude other cause.
- Use of two different methods for haemostasis shown to be more effective — options of heater probe, clips, adrenaline (1 : 10,000) injection.
- Assess risk of re-bleeding using Forest classification:
  - 1a — active spurting vessel, up to 100%
  - 1b — oozing vessel, 55 to 100%
  - 2a — visible vessel, 50%
  - 2b — clot, 25%
  - 3 — stable clot — no bleeding 5%
  - 4 — clean ulcer.

Possible scenarios and management

- If haemostasis achieved → transfer to ICU. Continue PPI infusion. Transfuse PRBCs with aim for Hb >90, monitor U/O, DVT prophylaxis.
- If re-bleed then for repeat endoscopy (no difference in outcome in repeat endoscopy vs surgery for first re-bleed).
- Unable to control bleeding, proceed to surgery.

OPERATIVE

- Duodenotomy and under-running of bleeding vessel (likely gastroduodenal artery) with multiple figure of 8 sutures around bleeding point.
- Close longitudinal duodenotomy transversely.
- Partial gastrectomy may be required.

ANGIOGRAM AND EMBOLISATION

Consider in scenario of ongoing bleeding but stable patient.

Note: must commence H. pylori eradication therapy prior to discharge irrelevant of antral biopsy result as often negative in setting of large amount of blood.

2.4.19 Complications after laparoscopic cholecystectomy

Question: you are asked to see a 53-year-old woman who underwent a laparoscopic cholecystectomy for acute cholecystitis the previous evening. A drain was placed intra-operatively and about 300 ml of bile has been observed from this in the last 12 hours. Outline your early management.

Answer

Plan

- ABC.
- Resuscitation/control sepsis.
- Need for re-laparoscopy/laparotomy.
- Determine injury: enteric, bile duct injury or leak from cystic duct without injury to bile ducts.
- Definitive Mx: drainage alone vs ERCP vs surgery.
- Surgery: hepatico-jejunostomy — late vs early.

INITIAL ASSESSMENT

- ABC approach. Supplemental O2. IV access, fluid resuscitation. Check FBC, EUC, LFT, Amylase, Coag, ABG.
- BP, pulse, postural drop, jaundice, hydration, pyrexia, signs of peritonism/shock.
- Drain fluid volume and nature — enteric or purely bilious? Blood?

IMMEDIATE MX

NPO. IV fluids. IV Abx if SIRS. Insert NGT. Urinary catheter to monitor U/O. Examine operation report: bleeding or bile seen intra-operatively — greater risk of bile duct injury. Was a cholangiogram performed? Cholangiogram satisfactory: ? distal obstruction, ? intra-hepatic biliary tree seen ? talk to surgeon.

DEFINITIVE MX

Depends:

- SIRS/shock/peritonitis — immediate return to OT for initial laparoscopic washout, examination of 'at risk' structures — duodenum, cystic duct stump. Further drains. Convert to laparotomy if required. Generally, goal is drainage and to ensure no enteric injury.
- No SIRS/shock/peritonitis. CT/US scan of abdomen to detect collection or other complications (perforated bowel).
  - If no collection or free fluid then CT cholangiogram if available immediately. HIDA more sensitive but less anatomic information:
    - CT cholangiogram shows bile duct transection: contact regional HPB surgery unit for transfer
    - CT cholangiogram: main bile duct intact or is indeterminate, then ERCP.
- Further management depends on ERCP findings:
  - cystic duct remnant leak +/– distal obstruction: stent and expectant management provided no sepsis and bile leak controlled
  - normal ER cholangiogram = probably duct of Luschka. Sphinterotomy +/– stent and expectant management
  - if signs of major bile duct injury (CBD, CHD or sectoral duct — usually right posterior sectoral) then consult with regional HPB unit
  - ECRP endoscopist unable to cannulate bile duct, then PTC and drainage if biliary tree dilated. Drainogram if bile ducts not dilated.
- Timing of surgery: early surgery (<7days) better if sepsis and general condition allow:
  - if sepsis and poor general condition, avoid early surgery
  - maintain nutrition, preferably enteral.
- Definitive surgery:
  - direct closure over T-tube or end-to-end anastomosis: high rate of primary failure and secondary stricture
  - most injuries require dissection of porta hepatis to determine extent of major vascular injury and re-construction with Roux-en-Y hepatico-jejunostomy.

2.4.20 Solid liver lesions

Question: a 57-year-old patient is found to have a solid liver lesion on CT scan. Outline your differential diagnosis and assessment.

Answer

Differential diagnosis

Solid liver lesions could be either benign or malignant.

- Benign solid lesions include:
  - haemangioma — most common benign tumour
  - focal nodular hyperplasia
  - hepatic adenoma.
- Malignant solid lesions:
  - hepatocellular carcinoma (90% of all liver primary tumours)
  - intra-hepatic cholangiocarcinoma
  - metastases:
    - colorectal (most common cause of liver metastases)
    - neuroendocrine tumours: carcinoid, pancreatic
    - gastrointestinal stromal tumours
    - gastrointestinal non-neuroendocrine: gastric adenocarcinoma, pancreatic adenocarcinoma, cholangiocarcinoma, oesophageal adenocarcinoma/SCC, tumours of the ampulla, small bowel adenocarcinoma
    - breast
    - melanoma
    - gynaecological: ovarian, endometrial
    - renal cell carcinoma, urothelial cancer.

Assessment

HISTORY

- Age and sex of patient.
- Symptoms:
  - abdominal pain
  - nausea/vomiting/anorexia
  - weight loss
  - fevers/sweats
  - alteration in bowel habit/per rectal bleeding.
- Past history:
  - hepatitis — risk factors including IVDU, previous transfusions, tattoos
  - cirrhosis or other liver disease (PSC, PBC)
  - previous malignancy including skin cancers (esp melanoma).
- Medications:
  - combined oral contraceptive pill
  - steroids.
- Social:
  - IVDU
  - alcohol
  - occupation.
- Family history of malignancy.

EXAMINATION

- Signs of jaundice/scleral icterus.
- Stigmata of chronic liver disease/portal hypertension.
- Abdominal examination for:
  - masses
  - hepatomegaly
  - splenomegaly.
- PR examination.
- Breast examination.
- Skin examination.

INVESTIGATIONS

- Bloods:
  - full blood count — Hb (anaemia), WCC, PLT
  - electrolytes, urea, creatinine
  - liver function tests (Bilirubin, albumin, protein, GGT, ALP, AST, ALT)
  - coagulation: PT/APTT
  - tumour markers: CEA, AFP, CA 19.9, CA 15.3, Chromogranin A, CA 125
  - hepatitis serology.
- Imaging:
  - ultrasound — differentiate between solid and cystic lesions
  - triple phase CT of abdomen and pelvis — appearance of the liver lesions on the different phases of CT is sensitive and specific for many liver tumours
  - MRI of liver with Gadolinium/Primovist — can be used to evaluate liver lesions which are equivocal on CT
  - FDG — PET
  - additionally consider the following as clinically indicated and suspicious of mets:
    - gastroscopy
    - colonoscopy
    - mammography
    - pelvic ultrasound.
- Histopathology — liver biopsy:
  - not used as a first line investigation due to risks of tumour seeding and complications including bleeding
  - may be used in selected cases where there remains diagnostic uncertainty or if the patient is not an operative candidate
  - can be performed as an image guided percutaneous procedure or laparoscopically if superficial as part of a diagnostic laparoscopy.

COMMON LESIONS

- Haemangiomas: usually asymptomatic; on contrast enhanced CT/MRI — peripheral enhancement with filling in on delayed images.
- Hepatic adenoma: usually female patient with history of OCP use, can present acutely with pain from haemorrhage, blood tests usually normal.
  - U/S: solid lesion, may have variable echogenicity due to haemorrhage.

  - CT: otherwise normal liver with lesion on pre-contrast images hypodense or isodense.
  - MRI: Increase signal on T1 and T2, Gadolinium — hypervascularity in arterial phase.
  - PET: negative.
- Focal nodular hyperplasia: asymptomatic lesions, on contrast enhanced CT and MRI have a central feeding arteriole.
- HCC: history of cirrhosis (viral/alcoholic), transaminases usually elevated, check hepatitis serology, Duplex U/S shows peritumoural arterial. Enhancement, contrast CT shows intense contrast enhancement on arterial phase with washout in the portal venous phase.
- Cholangiocarcinoma: jaundice may be present, LFTs may show cholestatic pattern, biliary dilation, hypodense on PV phase of CT, intrahepatic lesions have very similar appearance to colorectal metastases on MRI.
- Metastases: may have a history of malignancy or focal symptoms that point to an undiagnosed primary tumour (alteration of bowel habit or per rectal bleeding may indicate a colorectal malignancy), tumour markers may be elevated, CT shows a hypoattenuated mass.
  - Colorectal metastases: CT — hypodense in portal venous phase, small amount of peripheral rim enhancement on arterial phase. MRI — low signal on T1 and moderate signal intensity on T2. MRI is more sensitive for small lesions and for differentiating from simple cysts which are bright on T2.

2.4.21 Pancreatic mass

Question: a 57-year-old man presents with a 3 week history of progressive painless jaundice and pale stools. He is referred with a portal venous CT scan of the abdomen showing a 2.5 cm mass in the head of the pancreas and dilated bile and pancreatic ducts. Describe your approach to diagnosis, staging and management of this patient.

Answer

Plan

- Diagnosis: Hx, PE, bloods.
- Staging: triple phase CT, CT chest, EUS +/– Bx, PET, staging lap.
- Mx: MDT, ERCP + stent.
  - unfit/met: palliative Mx
  - borderline: neoadjuvant
  - resectable: counsel (10% risk not cancer; 5% risk death).

Diagnosis

- History:
  - weight loss, back pain, diarrhoea, vomiting, exercise.
- Physical examination:
  - supraclavicular lymphadenopathy, fitness for surgery.
- Bloods (biochemical):
  - CA 19.9, CEA, IgG4.

Staging

- Review imaging:
  - ? evidence of mets (liver mets, ascities)
  - ? local invasion (SMV/PV, SMA, coeliac axis and hepatic artery).
- Further imaging:
  - pancreatic protocol CT (assess arterial involvement, aberrant hepatic arterial anatomy)
  - CT chest and neck: intra-thoracic metastasis.
- FDG PET — changes management in 10% by detecting mets occult on CT.
- EUS biopsy: operator-dependant:
  - EUS FNA specific (99%) but not sensitive (60%). Negative result does not exclude cancer. Role for borderline resectable disease where neoadjuvant treatment required.
- Staging laparoscopy:
  - pick-up low (<5%). Only useful in avoiding a laparotomy e.g. if palliative bypass surgery for unresectable disease is not considered an option.

Management

- Discuss in MDT.
- Role of ERCP and stent: pre-operative stent does not reduce mortality or post-operative stay after pancreaticoduodenectomy (PD). Associated with increased infectious complications and ERCP complications. Not all centres have capacity for expeditious surgery without stenting.

PATHWAYS

- Unfit or metastatic — palliative management. Palliate jaundice, gastric outlet obstruction and pain. Endostents, bypass surgery, coeliac axis alcohol neurolysis (percutaneous or EUS), opiates and palliative chemotherapy.
- Fit but unresectable or borderline resectable: Neoadjuvant treatment (Chemo-RT). Main value is detecting patients with progressive disease on treatment. Down-staging achieved in some.
- Fit and resectable: counsel about risks of surgery. PJ leak, bleeding. In most studies there is a 10% risk that the lesion is not cancer. The patient must understand this.
- If unresectable at laparotomy options are bypass (biliary alone or double):
  - bypass surgery more durable than metal stents
  - most of morbidity is from laparotomy and bypass adds little to post-operative complications
  - benefit depends on life expectancy. If >6 months bypass is likely to improve QOL and reduce hospitalisation.

2.4.22 Venous thromboembolism prophylaxis

Question: a 58-year-old woman has been recently diagnosed with early stage rectal cancer which requires an anterior resection. She has been on HRT for her menopausal symptoms commenced by her gynaecologist. Outline your management plan to minimise the risk of DVT peri-operatively.

Answer

On the basis of the clinical information provided, this patient is at high risk of developing a DVT because of:

- age >40
- major abdominal surgery (which takes >45 minutes)
- diagnosis of cancer
- HRT.

To modify her risk peri-operatively

Risk stratify patient-risk from history:

- previous DVT, pulmonary emboli
- previous pelvic surgery, major trauma, pelvic fracture
- personal/FHx of thrombophilia
- venous insufficiency — varicose veins, oedema in lower limbs
- allergy to heparin or LMWH including history of HITTS (heparin induced thrombosis thrombocytopenia syndrome).

Evaluate risks of mechanical preventive devices:

- peripheral vascular disease (claudication, non-healing ulcer)
- lower limb deformity, skin graft or active skin pathologies.

To reduce the risk in the peri-operative period, appropriate strategies pre-, intra- and post-operatively as well as post-discharge should be considered.

- Pre-operative period:
  - cease HRT ideally 6 weeks prior to surgery. Involve gynaecologist in care to help manage menopausal symptoms
  - encourage regular exercise
  - maintain adequate hydration (important if using mechanical bowel preparation)
  - cease smoking tobacco, encourage healthy lifestyle
  - cease alcohol consumption
  - educate patient about DVT, risk factors and how to decrease the risks.
- To reduce the risk on the day of operation (NB: the following regimen presumes no contraindications):
  - one dose of unfractionated heparin or LMWH *before* surgery
  - intermittent pneumatic compression (IPC) device during surgery
  - graded compression stockings
  - adequate hydration during surgery.
- To reduce the risk post-operatively:
  - early mobilisation — remove IDC, drains as soon as possible
  - IPC for first 24 hours
  - graded compression stockings until fully mobilised
  - LMWH or UFH while in hospital.
- To reduce the risk post-discharge (NB: one-third of DVT occur post-discharge):
  - encourage physical activity
  - keep hydrated

  - continue LMWH for 4 weeks
  - avoid HRT until cancer treatment completed.

2.4.23 Leg ulcers

Question: a 78-year-old woman presents with an ulcer on the medial aspect of her right lower leg that has been present for 6 months and has failed to heal with simple dry dressings applied by a community nurse. List the possible causes of the ulcer and discuss your management of the patient.

Answer

Plan

CAUSES OF ULCERS

- Commonest: venous/arterial/mixed arteriovenous.
- Less common causes: 'TIN' (trauma; infective; neoplastic/neuropathic).

MANAGEMENT OF PATIENT

- History/examination: attempt to establish features of ulcer/possible aetiology.
- Investigation: basic blood Ix and objective vascular assessment (anatomical/functional).
- Treatment aims:
  - improve symptoms/promote healing:
    - general measures
    - specific treatment options dependent on aetiology (compression therapy/endovascular and surgical intervention)
  - prevent recurrence.

Causes of ulcers

- Venous disease (60%):
  - superficial incompetence
  - deep venous damage (post-thrombotic).
- Arterial ulcers (15%):
  - ischaemic — major vessel atherosclerosis
  - small vessel disease (rarer):
    - vasculitis/arteritis (Takayasu's, Buerger's disease, giant cell, polyarteritisnodosa, Wegener's granulomatosis)
    - vasospasm — primary or secondary to connective tissue disease (e.g. systemic sclerosis, SLE, RA etc.)
- Mixed arterial and venous disease (15%).
- Other (10%):
  - neuropathic ulcers (diabetes mellitus, peripheral neuropathy)
  - traumatic ulcers
  - neoplastic ulcers (squamous cell carcinoma and basal cell carcinoma)
  - infective (TB, syphilis).

Management of patient

History:

- ulcer duration/change/associated symptoms (pain)
- predisposing events (trauma etc.)
- Hx of claudication/chronic venous insufficiency
- PHx DVT/post-operative leg swelling.

Examination:

- site/size/shape/'BEDD' (base/edge/depth/discharge)
- full examination of venous system (see 3.5.10)
  - evidence of chronic venous insufficiency/varicosities
- full examination of arterial system (see 3.5.8)
  - assessment of peripheral pulses/doppler pressures (ABPI)
- full neurological examination of the lower limbs
  - peripheral neuropathy

Investigations:

- blood Ix
  - FBC, ESR/CRP, autoantibodies
- objective assessment of vascular tree (anatomical/functional)
  - duplex scan
    - venous: anatomy/reflux/DVT
    - arterial: waveform/segmental pressures (stenosis/occlusion)
  - arteriography/venography (if duplex equivocal)
  - plethysmography —measurement of venous function.
- Consider biopsy for histopathological analysis.

Treatment:

- best in multidisciplinary setting
- aims are (i) improve symptoms and promote healing and (ii) prevention of recurrence
- general measures (analgesia, antibiotics if infected, debridement, optimise dressing/wound care, prosthetics/orthotics)
- specific treatment options dependent on aetiology.

Venous

- Limb elevation/Rx comorbidities (CCF).
- Compression therapy — Charing Cross 4 layer elastic compression.
- Surgery:
  - superficial/perforator/deep venous surgery/reconstruction — Eschar trial — superficial venous surgery reduces recurrence but does *not* speed healing!
  - skin grafting.

Arterial

- Aggressive modification/normalisation of arterial risk factors:
  - quit smoking
  - optimise treatment of diabetes and other health conditions

    - exercise/weight loss
    - antiplatelet therapy.
- Need revascularisation:
    - radiological
    - surgical.

Mixed

- Severe arterial (ABPI <0.5) — Rx arterial first (as above) then elastic compression therapy.
- ABPI >0.85 *usually* tolerate compression.
- ABPI 0.5 — 0.85 *may* tolerate compression or revascularise first.

2.4.24 Needle stick injury

Question: while instilling local anaesthesia during a perianal procedure, you sustain a needle stick injury. Discuss your management.

Answer

This is an occupational health and safety issue. Each hospital/area health service will have established policies and protocols for the management and reporting of these events.

Aim is prevention through personal protective equipment, safe disposal of sharps and correct handling and use of sharps (sharps dish for scalpel blades/ making suture needles safe).

Serious pathogens: HBV, HCV, HIV, and in some areas HTLV1.

Risks:

- HBV most infectious 1:16–1:33
- HCV intermediate risk 1: 55
- HIV lowest risk 1:313
- hollow bore needles with penetration and obvious blood carry highest risk
- minimal risk when intact skin/mucosa receives body fluid splash.

Management includes the following.

- Prevention of further injury and exposure of the donor to the recipient's blood (e.g. the needle responsible for the injury should be removed from the operative field).
- Initial first aid — copious irrigation of the wound with water and expressing blood from the injured surface. No evidence for topical application of antiseptics or disinfectants. Dressing of the area.
- Determine the donor's risk factors for infection. Donor should be tested after informed consent obtained by another member of the treating team. (HBsAg, HCV antibodies, HIV antibodies— also need to assess if the source could be in a 'window' period.). Likelihood that donor is infected will determine whether post-exposure prophylaxis should be given to recipient.

- Baseline testing of the recipient — check for seroconversion if immunised to HBV (HBSAb), HCV, HIV 1 and HIV2, LFTs (used as a baseline to monitor for early signs of hepatitis).
- Post-exposure prophylaxis (PEP). Depends on:
  - type of exposure (high risk vs low risk)
  - infectious status of donor
  - immunisation.
- Counselling and monitoring for seroconversion.
- Reporting of the incident as per local guidelines:
  - workers compensation
  - may be important to identify ongoing risks and prevention of injury to others.

HBV

- Immunisation has reduced the incidence of infection (high rates of immunisation in the community and compulsory immunisation of staff members).
- If donor negative and not in a window period and if immunised and seroconversion proven then no further action required.
- If immunised and seroconversion unknown, administer dose of HBV vaccine immediately and dose of HBV immunoglobulin (within 24 hours).

HCV

- If donor negative and not in a window period then no further action is required.
- There is no active or passive immunoprophylaxis available.
- The recipient should be followed up with HCV RNA at 6 weeks and HCV antibodies and LFTs at 3 and 6 months.

HIV

- If the donor is negative and not in a window period no further action is required.
- Follow-up HIV antibody testing at 6 weeks, 3 months, 6 months.
- If determined that PEP should be given should be ideally commenced within 24 hours.
- Combination of two anti-retrovirals for low risk exposures — lamivudine and zidovudine for 4 weeks.
- For high-risk exposures (deep injury, hollow bore needle, late stage disease or high viral load in source) additional anti-retrovirals are given (lopinavir, ritonavir).
- PEP is usually given under the supervision of a HIV physician.

HTLV1

- Not routinely tested unless donor known to be infected.
- Post-exposure prophylaxis as per HIV recommended but efficacy is unknown.

Section 3

The clinical examination

Chapter 3.1

An approach to the clinical examination

If you have no critics you'll likely have no success.
(Malcolm Forbes, 1919–90)

The examination format

The clinical examination is the area where candidates are most likely to perform below par. Whilst this may be due to inadequate knowledge acquisition or missing an important clinical sign during the examination, it is more commonly because of insufficient practise and an inability of candidates to organise or communicate their own thoughts and comments. The clinical examination consists of medium cases and short cases. Candidates are notified of the venue and starting times of all such examinations about 1 month prior to the examinations and are usually sent a map of the venue. You will be marshalled to a 'pre-exam' waiting area. Make sure that you are on time. The medium cases are usually in the morning and the short cases are usually in the afternoon.

Exam technique

During the actual clinical examinations you need to demonstrate a sound clinical approach to each case. Imagine that you are in the out-patients clinic, in the emergency department or even on a ward round in your hospital. What would you think, do and say in your hospital if that was your patient? When tackling the questions posed by the examiners, present your answers from the perspective of a general surgeon with an emphasis on safe and sensible practice — just as you would in everyday clinical practice. Do not be tempted to deliver an answer detailing what another surgeon from another hospital would do. Further, you should avoid quoting practice that you are unfamiliar or not fully conversant with, since it is usually immediately obvious when candidates are out of their 'comfort/knowledge' zone! Of course, it is sound evidence-based practice to quote from the literature when asked to do so and to be able to demonstrate that you are aware of other investigations and treatment techniques that are, or may be, used elsewhere.

Remember to always speak in the first person when asked, 'how would you investigate or manage a patient or condition'. Construct answers that start with or include 'I would', 'I will', 'in my experience', and avoid second person pronouns such as 'you could', 'you would', 'some say'. You are trying to present yourself as a competent, but not overly confident, junior colleague to the examiners. The examiners will appreciate that you are not yet an expert in everything and that you have your whole career ahead of you to shape your own practice. However, they do want to see evidence that you are immediately capable of safe practice. As with the other oral examinations, you can only be awarded marks for what you say (and do). This sounds obvious but knowledge in your brain that you have not been able to demonstrate or communicate to the examiners will *not* score you marks.

As well as listening to your answers, the examiners will be watching your actions and body language. This is crucially important in the clinical examinations, as you will have an opportunity to impress the examiners (and score points) by demonstrating a caring, polite approach to patients, as well as your confidence with various examination techniques to maximise your chances of eliciting subtle clinical signs.

It is customary to bring a torch, stethoscope and small measuring rule to the exam. Make sure you wash your hands between each case in the shorts and mediums, either using the alcohol wash provided or at a sink. You will fail if you don't. You may put gloves on when appropriate (e.g. during scrotal examination) in the short cases.

Preparation and practising

The need for adequate, appropriate practise when preparing for the clinical examinations cannot be overstated. Most successful candidates have spent several months seeing and examining a wide range and large number of short and medium cases. This is best done in front of a range of mentors/bosses to allow your style/technique to be critiqued so that your performance for the actual examination can be optimised. Whilst a diverse range of opinions is very useful when trying to improve your performance, be alert to the fact that you will receive many conflicting opinions about how you should approach certain cases. Some candidates become confused, disorientated and less confident as a consequence. However, our advice is to absorb each of these varied opinions and distil them into *your* preferred approach. Often, these differences relate to style only and the detail/content of the various examinations are surprisingly similar. Also, make use of practising in front of your peers/members of your study group. It is particularly helpful if you belong to a study group with candidates from different hospitals, as this will provide access to unfamiliar hospital environments and consultants and will better simulate the examination itself. If you intend to take *B*-blockers because of anxiety, do not prescribe them yourself. Instead, you should see an appropriate expert and seek advice about their appropriateness/safety and make sure you have a trial run using them before the actual day of the examination.

With regard to dress, most candidates will present wearing conservative, dark (blue/black/grey) suits — both men and women. This was true when we sat our examinations and still holds true today. On that basis, it is ill advised to model your latest attire if it doesn't conform to this traditional look; no matter how good you may look in it! Make sure that you have a good night's sleep before all examinations and that you are not staying too far away from the examination venue, especially if you don't live in the city of the examination. Make sure you arrive at least 30 minutes before your commencement time in case there are delays on your way to the venue, especially if you are travelling in an unfamiliar city.

Chapter 3.2

The medium case clinical examination

Common sense is not common practise. (Stephen Covey, 1932–2012)

The examination format

The medium case clinical examination lasts 40 minutes and comprises two medium cases of 20 minutes each. These usually take place in a hospital out-patient or clinic setting. Certain patients and cases are suited to the medium cases. The pool of pre-operative patients is diminishing, which means that the majority of patients are post-operative inpatients or out-patients that have been brought along to the exam. Most medium case patients can give a good history as they have been vetted to make sure they are suitable for inclusion in the exam. This means that there is often a narrow range of patients who are used for medium cases. Clearly, they can't be too unwell or suffering with an acute condition, as they would already be in surgery. Certain hospitals have a reputation for practice in a particularly area, such as the melanoma units at PAH in Qld and RPAH in NSW. If you are going to such hospitals, you would be foolish to have not practised such cases. Do your research ahead of the exam and prepare predictable topics thoroughly.

After the bell rings the two examiners take you to the first patient and make a statement such as 'this is Ron B, would you like to take a history and perform an examination'. Occasionally, they will have a more detailed introduction, depending on how good a historian or how complex the patient is.

Exam technique

You have 10 uninterrupted minutes to take a history and examine the patient. The examiners quietly observe you and may stand closer when you examine the patient to observe if you examine and elicit the signs correctly. Many candidates don't have time to write notes. Nevertheless, it is still a good idea to take a pen and piece of A4 paper, folded in four so that it fits neatly into a pocket, into the examination in case you have time to make notes.

The history

It is important to use a structured approach to history taking. Whilst there are many ways of doing this, one method uses the following structure.

1. Introduction and orientation.
    - After introducing yourself to the patient, ask the patient what is the matter with them. Use phrases such as 'what was the problem that brought you to the hospital' or 'what was wrong that made you come to the hospital'. Often, patients will ask if they are allowed to tell you what is the matter with them, to which you should confidently reply 'yes'.
    - Establish if the patient is an inpatient or out-patient.
    - Establish the patient's function, especially if post-operative.
    - Establish the patient's age, occupation and marital/social status.
2. The presenting symptoms and history of presenting complaint.
    - Detailed enquiry about the presenting symptoms:
        - when did they start
        - characterisation of pain (SOCRATES):
            - **s**ite
            - **o**nset: when did the pain start, and was it sudden or gradual? progressive or regressive?
            - **c**haracter
            - **r**adiation
            - **a**ssociations: any other signs or symptoms associated with the pain?
            - **t**ime course: does the pain follow any pattern?
            - **e**xacerbating/relieving factors
            - **s**everity: how bad is the pain?
        - quantification of bleeding/weight loss etc.
    - Associated symptoms of the 'diseased system' (e.g. GI system).
    - Associated symptoms:
        - from anatomically related viscera (urogenital/gynaecological in pelvic disease.
        - systemic (weight loss etc.).
    - Who has the patient seen?
    - Investigations that have been performed — when and what was found?
    - Treatments to date, specifically any operations — what, when, outcome:
        - what are the future plans of the attending medical officers?

Patients will, again, often ask are they allowed to tell you what investigations and operations they have had and you should once again answer in the affirmative.

3. Risk factor assessment for cancers/vascular disease, if relevant.
4. Past medical/surgical history.
    - Check each of the major systems.
    - Remember you are assessing fitness for surgery. Additional questions such as 'do you get short of breath when you walk?', 'how far can you walk?', 'can you walk up a flight of stairs?' also provide information about functional status.
5. Drug history.
    - Ask specifically about anti-platelet and anti-coagulant medication.
    - Check for allergies.

6. Family and social history.
   - Identification of pertinent risk factors.

Try to avoid leading closed questions, particularly if the desired response is in the negative. For example, 'you don't have x, do you?'.

The examination

The examiners leave it up to you to decide when to begin examining the patient. Listen to the examiners' instructions carefully. If they instruct you to examine the gastrointestinal *system* ensure that you begin with the hands. By contrast, if they instruct you to examine the abdomen then begin with the inspection of the abdomen itself and do *not* start with the hands. If there is no specific direction, begin with the hands and attempt to perform a total body examination if you can. The examiners will often get you to focus your examination if there are time constraints.

It is crucial to have a system that you can apply to any medium case and that will provide you with a framework that you can use in the examination. Such a system is critically important if you are faced with an unfamiliar case or lose your composure during the exam (it can and does happen!). We recommend the sequence in the top tip below.

TOP TIP

FRAMEWORK FOR CLINICAL EXAMINATION OF ANY MEDIUM CASE

Preparation — the 5 Ps:

place your hands in the sink or under the hand sanitiser
permission to perform the examination
position the patient
preserve the patient's dignity during exposure
progress to the foot of the bed.

General examination from the end of the bed:

overall condition
drains, tubes, infusions etc.

Assessment for peripheral signs, unless instructed otherwise:

vital signs.

Examination of the system of interest:

inspection
palpation
percussion
auscultation.

Conclusion — reverse sequence to preparation!

Cover the patient.
Reposition the patient.
Thank the patient.
Clean your hands again.
Only now turn to face the examiners.

The presentation summary

After 10 minutes the examiners will stop you and will want to discuss the case. You then sit down and talk about the case with the examiners. If you do not start speaking and summarising the case, the examiners will begin the discussion with something like 'would you provide a summary of the case?'. The way that you present the case summary depends on whether the patient:

(a) is post-operative or pre-operative
(b) if pre-operative whether they have a known diagnosis or
(c) has symptoms and/or signs that still require investigation or treatment.

TOP TIP

- *Begin* your presentation with a strong introductory phrase.
- *Maintain* momentum and a good level of performance throughout.
- *Finish* even stronger, with a succinct summary, indicating that you have finished.

All too often, candidates make the mistake of not finishing strongly enough and the presentation fades towards the end, often leaving the examiners uncertain as to whether the candidate has finished.

Ensure that you get off to a good start, maintain momentum throughout and aim to finish as strongly as you started. Attempt to talk directly to the examiners when you begin to present the case. For example, if the patient is:

- post-operative (simple): 'I should like to present Mr B, who is a 24-year-old man who is 8 weeks post-operative following a laparotomy and small bowel resection for....'
- post-operative (more involved): 'Mrs Jones is a 56-year-old woman who 4 months ago had a left breast wide local excision and sentinel lymph node biopsy. She then went on to have a mastectomy and axillary lymph node clearance 4 months ago. She underwent post-operative radiotherapy and is currently receiving adjuvant chemotherapy treatment
- pre-operative with known diagnosis: 'I had the pleasure of seeing Mr B, who is a 24 year-old man with a small bowel tumour who is booked for surgery next week
- pre-operative with unknown diagnosis who may require surgery: 'Mr B is a 24-year-old inpatient with a 3 month history of recurrent abdominal pain who is currently being investigated to establish a formal diagnosis for his symptoms'.

The examiners may interrupt during your presentation to clarify specific points. If you are presenting well, you may end up speaking without interruption. If so, be prepared to summarise the sequence of events and the current issues and focus on pertinent investigations and treatment issues.

TOP TIP

FRAMEWORK FOR CASE PRESENTATION

- Introductory statement.
- Setting (out-patient/inpatient).
- History of the presenting illness:
  - detailed symptom description (e.g. characterisation of pain/quantification of bleeding)
  - associated symptoms of the 'diseased system' (e.g. GI system)
  - investigations — which, results or planned
  - treatment — done: what? when? or planned: what?, when?
- Risk factor assessment (if relevant).
- Past medical/surgical history/fitness for surgery:
  - relevant comorbidities/diagnoses/drugs.

Once you have finished presenting, the examiners will form questions based on the case and the scenario. The discussion usually focuses on patient and disease factors; for example, the fitness of the patient and the stage of the tumour when faced with cases of cancer. Remember to expect multiple questions and abrupt changes in the flow/direction of questions. If you do not know an answer to a question simply state, 'I do not know', rather than having long, painful pauses.

Occasionally, the examiners may allow you to initiate and direct the discussion. If so, it is useful to have a framework for discussion of the medium cases. An example is presented in the following top tip.

TOP TIP

FRAMEWORK FOR CASE DISCUSSION

- Disease factors:
  - if benign disease
    - extent/severity, symptoms, indications for surgery
  - if malignant disease
    - stage, symptoms, curative or palliative intent (what are the goals of surgery), indications for surgery.
- Patient factors:
  - fitness for surgery
  - what the patient wants, e.g. conservation of an organ, avoidance of a stoma.
- Investigations:
  - what they are and how they work
  - interpret specific scans and images.
- Treatment:
  - explain your preferred treatment option and why
  - detail the risks, benefits and alternatives of each treatment option.

Many of these techniques will be demonstrated in the model answers in Chapter 3.3.

Preparing and practising

As previously stated, frequent practise is essential. You have 10 minutes to obtain a history and examine the patient. It is immediately obvious if you have not repeatedly practised and you will fail. Look at the list of common medium cases listed in Chapter 1.3 and add to it with reports from previous exam candidates of what medium cases they encountered in their examinations. Find these cases in your hospital and practise them. Succinctly summarising cases requires mental and verbal practise and repetition. Getting used to openly discussing patient investigation and treatment, a common and frequent facet of consultant practice; this also requires repetition.

The fellowship examination examines the skills required in clinical practice and nowhere is this more true than in the medium case clinical examination. To this day, the authors still employ many of the same strategies as outlined above when seeing new patients in the office.

Chapter 3.3

Common medium cases

3.3.1 Breast cancer

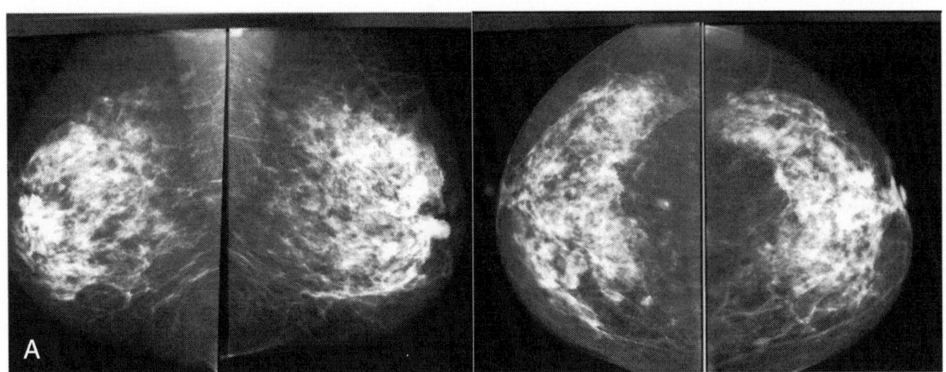

Figure 3.3.1A

Mammogram with possible microcalcification in left breast, MLO views on left, CC views on right

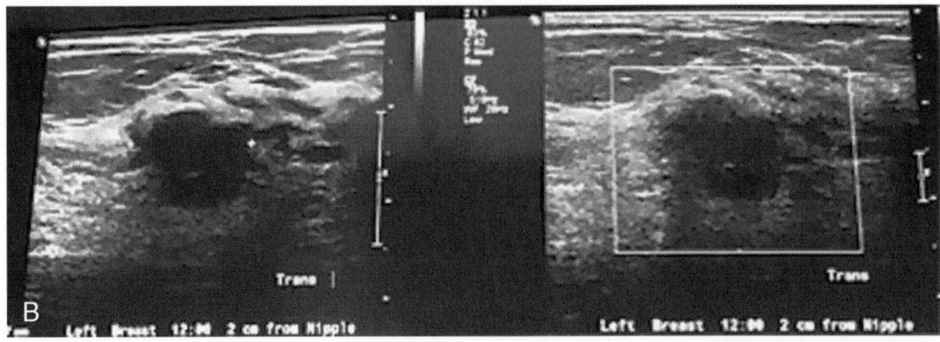

Figure 3.3.1B

Ultrasound of solid breast mass

One in nine Australian women will develop breast cancer before the age of 85 years, so breast cancer cases are common. Typical cases include women who have had recent surgery or who are in the middle of or have just completed multidisciplinary complex treatment. You may well get a complete structured history from a single open question. Allow time for the patient to talk and it will become obvious whether or not this is the case. If it seems that information is missing, then some prompting will be required. The patients are usually surprisingly well-informed and will often use jargon accurately such as sentinel node or DCIS.

You may be introduced to a woman sitting in a clinic room as follows: 'This is Mrs Jones, would you please take a history from her and perform an appropriate examination'.

The history

- Introduce yourself and ask the patient what has been going on. The patient may indicate that she has had a breast cancer removed 4 months ago, for example.
- Try to maintain a structure to your history, using the framework above. After orientation, ask questions specific to the breast problem.
- The presenting symptoms and history of presenting complaint:
  - *presentation*: presenting clinical symptoms (presence of a lump, pain, breast skin change, nipple change or discharge), or asymptomatic detection during regular check-up or screening mammogram
  - *investigations*: radiology/biopsy
  - *treatment:*
    - Was neo-adjuvant treatment required or discussed?
    - What surgery did she have done? Establish whether the initial operation was mastectomy or lumpectomy and method of axillary staging. Has a re-operation been performed (cavity re-excision or mastectomy or axillary lymph node clearance). If so, ask why re-operation was required (positive margin or positive sentinel node).
    - Did she undergo any breast reconstruction?
    - Were there any complications (seroma, shoulder pain or lymphoedema)?
    - What adjuvant treatment was required (radiotherapy or chemotherapy)? What chemotherapy? Is she taking tamoxifen or other hormonal therapy?
    - What follow-up imaging has she had?
- Risk factor assessment:
  - oestrogen and reproductive history: age at menarche, menopause, number of children, contraceptive and hormone replacement therapy.
- Past medical history.
- Surgical history including previous breast lumps or breast cancer.
- Drug history and allergies.
- Family history — particularly of breast or ovarian cancer.
- Social history: occupation, home circumstances, smoking tobacco and alcohol consumption.

The examination

- Preparation — (see above):
  - position: edge of the bed
  - remove upper garments including brassiere.

- Breast examination:
  - Inspection:
    - breast asymmetry/skin changes, including nipples and areolar
    - scars from the previous surgery breast/axilla
    - tattoos from radiotherapy (usually on sternum and lateral chest wall)
    - evidence of chemotherapy port on the chest wall
    - the back of the chest for a scar from a latissimus dorsi flap
    - enhance inspection with movement: ask the woman to put her hands on her hips and squeeze her hips together
    - ask her to raise her hands above her head and look for tethering of the skin.

Position change: ask the woman to lie down on slightly reclined couch (if available).

  - Palpation:
    - each breast and ipsilateral axilla, including nipples and areolar
    - the supraclavicular fossa bilaterally
    - with the patent still recumbent, examine the abdomen briefly by inspection (looking for scars from TRAM flap) then palpation of the liver edge.
  - Auscultation:
    - sit the patient forward and auscultate to the lung bases.
- Conclusion:
  - thank the patient for taking the time to come to help with your exam
  - help her off the couch if required and to find her clothing if necessary
  - wash or sanitise your hands again at the end of the examination if possible.

The examiners will then commence discussion in the same room or another room, depending on the venue.

The discussion

Breast cancer diagnosis is best achieved using triple assessment:

- clinical
- imaging: mammogram and ultrasound
- pathological: FNAC or core biopsy.

INVESTIGATIONS

- Imaging — mammography.
  - The standard for mammography is a bilateral mediolateral oblique (MLO) and cranio-caudal (CC) view.
  - These are low energy x-rays (30 kVp) obtained by parallel plate compression to even the thickness of the breast tissue.
  - The images are assessed for symmetry, architectural distortion, masses, calcifications and densities.
  - Fig 3.3.1A shows a bilateral mammogram with MLO and CC views. The MLO is shown on the left and is distinguished by the pectoral muscle shadow. The convention is to arrange them on the viewing box as shown.
  - For any mass describe the shape, margin, density and associated microcalcifications. Round or oval shapes are typically benign (fibroadenoma or cyst). Lobulated or irregular masses are typically malignant. Margins that are circumscribed are benign, whereas microlobulated, obscured, indistinct or spiculated outlines are suspicious for malignancy. For calcifications describe the shape, location, number and distribution. There are a variety of typically benign calcifications such as skin, vascular, popcorn-like, rod-like, round, punctate, milk of calcium, eggshell, dystrophic and suture. Of intermediate concern are amorphous or indistinct

calcifications. Microcalcifications that are pleomorphic or heterogeneous, fine/linear and fine or linear/branching calcifications have a high probability of malignancy.

- Imaging — ultrasound.
  - Breast ultrasound uses higher frequency sound waves (typically 8–13MHz) than used for abdominal ultrasound, offering greater resolution but less penetration.
  - Benign features include ellipsoid shape, hyperechogenicity or anechoic, and smooth, well-circumscribed margins. Cysts are oval or round, well circumscribed, anechoic with posterior acoustic *enhancement*. Features of malignancy are irregular margins, hypoechoic to the surrounding tissue, with posterior acoustical *shadowing*. Malignant masses are usually taller than they are wide.
  - Fig 3.3.1B shows an ultrasound of a breast mass demonstrating many of the features of malignancy.
- Pathological: FNAC.
  - FNA uses a 22G needle and a syringe (aspirated to include several ml of air), which is passed into the mass if clinically apparent or using ultrasound guidance.
  - It has a false positive rate <1%, a false negative rate <10%. Insufficient material for diagnosis occurs in about 10% of cases.
  - The presence of carcinoma cells does not differentiate between invasive and in situ breast cancer.
  - FNA results are reported as:
    - C1 — inadequate/acellular
    - C2 — benign
    - C3 — atypical
    - C4 — suspicious or
    - C5 — malignant.
- Pathological: core biopsy.
  - Conventional core biopsy uses a spring-loaded biopsy gun unseeing a double-action needle (typically 14G) consisting of an inner trocar with a sample notch and an outer cutting cannula.
  - To obtain the specimen the needle must be withdrawn. Usually, 4–6 samples are taken (4–6 insertions).
  - Core biopsy provides a diagnosis of histological type, grade, hormone receptor status, HER2 expression.
  - Core biopsy differentiates ductal carcinoma in situ (DCIS) from invasive cancer.

TREATMENT

- Treatment should be discussed at an MDT with medical and radiation oncologists involving review of the pertinent radiology and pathology.
- It should be considered within three dimensions: (1) treatment of the breast; (2) staging and treatment of the axilla; and (3) systemic treatment.

Treatment of the breast

- Options are mastectomy (with/without immediate or delayed reconstruction) or wide local excision (WLE) to clear margins combined with post-operative radiotherapy (XRT).
- The risk of local recurrence with WLE alone is 30–40%. The risk of local recurrence may be higher with breast conservation and XRT than mastectomy but the long-term survival is the same.
- Breast conservation should be considered if a satisfactory cosmetic result can be achieved (which is less likely when > 10–20% of breast volume is removed).

- If the woman has a large breast, especially if upper/outer quadrant, WLE is often a good option. For a woman with a smaller breast cosmetic outcome may be unsatisfactory. Oncoplastic techniques can be used to facilitate reconstruction of the conserved breast (possibly combined with contralateral balancing procedure).

Staging and treatment of the axilla

- Lymph node status is the strongest prognostic determinant in early breast cancer.
- If the axilla is clinically positive with palpable nodes, then a core biopsy or FNA should be performed. If cancer is confirmed then axillary lymph node dissection (ALND), generally to level III, will be required.
- If the axilla is clinically and radiologically negative then a staging procedure is required. Options are: sentinel lymph node biopsy (SLNB) and axillary lymph node dissection.
- SLNB is performed using radio-labelled colloid and/or blue dye. SLNB has a <10% false negative rate in experienced hands. This is an acceptable staging procedure for the axilla. If positive then ALND is performed either at the time (if frozen section is used) or after definitive pathology is available. In 80% of cases where SLNB is positive for malignancy, the SLN is the only positive node found in the axilla.
- The benefit of completion ALND is currently the subject of RCTs. There are four large RCT of SLNB (NSABP B-32, Almanac, SNAC and Milan study). These have enrolled patients with clinically negative axillae and cancers less than 3 cm. The follow-up of these studies is currently relatively short and most demonstrate only the false negative rate (negative SLNB where subsequent ALND showed lymph node metastasis), usually of 5–15%. The oncological implications of the false negative rate are currently unknown. Most studies have identified reduced short-term morbidity (pain, shoulder stiffness and lymphoedema) with SLNB.
- Traditionally, ALND to level II or even level I (node sampling) has been performed in the clinically negative axilla for staging. This has been replaced by SLNB in many centres but remains a treatment of proven efficacy where skills or equipment for SLNB are not available.
- ALND should be omitted in cases of DCIS as rates of metastases is <1%.

Systemic treatment

- Adjuvant systemic treatment involves the use of cytotoxic or endocrine therapy after local treatment of breast cancer to eliminate clinically occult micrometastases, to prevent local recurrence and improve survival.
- Adjuvant endocrine therapy reduces local recurrence and contralateral breast cancer development by 50% and mortality by 25%.
  - Tamoxifen is generally offered if the cancer is ER/PR positive and should be taken for 5 years. Its use is associated with increased risk of endometrial cancer (excess mortality 1–2/1000), DVT/PE, stroke, flushing, vaginal dryness, weight gain, nausea, disturbances hair and nail growth and reduced metabolism of warfarin.
  - GnRH agonists (zoladex) overstimulate and subsequently down-regulate GnRH receptors to achieve postmenopausal levels of estrodiol and can be used in *pre*-menopausal women.
  - Aromatase inhibitor (such as anastrozole) may be used in *post*-menopausal women upfront (better than tamoxifen), switching from tamoxifen (better than tamoxifen) or after tamoxifen (better than placebo). They increase GnRH in pre-menopausal women with the undesired effect of increasing oestrogen levels.

- Chemotherapy produces a relative risk reduction (RRR) of recurrence of 20–35%, and of death by 10–30%. The same proportional RRR is seen in all subtypes of breast cancer. However, the absolute benefit depends on the risk of recurrence or death for that patient with those with the highest chances of recurrence receiving greatest absolute benefit.
  - Women under 70 years with node-positive disease should be offered adjuvant chemotherapy, but the benefit is greatest in women under 50 years.
  - Taxanes are preferred agents.
  - In patients with lower risk of recurrence and death the absolute benefit is lower and the risks and side effects of chemotherapy may exceed its benefits. However, there is a group of patient with node-negative disease who may benefit form adjuvant chemotherapy. These include: (a) tumour > 2 cm; (b) Grade II/III; (c) Lymphovascular or perivascular invasion present; (d) age <35; (e) ER/PR negative; and (f) HER-2 +ve.
- Signal transduction inhibitors:
  - trastuzumab (Herceptin) for at least 1 year in HER-2 positive disease
  - achieves a 50% reduction in risk of recurrence and 33% reduction in risk of death.
- Metastatic systemic therapy:
  - bisphosphonates decrease skeletal events in metastatic disease but do not reduce rate of bone metastases in early breast cancer
  - signal transduction inhibitors (trastuzumab — Herceptin) are effective in HER-2 positive tumours and is usually given with chemotherapy.

Extra notes

INVASIVE CANCER

Ductal (no special type) carcinomas account for 70–80% of breast cancers, lobular carcinoma account for 20% and the remaining 10% are mucinous, tubular or medullary.

IN SITU CANCER

- DCIS is a pre-invasive, in situ lesion of the breast where malignant epithelial cells are found confined within the basement membrane. The architectural types of DCIS are comedo, solid, cribriform and papillary/micropapillary.
- When a few cells penetrate the BM with no focus of invasion >1 mm, the disease is deemed 'microinvasive'.
- DCIS represents 5% of all symptomatic breast cancers, but 20% of screened breast cancers.
- About two-thirds of invasive breast cancers have associated DCIS. The risk of invasive breast cancer in patients with DCIS is 10x the normal population, the majority in the ipsilateral breast.
- On mammography, DCIS tends to be present as clustered, pleomorphic and branching or linear calcifications. Given that FNA cannot differentiate invasive carcinoma from DCIS, a tissue biopsy should be used for treatment planning of suspected DCIS.
- The vast majority of DCIS is not palpable, so tissue diagnosis must be obtained using hookwire localisation or stereotactic core biopsy (when a carbon tack is placed to mark the site).
- Small, localised areas of DCIS (<4 cm) should be treated by breast-conserving surgery with or without radiotherapy. Impalpable lesions require radiological localisation pre-operatively.
- The NSABP B-17 and EORTC 10853 studies showed that RXT reduces the risk of local recurrence of DCIS by about 50% compared with excision alone and reduced

the proportion of recurrence with invasive pathology. The Van Nuys prognostic index (VNPI) is a scoring system, which generates a score based on these factors to help guide appropriate treatment based on the risk of recurrence, but has not been validated in a prospective trial.

- Mastectomy is indicated for widespread contiguous or multi-focal DCIS, where adequate excision cannot be achieved with a cosmetically acceptable wide excision. Widespread microcalcification (on pre-operative mammogram) in the presence of proven DCIS, or persistent positive margins when attempting to excise DCIS are also indications for mastectomy.
- Positive axillary lymph nodes are seen in <1% and thus axillary staging can be avoided.
- Lobular carcinoma in situ (LCIS) is a monomorphic proliferation of cells in one or more terminal ducts or acini.
- It is uncommon and usually found incidentally at histology (about 1% of breast biopsies) and is usually found in perimenopausal women (median age 40–45 yrs), and has a decreasing incidence after menopause.
- It is multicentric and/or multifocal and/or bilateral in up to 60%. It is considered to be an index of risk for invasive cancer in either breast, rather than a premalignant lesion, with a 25 to 30% long-term cancer risk over 20 years.
- If LCIS is picked up on biopsy, excision and clear margins are probably unnecessary, as the abnormality cannot be imaged, and there is multicentricity and bilaterality. Need to consider excision to clear margins in cases of pleomorphic LCIS (histologically aggressive variant), especially in young patients. Follow-up involves lifelong surveillance, including annual mammography (at least for 10 yrs until age 50) and examination, including the axilla.

For breast cancer please also see 2.2.2, 2.2.4, 4.2.2, 4.4.3, and 4.6.1.

3.3.2. Rectal cancer

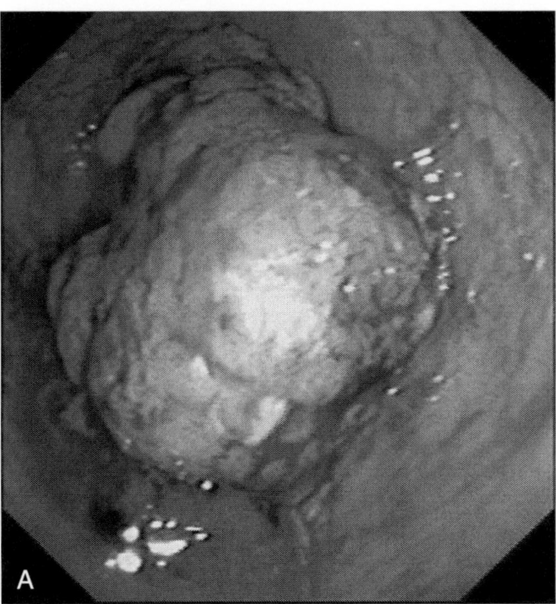

Figure 3.3.2A
Rectal cancer colonoscopic image

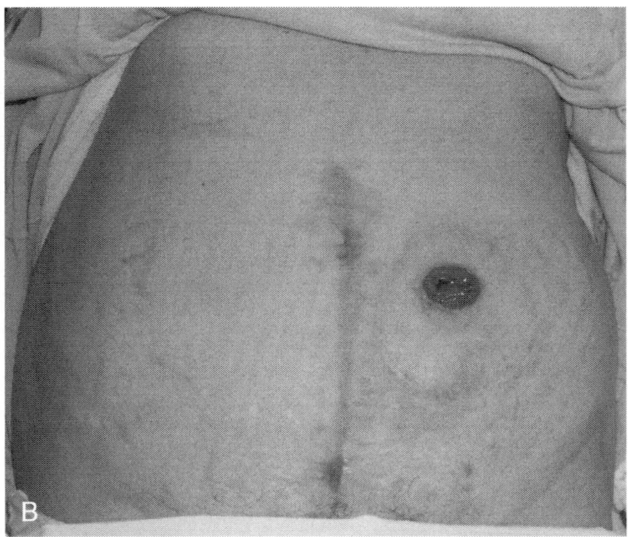

Figure 3.3.2B
End colostomy

One in 12 Australians will be affected by large bowel cancer by the age of 85 years, so colorectal cancer cases are common.

You may be introduced to a man sitting in a clinic room as follows: 'This is Mr Jones. Would you like to take a history from him and examine him as is appropriate'.

The history

- Introduce yourself and ask the patient what has been going on. The patient may indicate that he had an operation for rectal cancer recently and has had a stoma bag for 3–6 months.
- Try to maintain a structure to your history, using the framework above. Begin by orientating yourself.
- The presenting symptoms and history of presenting complaint:
  - *presentation* — bleeding per rectum (PR) and its detail; altered bowel habit (constipation/ diarrhoea/both); tenesmus; mucous discharge per rectum; abdominal pain (SOCRATES) or distension
  - *associated symptoms of the diseased (GI) system*: nausea; vomiting; jaundice
  - *other associated symptoms — systemic*: weight loss; anorexia; malaise; shortness of breathe
  - *other associated symptoms — pelvic*: pneumaturia; UTI; haematuria
  - *investigations*: colonoscopy/staging radiology (CT/MRI)/biopsy.
  - *treatment:*
    - Was the patient admitted electively or acutely?
    - What procedure was performed?
    - Was neo-adjuvant treatment required or discussed?
    - Were there any complications after the operation?
    - Current status of the patient (diet, mobility, bowel function, expected date of discharge).
    - Will adjuvant treatment be required (radiotherapy or chemotherapy)?

- Risk factor assessment:
  - personal or family history of polyps/colorectal cancer/inflammatory bowel disease.
- Past medical history.
- Surgical history.
- Drug history and allergies.
- Family history — particularly of endometrial/gastric/ovary/urothelium (HNPCC).
- Social history: occupation, home circumstances, smoking tobacco and alcohol consumption.

The examination

- Preparation — see above:
  - position the patient flat with one pillow under the head
  - expose the abdomen from nipples to pubic symphysis but state that ideally you would like to expose the patient to mid-thigh.
- General examination from the end of the bed:
  - overall condition
  - drains, tubes, infusions, TPN, IDC, oxygen etc.
- Assessment for peripheral signs, unless instructed otherwise:
  - vital signs
  - hands: stigmata of gastrointestinal disease — anaemia/clubbing/malnutrition
  - head and neck: cachexia (wasting of temporalis)/jaundice/pallor/lymphadenopathy.
- Examination of the abdomen:
  - inspection: moving with respiration; distension; scars; drains; stomas; dressings; bruising. Inspect wounds for signs of infection. Look at drains, stomas and urine bag if present
  - palpation: ask if there is any pain. Soft; tender; organomegaly; ascites. Assess groin and incision for evidence of a cough impulse. Palpate the testicles
  - percussion: not usually relevant post-operatively unless distended and you want to determine if it is gaseous or fluid (ascites/ileus). Percussion for shifting dullness; fluid thrill
  - auscultation: listen in four quadrants for the character of borborygmi, bruits over the renal arteries, aorta and liver.
- Conclusion:
  - say that you would do a digital rectal examination in the pre-operative setting (distance of cancer from the anal verge; prostate; sphincter tone)
  - cover the patient
  - reposition the patient
  - thank the patient
  - clean your hands again
  - only now turn to face the examiners.

The discussion

- The examiners may ask you to tell them what you found. An example of a succinct summary for this case would be as follows, 'Mr Jones is a 64-year-old man who had a rectal cancer found at colonoscopy after presenting with 3 months of rectal bleeding. He was found to have a low rectal cancer and after CT scan of his abdomen and pelvis and a MRI he proceeded to have pre-operative radiotherapy for 6 weeks followed by an ultra-low anterior resection and a diverting loop ileostomy one week ago.'

- Investigation of a patient with rectal cancer
  - Blood tests:
    - FBC, EUC, LFTs, CEA.
  - Colonoscopy:
    - to exclude synchronous colonic neoplasms.
  - CT scan chest, abdomen and pelvis — staging to detect metastatic disease.
  - TRUS/MRI pelvis and PET scans where indicted.
    - TRUS/MRI determine the depth of invasion through the bowel wall (T staging) and spread to adjacent nodes to help decide which patients need neo-adjuvant therapy.
  - Examination under anaesthetic:
    - tumour location (anterior/posterior/circumferential), height (from anal verge), relationship to the anal sphincters and depth of penetration (T stage) can be estimated. Superficially invasive tumours are mobile, whereas more advanced lesions become tethered and fixed with increasing depth of penetration.
- Benefits of TRUS versus MRI:
  - TRUS is superior in assessing early T stage (T1/T2) cancers. TRUS offers excellent delineation of the relationship between a tumour, the mucosa, the muscularis propria, and tumour extension beyond the muscularis propria
  - MRI is superior to TRUS:
    - for assessment of the circumferential resection margin to determine whether it is threatened by tumour
    - for providing a larger field of view and more detail about proximal tumours
    - as it tends to be less operator and technique dependent
    - as it allows assessment of obstructing cancers (TRUS not possible)
  - In practice, the information obtained from TRUS and MRI is often complementary and, at many institutions, both procedures are done pre-operatively particularly for patients whose tumours extend beyond T2. For early staging of T1 and T2 lesions, TRUS offers excellent delineation of the relationship between a tumour, the mucosa, the muscularis propria, and tumour extension beyond the muscularis propria. However, TRUS is clearly limited in terms of tumours that extend deeply into the pelvic side-wall, into additional pelvic structures, or for the detection and characterisation of adenopathy in the internal and external iliac distribution.
- Indications for neo-adjuvant treatment in rectal cancer:
  - some controversy exists and the indications are constantly changing
  - employed in:
    - resectable cancers to reduce local recurrence rates (typically by 50%) — usually short-course pre-operative radiotherapy (SCPRT)
    - non-resectable tumours to achieve 'down-staging' prior to surgery — usually long course chemoradiotherapy.
- Large RCTs suggest 50% local reduction rates with a policy of routine short course pre-operative radiotherapy compared to selective post-operative radiotherapy (UK MRC07, *Lancet* 2009) for all tumour stages and heights. However, benefit is most pronounced for:
  - T3/4 tumours
  - clinically node-positive T1/2 tumours
  - more distal rectal tumours (mid- and lower-third tumours)
  - men

- anterior tumours
- when the circumferential resection margin is threatened; that is, cancer invading or are in close proximity to the mesorectal fascia on *pre*-operative imaging.

- Difference between short-course and long-course radiotherapy
  - SCPRT gives 25 Gy over 5 days and is followed by immediate surgery
  - long course radiotherapy gives 50 Gy over 5 weeks and is combined with chemotherapy (infusion of 5-FU for 5 days on weeks 1 and week 5), then surgery 6–8 weeks post-treatment
  - the advantage of *pre*-operative radiotherapy is that the pelvic anatomy is undisturbed and there is less chance of the small bowel getting irradiated. The tissues are likely to be well oxygenated which increases radiosensitivity. It also enables assessment of the tumour response on histopathology enabling prognostication and need for adjuvant treatment.
- Surgery for rectal cancer
  - Depends on the location of the tumour, its relationship to the anal sphincters and the ability to get an oncologically clear distal margin.
  - In general, a 5 cm margin of distal clearance is preferred for poorly differentiated cancers. However, for other differentiated rectal cancers a 1.5–2 cm margin of clearance has been shown to be oncologically safe.
  - In rectosigmoid or upper rectal cancers 5 cm of distal clearance is easily achievable, allowing construction of a colorectal anastomosis to the mid-third of the rectum.
  - In mid- and lower-third rectal cancers, total mesorectal excision is necessary for complete oncological control. As a result, most surgeons would accept a distal clearance of 1.5 to 2 cm to allow GI restoration. This is supported by the available evidence. Due to the leak rate of distal anastomoses, most surgeons defunction with a loop ileostomy.
  - Tumours adjacent to (where not possible to get adequate distal clearance) or involving the sphincter require abdominoperineal excision of the rectum, although sphincter-saving surgery, involving inter-sphincteric dissection is performed in specialist centres in selected cases.
  - In order to preserve continence, it is necessary to have good sphincter function and an adequate reservoir. With complete removal of the rectum a reservoir can be reconstructed by creating a 5–8 cm colonic J pouch. Straight coloanal anastomosis result in fairly poor function for up to 2 years and have been reported to have a higher leak rate than colonic pouch anastomosis. More importantly, there have been a number of studies that demonstrate that early function with a colonic J pouch is superior to straight coloanal anastomosis, particularly in the elderly with compromised anal sphincters.
  - Accordingly, the options are:
    - high anterior resection — for upper rectal tumours, that is within 10–15 cm of the anal verge
    - low anterior resection (± colonic J pouch ± loop ileostomy) — for mid to upper rectal tumours i.e. within 6–10 cm of the anal verge
    - ultra-low anterior resection (ULAR) (± colonic J pouch) and loop ileostomy — for tumours within the mid to low rectum in which distal clearance of 1 cm can be achieved
    - abdominoperineal excision of the rectum and anus — for low rectal tumours in which a distal clearance of 1 cm cannot be achieved or in which there is involvement of the anal sphincters.

- High versus low ligation of the inferior mesenteric artery (IMA):
  - high ligation involves ligation of the IMA flush with the aorta; low ligation involves ligation of the IMA at the sacral promontory preserving the left colic artery
  - there is no evidence that high ligation confers a better oncologically result or cancer survival. However, most surgeons would perform a high ligation in order to achieve adequate length of the proximal bowel to perform a tension free colorectal anastomosis following low anterior resection/ULAR.
- Anatomy of the pelvic nerves (see 2.4.2).
- Indications for a defunctioning ileostomy:
  - patients who have had neo-adjuvant radiotherapy and an ULAR
  - anastomotic leak rates as high as 10–20% have been reported after ULAR
  - while a defunctioning ileostomy does not absolutely prevent an anastomotic leak, it usually minimises the degree of sepsis and avoid the need for repeat surgical intervention should it occur
  - other cases where there is concern about the anastomosis; for example:
    - evidence of an air leak after anastomosis testing with air and water
    - incomplete donuts in the circular stapling device
    - tension, or if the blood supply was questionable
    - difficult dissection and anticipation of problems post-operative (relative).

3.3.3. Colon cancer

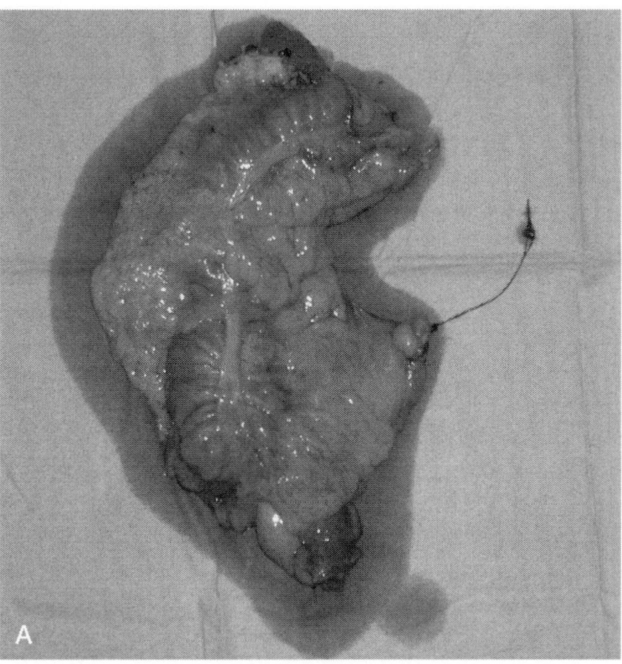

Figure 3.3.3A
Right hemicolectomy specimen

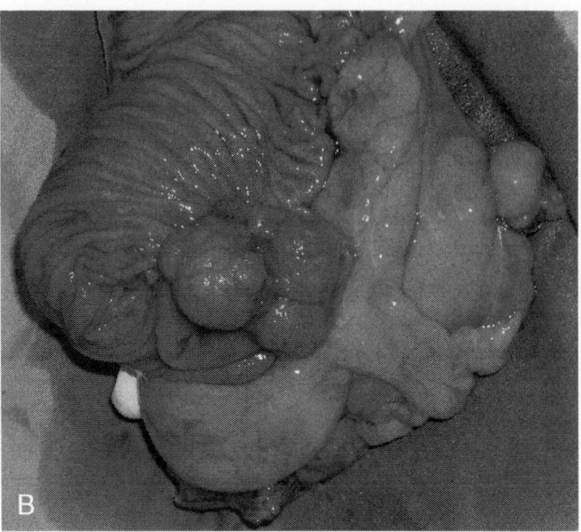

Figure 3.3.3B
Caecal cancer

As previously stated, colorectal cancer cases are common.

You may be introduced to a man sitting in a clinic room as follows: 'This is Mr Smith. Would you please take a history from him and perform an appropriate examination'.

The history

- Introduce yourself and ask the patient what has been going on. The patient may indicate that he had a bowel cancer removed 4 months ago.
- Try to maintain a structure to your history, using the framework above. Begin by orientating yourself.
- The presenting symptoms and history of presenting complaint:
  - *presentation*: asymptomatic after a positive faecal occult blood test or during surveillance colonoscopy. Symptomatic: bleeding per rectum (PR) and its detail; altered bowel habit (constipation/diarrhoea/both); abdominal pain (SOCRATES) or distension
  - *associated symptoms of the diseased (GI) system*: nausea; vomiting; jaundice
  - *other associated symptoms — systemic*: weight loss; anorexia; malaise; shortness of breath
  - *other associated symptoms — anaemia*: palpitations, weakness, SOB, CCF
  - *investigations*: colonoscopy/staging radiology (CT/MRI)/biopsy.
  - *treatment:*
    - Was the patient admitted electively or acutely?
    - What procedure was performed?
    - Which part of the colon was removed (right, left, all)?
    - Were there any complications after the operation?
    - Current status of the patient (diet, mobility, bowel function, expected date of discharge).
    - Will adjuvant treatment be required (radiotherapy or chemotherapy)?
- Risk factor assessment:
  - personal or family history of polyps/colorectal cancer/inflammatory bowel disease.
- Past medical history.

- Surgical history.
- Drug history and allergies.
- Family history — particularly of endometrial/gastric/ovary/urothelium (HNPCC).
- Social history: occupation, home circumstances, smoking tobacco and alcohol consumption.

The examination

- Preparation — see above:
  - position the patient flat with one pillow under the head
  - expose the abdomen from nipples to pubic symphysis but state that ideally you would like to expose the patient to mid-thigh.
- General examination from the end of the bed:
  - overall condition
  - drains, tubes, infusions, TPN, IDC, oxygen etc.
- Assessment for peripheral signs, unless instructed otherwise:
  - vital signs
  - hands: stigmata of gastrointestinal disease — anaemia/clubbing/ malnutrition.
  - head and neck: cachexia (wasting of temporalis)/jaundice/pallor/ lymphadenopathy.
- Examination of the abdomen:
  - inspection: moving with respiration; distension; scars; drains; stomas; dressings; bruising. inspect wounds for signs of infection. look at drains, stomas and urine bag if present
  - palpation: ask if there is any pain — soft; tender; organomegaly; ascites. Assess groin and incision for evidence of a cough impulse; palpate the testicles
  - percussion: not usually relevant post-operatively unless distended and you want to determine if it is gaseous or fluid (ascites/ileus); percussion for shifting dullness; fluid thrill
  - auscultation: listen in four quadrants for the character of borborygmi, bruits over the renal arteries, aorta and liver.
- Conclusion:
  - say that you would do a digital rectal examination
  - cover the patient
  - reposition the patient
  - thank the patient
  - clean your hands again
  - only now turn to face the examiners.

The discussion

- The examiners may ask you to tell them what you found. An example of a succinct summary for this case would be as follows, 'Mr Smith is a 54-year-old man who had a colonic cancer detected on a screening colonoscopy following positive FOBT. He has a family history of colonic cancer. His brother died of colon cancer aged 44 and his father had two colon cancers treated in his 50s and 60s before he died of a heart attack. The history and physical examination suggest he underwent an uncomplicated laparoscopic right hemicolectomy. He was told it had spread to the lymph glands and he has had chemotherapy. He has one son and one daughter and has seen a genetic counsellor.
- Average risk of developing colonic or rectal cancer in Australia:
  - bowel cancer affects 1 in 12 before the age of 85 years (Cancer in Australia 2010. Australian Institute of Health & Welfare).

- Causes of colonic and rectal cancer:
  - certain conditions predispose to the development of colorectal cancer, including IBD, acromegaly, history of uretero-colostomy and radiation therapy also increase risk
  - increasing age is a strong risk factor
  - it is a multi-factorial disease; in approximately 5%, there is an overwhelming genetic/inherited contribution (HNPCC/FAP — see below)
  - there are well-defined environmental factors, the most important are probably dietary
  - there is a correlation of consumption of total fat, saturated fat and cholesterol with increased cancer risk
  - dietary fibre is associated with reduced risk — it increases bulk to dilute potential carcinogens, speeds their transit through the colon, binds certain mutagens and favourably changes faecal pH
  - lack of physical activity, diabetes, increased concentration of insulin and IGF1 are associated with increased risk. There is a modest association with smoking.
- What is HNPCC?
  - It is an autosomal dominant inherited condition associated with an increased risk of colorectal cancer. Microsatellite instability (MSI) is the hallmark of HNPCC tumours. It is also known as Lynch syndrome.
  - It is due to germ-line mutations in mismatch repair genes. The involved genes include hMLH1, hMSH2, and hMSH6. hMSH2 and hMLH1 and together account for > 90% of identifiable mutations.
  - 20% of cases are spontaneous germ-line mutations with no family history.
  - HNPCC is diagnosed on the basis of genetic testing. Given the expense involved, individuals fulfilling the Amsterdam criteria and tumours meeting the Bethesda criteria are tested.
    - Amsterdam criteria can be remembered by '3, 2, 1 rule'; that is, *three* relatives affected with an HNPCC cancer (colorectal, endometrium, small bowel, urothelium), over *two* successive generations, with *one* cancer under the age of 50 years. These criteria are neither sensitive (79%) nor specific (61%) for the diagnosis.
    - The *Bethesda* criteria are used to determine whether to test for MSI. They can be remembered using Bet**hesda**:
      - **bet**
      - **h**istopathological characteristics of MSI in pts <60 yrs
      - **e**xtra HNPCC cancers (synchronous/metachronous)
      - **s**ingle (≥1) 1st degree relative <50 yrs
      - **d**ouble (≥2) $1^{st}/2^{nd}$ degree relative HNPCC cancer
      - **a**ge <50 yrs.
  - Tumours can be MSI-high (> 2 loci show band-shifts), MSI-low (1 locus shows band shifts), MS-stable (no band shifts). Almost all HNPCC cancers and about 70% of adenomas are MSI-high. However 15% of sporadic colorectal cancers are MSI-High.
  - Immunostaining for loss of expression of hMLH1, hMSH2, hMSH6 or hPMS2 may be an indicator of a germ-line mutation in the gene coding for that protein and has 76% sensitivity in predicting MSI status and is 100% specific. Diagnosis by germ-line genetic testing allows identification of the causative germ-line mutation in an affected individual. This also means that other at-risk family members can be offered predictive testing.

- Investigation and staging of a patient with colon cancer
  - Blood tests:
    - FBC, EUC, LFTs, CEA.
  - Colonoscopy:
    - for (histopathological) diagnosis
    - to exclude synchronous colonic neoplasms
    - barium enema/virtual colonography remain alternatives.
  - CT scan chest, abdomen and pelvis:
    - assessment of tumour (local advanced) and complications
    - staging to detect metastatic disease.
- Management of colon cancer
  - Stage the cancer.
  - Determine intent (curative/palliative).
  - Determine patient's wishes.
  - Assess patient's fitness for surgery.
  - Discuss in MDT setting (if elective presentation).
  - Discuss operative approach (Laparoscopic vs Open colectomy).
  - Complete clinicopathological staging post-operatively to determine need for adjuvant therapy:
    - stage III cancers and high risk stage II disease (T4, poor histologic grade, peritumoural lymphovascular involvement, obstruction, T3 with local perforation, and close or positive margin).
- Staging of colon cancer — TNM AJCC (clinicopathological staging)
  - Primary tumour (T):
    - Tis, carcinoma in situ: intraepithelial or invasion of the lamina propria
    - T0, no evidence of primary tumour
    - T1, tumour invades submucosa
    - T2, tumour invades muscularis propria
    - T3, tumour invades through the muscularis propria into the subserosa or into non-peritonealised pericolic or perirectal tissues
    - T4, tumour directly invades other organs or structures and/or perforates visceral peritoneum
  - Regional lymph nodes (N):
    - N0, no regional lymph node metastasis
    - N1, metastasis in one to three regional lymph nodes
    - N2, metastases in four or more regional lymph nodes
  - Distant metastasis (M):
    - M0, no distant metastasis
    - M1: distant metastasis.
- 5-year survival rate:
  - stage I (T1/2, N0) 85–90%
  - stage II (T3/4,N0 66%
  - stage III (N+) 40–50%
  - stage IV (M+) 0–10% (increased to 30% if metastectomy).
- Evidence for laparoscopic compared to open colectomy
  - Surgery is the only potentially curative modality of treatment — the aims must be the same, irrespective of the approach:
    - achieve an R0 resection by resecting the affected segment of bowel with at least 5 cm of proximal and distal clearance along with its draining lymphovascular pedicle

    - restore bowel continuity if possible.
    - Laparoscopic surgery has been shown to be non-inferior to open resection in three large RCTS (COST/CLASSIC/COLOR). Laparoscopic surgery may be superior in terms of: (a) decrease length of stay; (b) quicker return of bowel function; and (c) less post-operative pain.
- What is the strategy of treatment for primary colon cancer?
  - Surgery for primary colonic cancer requires removal of primary tumour with adequate margins and regional lymphadenectomy with restoration of the colonic continuity.
  - The nature of the segmental colonic resection required depends on the location of the primary. Surgery involves resection of the affected colonic segment with itys lmyphovascualr pedicle, resulting in an en bloc lymphadenectomy. This ligation of the artery will in turn usually determine the minimum amount of bowel that must be resected to leave well vascularised bowel for anastomosis.
  - The resections for a right-sided cancer include right hemicolectomy or extended right hemicolectomy (hepatic flexure cancers). Transverse colon cancers can be treated by extended right hemicolectomy, left hemicolectomy or subtotal colectomy (Note: transverse colectomy is not recommended as it is not oncological and blood supply and tension issues can increase rate of anastomotic leak. Left sided lesions can be treated by extended left hmicolectomy, high anterior resection or Hartmann's procedure. Synchronous lesions can be treated with synchronous resections (and 2 anastomoses), although subtotal colectomy is preferred, particularly in the setting of HNPCC/mucosa field change.
- Role of adjuvant treatment of colon cancer
  - The goal is to eradicate micrometastases, reducing the likelihood of disease recurrence and distant metastases.
  - 30–70% of stage III (node-positive cancers) patients develop recurrence and its use is best established in such patients.
  - Standard (5FU/folinic acid) chemotherapy confers a survival benefit of 5–6% in node-positive cancers (Dukes C, stage III) compared to no adjuvant therapy.
  - However, a (unidentifiable) proportion will be cured by surgery alone and will *only* be exposed to the risks of chemotherapy *without* benefit. Additionally, a (unidentifiable) proportion will relapse despite chemotherapy and will succumb to their disease.
  - The MOSAIC trial (NEJM 2004) suggested improved survival advantage with addition of Oxaliplatin to standard regime of 5FU/folinic acid, giving rise to FOLFOX schedules (FOL— Folinic acid; F — Fluorouracil [5-FU]; OX — Oxaliplatin).
  - Current recommendations state that all medically appropriate node-positive patients receive adjuvant chemotherapy for 6 months after resection.
  - Possible benefit to high-risk stage II (debated): (a) T4 tumours; (b) poor histologic grade; (c) peritumoural lymphovascular involvement; (d) obstructing tumour; (e) T3 with local perforation; (f) close or positive margins.
  - However, standard chemotherapy confers an absolute survival advantage of 1.5% (UK QUASAR II) and FOLFOX confer an absolute survival advantage of 3% in node-negative (Dukes B) cancers.
  - Radiation therapy has no defined role in current guidelines for treatment of colon cancer.
  - Median survival is increased from a median of 6 months (no chemotherapy) to 12 months with standard regimens and up to 18–20 months with FOLFOX in non-resectable stage IV patients (metastatic disease). However, the response rate is only 20%.

- Complications of colon cancer and their surgical treatment
  - Perforation, obstruction and bleeding are the most common complications of colon cancers requiring emergency treatment
  - Obstructing lesions in the distal colon (and rectum) can have deleterious effects on the proximal/entire colon (the caecum is particularly vulnerable) if the ileo-caecal valve is competent and a closed loop obstruction ensues. This can result in caecal ischaemia, compromise, damage and perforation. This will change the operation that is necessary.
- Hepatic metastases (for assessment see 2.4.20; for selection and treatment see 3.3.7).
- Colonic polyps, Haggit's levels, adenoma-carcinoma sequence, FAP (see 4.6.2).

Table 3.3.3 Indications, advantages and disadvantages for different surgical options in malignant large bowel obstruction

OPTION	INDICATION	ADVANTAGE	DISADVANTAGE
Defunctioning proximal colostomy without resection	High risk patient Elderly or frail Palliation	No anastomosis Shorter procedure	Burden of colostomy. Primary resection should be performed whenever possible
Hartmann's procedure	High risk patient. Inexperienced surgeon	No risk of anastomosis	Need for further surgery Stoma never reversed in > 50%
Resection with on-table colonic irrigation and primary anastomosis	Allows one stage resection in unprepared bowel	Addresses the issue of bowel preparation	Cannot use if damage to proximal colon Increased operating time
Colonic stent	Palliation, bridge to surgery	Lower colostomy rate, allows elective resection	Uncertain long term outcome in bridge to surgery group Expensive Limited availability Technical failure rate
Subtotal colectomy	Synchronous tumours and proximal bowel damage	As safe as segmental resection	Suboptimal functional outcome Extensive surgery

3.3.4 Ulcerative colitis

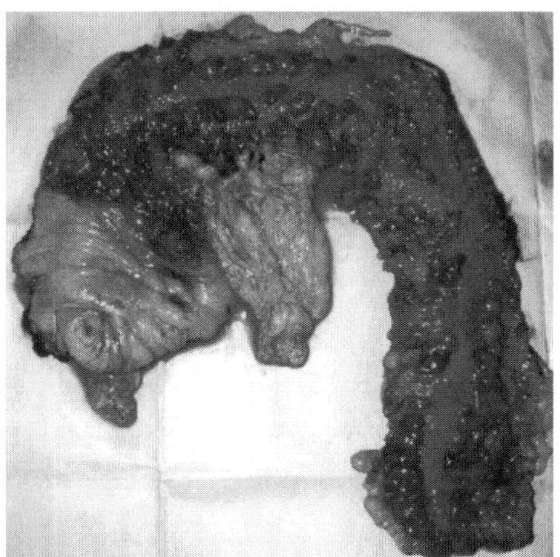

Figure 3.3.4
Ulcerative colitis

Such cases are likely to be post-operative, but an inpatient or out-patient with UC who is booked for, or contemplating, elective surgery may be presented.

Extent of disease is usually:

- proctitis 50%
- proctocolitis 30% (extends to left colon)
- extensive colitis 20% (beyond splenic flexure).

The history

- Introduce yourself and ask the patient what has been going on.
- Try to maintain a structure to your history, using the framework above. Begin by orientating yourself.
- The presenting symptoms and history of presenting complaint:
  - *presentation*: cardinal symptoms of *abdominal pain and bloody diarrhoea*. Abdominal pain (SOCRATES) and distension (toxic dilatation). Bleeding per rectum (PR) and diarrhoea — amount of blood, stool frequency, relative amounts of blood/stool. Mucous discharge per rectum; faecal incontinence; tenesmus
  - *associated symptoms of the diseased (GI) system*: nausea; vomiting; jaundice (PSC)
  - *other associated symptoms — systemic*: weight loss; anorexia; malaise; anaemia
  - *other associated extracolonic manifestations:*
    - *urinary*: calculi
    - *skin*: erythema nodosum/multiforme, pyoderma gangrenosum
    - *musculoskeletal*: arthritis, ankylosing spondylitis — independent of IBD activity
    - *eyes*: uveitis, chorioretinitis, iridocyclitis
  - *investigations*: bloods/radiology/colonoscopy/biopsy.
  - *treatment:*
    - if the patient is post-operative, what was the indication for surgery?
    - any acute severe attacks (toxic dilatation, perforation, bleeding, unresponsive to medical treatment)?
    - chronic active disease problems: steroid dependence/failed medical treatment/recurrent acute attacks, growth retardation, dysplasia associated lesion or mass (DALM)/ malignancy?
    - if the patient is post-operative, which operation was performed:
      - acute attack — subtotal colectomy/mucous fistula and end ileostomy (about 65%)
      - chronic disease — (a) total colectomy/mucous fistula and end ileostomy; (b) proctocolectomy and end ileostomy; or (c) proctocolectomy and ileal pouch anal anastomosis
    - were there any complications after the operation
    - current status of the patient (diet, mobility, bowel function, expected date of discharge)?
- Past medical history.
- Surgical history.
- Drug history and allergies.
- Family history.
- Social history: occupation, home circumstances, smoking tobacco and alcohol consumption.

The examination

- Preparation (see above):
  - position the patient flat with one pillow under the head

  - expose the abdomen from nipples to pubic symphysis but state that ideally you would like to expose the patient to mid-thigh.
- General examination from the end of the bed:
  - overall condition — pale/jaundice/malnourished/Cushing appearance
  - drains, tubes, infusions, TPN, IDC, oxygen etc.
- Assessment for peripheral signs, unless instructed otherwise:
  - vital signs
  - hands: stigmata of gastrointestinal disease — anaemia/clubbing/malnutrition
  - head and neck: cachexia (wasting of temporalis)/jaundice/pallor/lymphadenopathy
  - eyes: uveitis, chorioretinitis, iridocyclitis
  - legs: erythema nodosum, pyoderma gangrenosum, arthritis of knees, ankylosing spondylitis.
- Examination of the abdomen:
  - inspection: moving with respiration; distension; scars; drains; stomas (mucus fistula); dressings; bruising. Inspect wounds for signs of infection. Look at stoma and urine bag if present
  - palpation: soft; tender; organomegaly; ascites. Assess groin and incision for evidence of a cough impulse. Palpate the testicles
  - percussion: not usually relevant post-operatively unless distended and you want to determine if it is gaseous or fluid (ascites/ileus). Percussion for shifting dullness; fluid thrill
  - auscultation: listen in four quadrants for the character of borborygmi, bruits over the renal arteries, aorta and liver.
- Conclusion:
  - say that you would do a digital rectal examination (depending if pre-op or post-op and no low anastomoses)
  - cover the patient
  - reposition the patient
  - thank the patient
  - clean your hands again
  - only now turn to face the examiners.

The discussion

- Confirmation of a diagnosis of ulcerative colitis
  - The diagnosis is made on the basis of clinical, luminal imaging (endoscopy/radiology) and pathology.
  - Investigations contribute to the diagnosis and also allow assessment of disease severity.
  - Full history and examination to exclude other causes of colitis (see 2.2.7 Colitis) and to establish GI and extra GI involvement to provide information of UC Vs Crohn's (see below).
  - Stool culture sample to exclude infectious cause.
  - Bloods — FBC (anaemia/ leukocytosis), ESR, CRP, LFTs, (inc. Albumin).
  - Radiology — AXR for toxic dilatation and signs of inflammation (granularity, loss of haustra causing lead-pipe appearance).
  - Flexible sigmoidoscopy/colonoscopy — rectum is almost always involved. Features include loss of vascularity, mucosal oedema, granularity, erythema, contact bleeding and frank ulceration, pseudopolyps (from previous attacks and regeneration). Findings are usually confluent unlike Crohn's disease which is characterised by skip lesions and patchy disease. Define proximal extent of the disease.

- Biopsies — demonstrate mucosal and submucosal involvement, Crypt of Lieberkuhn abscesses, absence of (non-caseating) granulomas.
- Clinical and histopathological differences between UC and Crohn's disease. (Please also refer to 4.6.3.)

Table 3.3.4 Clinical and histological features of ulcerative colitis and Crohn's disease

	ULCERATIVE COLITIS	CROHN'S DISEASE
Clinical Feature		
Distribution	Colon and rectum	Entire GI tract
Appearance	Superficial and disease areas are confluent	Skip lesions Cobblestone appearance — linear deep fissuring ulcers (serpiginous) with islands of oedematous mucosa in between Inflammatory polyps
Rectal involvement	Always	Rarely
Strictures	Rarely	Common
Fistulae	Rare	Common
Anal involvement	Rare	Common
Malignancy risk	10% at 20 yrs	10% at 20 yrs
Histological		
Bowel wall	Mucosa and submucosa	Full thickness
Non-caseating granulomas	Absent	Present 60–70%
Crypt abscesses	Common	Rare
Goblet cell	Depleted	Preserved

- Extra-intestinal manifestations and intestinal complications of UC/IBD
  These can be easily remembered using the acronym **ULCERATIVE COLITIS**.
  - Extra-intestinal manifestations:
    U Urinary calculi: especially oxalate (Crohn's disease)
    L Liver: cirrhosis, sclerosing cholangitis, fatty liver
    C Cholelithiasis: decreased bile acid resorbtion
    E Epithelium: erythema nodosum/multiforme, pyoderma gangrenosum
    R Retardation of growth and sexual maturation — especially in kids
    A Arthralgias — arthritis, ankylosing spondylitis — independent of IBD activity
    T Thrombophlebitis — migratory
    I Iatrogenic: steroids, blood transfusions, surgery
    V Vitamin deficiencies
    E Eyes: uveitis, chorioretinitis, iridocyclitis
  - Intestinal complications:
    C Cancer: increased by long duration/early onset, pancolitis
    O Obstruction: rare with UC, common in Crohn's especially post-surgery
    L Leakage (perforation): can form abscess especially in Crohn's (20%)
    I Iron deficiency: haemorrhage
    T Toxic megacolon: 3% (more often in UC)
    I Inanition: severe wasting due to malabsorption and decreased oral intake
    S Stricture/fistulas (40% of Crohn's), perianal abscesses

- Principles of treatment of ulcerative colitis
  - Depends on the severity of disease.
  - The majority of cases are treated medically unless complications arise. 70% of patients with UC are managed medically. 30% of patients will require surgical intervention that is usually curative.
  - The goal of treatment is to induce remission and maintain disease in this state. IBD needs to be managed in collaboration with a gastroenterologist/nutritionist/stoma therapist when and where indicated.
  - Assessment of severity — severe disease Truelove and Witt criteria:
    - No. bloody stools/day > 6
    - pulse rate >90
    - temperature >37.8
    - haemoglobin <105 g/L
    - ESR/CRP >30
- Treatment of acute severe ulcerative colitis
  - Medical treatment:
    - admit to hospital
    - resuscitate and correct electrolytes; nutritional support
    - IV hydrocortisone 100 mg QDS
    - stop NSAIDs, anticholinergics, antidiarrheals (increase toxic dilatation)
    - transfuse PRC to keep Hb >100 g/L
    - aim maximum 5 day therapy — 70% response rate
    - serial clinical/serological/radiological examinations to detect complications
    - unresponsive:
      - 2nd line: cyclosporine/tacrolimus or infliximab
      - colectomy.
  - Surgical treatment:
    - indications — **BUMP**:
      - **b**leeding
      - **u**nresponsive to medical Rx
      - **m**egadilation (toxic dilation)
      - **p**erforation
    - operation of choice: subtotal colectomy, ileostomy ± mucus fistula.
- Treatment of chronic ulcerative colitis
  - Medical treatment:
    - proctitis: topical 5-ASA (mesalzine 1G OD). Escalate to addition of topical steroid or oral 5-ASA
    - left-sided disease: topical 5-ASA and oral mesalazine (2G/day)
    - no response — oral steroids with a reducing dose over 8 weeks
    - extensive disease: as for left-sided but lower threshold for use of steroids.
  - Surgical treatment:
    - indications — **3Ms**:
      - **m**alignancy/severe dysplasia/DALM
      - **m**edical treatment failure
      - **m**aturation (growth/nutrition) failure
    - operations to consider:
      - the 'gold standard' is a panproctocolectomy and permanent ileostomy formation
      - restorative proctocolectomy and ileal J-pouch anal anastomosis (IPAA) for those who wish to avoid a stoma

    - colectomy with ileorectal anastomosis in highly selected cases with relative rectal sparing
    - colectomy with ileostomy and rectal preservation (so IRA is possible later).
- Complications of IPAA — **4Ps**
  - **P**ouch failure occurs in 5–10%. Reasons include:
    - pelvic sepsis (50%) from leak or infected haematoma
    - poor function (30%)
    - pouchitis (10%).
  - **P**ouchitis — aetiology is unknown but related to the original disease process, symptoms include frequency and urgency of stool. Need endoscopic confirmation of inflammation to confirm. Treatment is antibiotics (metronidazole, ciprofloxacin or augmentin). Long-term effects of chronic pouchitis predisposes to dysplasia.
  - **P**ost-operative complications — **4Ss**:
    - **s**mall bowel obstruction
    - **s**epsis (pelvis)
    - **s**tricture of anastomosis — occurs in 5–20%; may require surgical intervention if intestinal obstruction (dilatation/ revision)
    - **s**inus — pouch vaginal/perineal.
  - **P**oor function
    - normal function is 6–8 bowel motions per day; however, nocturnal frequency and incontinence are better markers of poor function. Trial of antidiarrheals should be given to improve function. There is a tendency for function to improve over time.

3.3.5 Oesophageal carcinoma

The history

- Introduce yourself and ask the patient what has been going on. The patient may indicate that he has had or is some way through treatment for oesophageal cancer.
- Try to maintain a structure to your history, using the framework above. Begin by orientating yourself.
- The presenting symptoms and history of presenting complaint:
  - *presentation*: dysphagia (difficulty) or odynophagia (pain) with full quatification (liquids/semi-solids/solids) and progression; haematemesis; previous reflux; abdominal pain (SOCRATES) or distension
  - *associated symptoms of the diseased (GI) system*: nausea; vomiting; jaundice
  - *other associated symptoms — systemic*: weight loss; anorexia; malaise
  - *other associated symptoms — chest*: SOB; cough; pneumonia
  - *investigations*: upper GI endoscopy/barium swallow; staging radiology (CT/MRI/PET scan)/endoluminal ultrasound/biopsy.
  - *treatment:*
    - Was a staging laparoscopy performed?
    - Was neo-adjuvant treatment required or discussed?
    - What surgery was performed? Separate neck/chest/abdominal incisions?
    - Were there any complications after the operation?
    - Current status of the patient (diet, mobility, bowel function, expected date of discharge).
    - Will adjuvant treatment be required (radiotherapy or chemotherapy)?

- Risk factor assessment:
  - personal history of preceding Barrett's disease.
- Past medical history.
- Surgical history.
- Drug history and allergies.
- Family history.
- Social history: occupation, home circumstances, smoking tobacco and alcohol consumption.

The examination

- Preparation (see above):
  - permission — ask to examine the patient's neck, chest and abdomen
  - position the patient flat with one pillow under the head
  - expose the neck, chest and abdomen (to pubic symphysis but state that ideally you would like to expose the patient to mid-thigh).
- General examination from the end of the bed:
  - overall condition
  - drains, tubes, infusions, TPN, IDC, oxygen etc.
- Assessment for peripheral signs, unless instructed otherwise:
  - vital signs
  - hands: stigmata of gastrointestinal disease — anaemia/clubbing/ malnutrition
  - head and neck: neck scars and supraclavicular lymphadenopathy; cachexia (wasting of temporalis)/jaundice/pallor.
- Examination of the chest/abdomen:
  - inspection: look for previous scars and presence of a portacath — get the patient to point out scars. (Note: most patients will have a right thoractomy and midline laparotomy. Some will also have a left-sided neck incision; patients who have had a minimally invasive oesophagectomy may have port site scars that are hard to see); drains; dressings; bruising. Inspect wounds for signs of infection
  - palpation: soft; tender; organomegaly — especially the liver edge; ascites. Assess groin and incision for evidence of a cough impulse. Palpate the testicles
  - percussion: not usually relevant post-operatively unless distended
  - auscultation: listen to the chest and all four quadrants in the abdomen for the character of borborygmi, bruits over the renal arteries, aorta and liver.
- Conclusion:
  - say that you would do a digital rectal examination in the pre-operative setting (distance of cancer from the anal verge; prostate; sphincter tone)
  - cover the patient
  - reposition the patient
  - thank the patient
  - clean your hands again
  - only now turn to face the examiners.

The discussion

- The examiners may ask you to tell them what you found. An example of a succinct summary for this case would be as follows, 'Mr X is a 54-year-old man who had a distal oesophageal adenocarcinoma detected on a screening endoscopy performed because of a history of Barrett's oesophagus. He received pre-operative chemotherapy and underwent an uncomplicated Ivor-Lewis oesophagectomy. He was told it had spread to the lymph glands and he has had further post-operative chemotherapy.'

- Investigation of a patient with symptoms suggestive of oesophageal malignancy:
  - bloods: FBC (anaemia), iron studies (iron deficiency), CEA (baseline for follow-up)
  - upper GI endoscopy:
    - the endoscopy should focus on definition of the location of the lesion as precisely as possible, using both distance from incisors and internal and external land marks
    - biopsy is essential to differentiate adenocarcinoma and squamous cell carcinoma as the management can be very different
    - a complete survey for other lesions and biopsy of mucosa around the lesion may give information about adjacent, non-invasive disease
  - endoscopic US provides valuable information about the depth of invasion of the primary and potential regional nodal metastasis
  - CT of the neck, chest, abdomen and pelvis is essential
  - FDG-PET — will up-stage patients (who seem to be candidates for surgery on all other grounds) by about 25% by detection of occult systematic metastasis. This may help avoid resection in these patients
  - the greatest accuracy of staging appears to be achieved when CT is combined with EUS (Table 3.3.5)
  - for those with tumours of the middle or lower third of the oesophagus, diagnostic laparoscopy will detect occult peritoneal or liver disease in a small percentage.

Table 3.3.5 The accuracy of staging modalities in oesophageal cancer

MODALITY	T STAGE	N STAGE	M STAGE	OVERALL STAGING ACCURACY
CT	40	50	85	45
EUS	85	40	40	70
CT + EUS	90	90	90	90

- What is the epidemiology and aetiology of oesophageal malignancy?
  - The disease is five times more common in men with a peak age of presentation of 50–70. There are marked geographic variations in the incidence of oesophageal cancer.
  - Oesophageal cancer is really two different disease entities with different epidemiology and management.
  - SCC is predominant worldwide (90%), but adenocarcinoma is more common (60%) is the Western world.
  - SCC is linked with excess alcohol intake, smoking, HPV (16 and 18). Predisposing factors include: achalasia (6–30x risk), alkaline stricture (22x risk), peptic stricture, Plummer Vinson syndrome (web in post-cricoid region and iron-deficient anaemia), Zenker's diverticulum.
  - SCC is located predominantly in the middle third (50%), with about 35% in the lower third and 15% in the upper third of the oesophagus.
  - The vast majority of adenocarcinoma are found in the lower third of the oesophagus. Adenocarcinoma has a rising incidence in industrialised nations. It has epidemiological similarity to cancer of the cardia of the stomach.
  - The predominant aetiological factor is gastro-oesophageal reflux, which leads to metaplastic change with progressive dysplasia and eventual adenocarcinoma.

- The risk of oesophageal adenocarcinoma is 30–50x higher with Barrett's oesophagus.
- Tumours around the OGJ have been classified into three types (Siewart):
  - type I tumours are adenocarcinoma of the distal oesophagus usually arising from Barrett's oesophagus which may have infiltrated the GOJ junction from above
  - type II lesions are true carcinoma of the cardia arising from the cardiac epithelium or short segments with intestinal metaplasia at the oesophago-gastric junction
  - type III junctional cancers are subcardial gastric carcinoma, which infiltrates the oesophagogastric junction and distal oesophagus from below
  - the type II cancers have demographic and pathological features similar to the adenocarcinoma found in Barrett's oesophagus. Compared to type III cancer they display aggressive behaviour, worse prognosis, greater propensity to serosal invasion and lymph node metastasis at presentation and not being associated with atrophic gastritis or intestinal metaplasia of the stomach.

- How is oesophageal cancer staged?
  - The AJCC (7th edition) staging system for oesophageal and junctional tumours has been recently updated (Ann Surg Oncol (2010) 17:1721–1724). This classification pertains to oesophageal tumours and tumours of the GOJ. It includes both SCC and adenocarcinoma. The junctional tumour group includes 'cancers whose epicentre is in the distal thoracic oesophagus, esophagogastric junction, or within the proximal 5 cm of the stomach (cardia) that extend into the esophagogastric junction or distal thoracic oesophagus (Siewert III)'.
  - The upper, middle and lower thirds of the oesophagus are defined according to distance from the incisor teeth at 20–25 cm, 25–30 cm and 30–40 cm respectively.
  - T stage:
    - Tx primary tumour cannot be assessed
    - T0 no evidence of primary tumour
    - Tis high grade dysplasia
    - T1 tumour invades lamina propria or submucosa
    - T2 tumour invades muscularis propria
    - T3 tumour invades adventitia
    - T4a: resectable cancer invades adjacent structures such as pleura, pericardium, diaphragm
    - T4b: non-resectable cancer invades adjacent structures such as aorta, vertebral body, trachea.
  - N stage:
    - Nx regional lymph nodes cannot be assessed
    - NO no regional lymph node metastasis
    - N1 1 to 2 positive regional lymph nodes
    - N2 3 to 6 positive regional lymph nodes
    - N3 7 or more positive regional lymph nodes.
    - the definition of a regional lymph node metastasis now includes any periesophageal node from cervical to celiac, irrespective of the location of the primary.
  - M stage:
    - Mx distant metastasis cannot be assessed
    - M0 no distant metastasis
    - M1 distant metastasis.

- Principles of oesophageal cancer treatment
  - Treatment is dictated by disease-related factors (mainly stage) and patient-related factors (fitness for surgery and wishes).
  - Due to improved surveillance of Barrett's oesophagus, early cancers are increasingly being recognised. Endoscopic mucosal resection (EMR) is generally an acceptable definitive treatment with cancer not entering the submucosa (Tis and T1a), as there is a rate of lymph node metastasis (<3%) lower than the mortality of oesophagectomy. However, where the EMR specimen shows invasion into the submucosa (T1b), the risk of lymph node metastasis is higher (15–20%) and surgery is generally recommended for a fit patient.
  - A patient should only be considered for surgery if there is a reasonable chance of resection without excess morbidity or mortality (not invading aorta, vertebra or heart) and there is likely to be oncological benefit. For patients with systemic metastasis (such as liver, lung or bone), peritoneal disease or lymphatic metastasis outside of the field of resection (such a supraclavicular metastasis in a GOJ cancer), the disease course is unlikely to be altered by resection of the primary and peri-oesophageal lymph nodes. For these patients, in additional to those who are unfit for or decline surgery, palliative treatments are indicated.
- Multimodal treatment of oesophageal cancer
  - For patients who are to undergo surgery, the standard practice in Australia is to offer pre-operative chemotherapy (5-FU and Cisplatin) according to the MRC OEO2 (MAGIC) protocol. If feasible, this is then followed by further post-operative chemotherapy.
  - Generally, there are few trials (except MRC OEO2) examining post-operative adjuvant chemotherapy. The absolute survival benefit of this protocol is 5–10% compared with surgery alone. The benefit is similar for SCC and adenocarcinoma.
  - There is little evidence to support radiotherapy (RT) alone in the adjuvant or neo-adjuvant setting. However, neo-adjuvant chemo-RT may be offered in stage II and III oesophageal cancer. The potential advantages include, down-staging and debulking, earlier treatment of micrometastases, decreased tumour seeding at surgery and increased radio-sensitivity due to increased tumour oxygenation before surgery. Also, there is the potential for biological selection (avoiding surgery for patients who progress on treatment) thus avoiding unnecessary radical surgery.
  - Neo-adjuvant Chemo-RT trials show an absolute survival advantage in the order of 10–15% when compared to surgery alone. SCC of the proximal third of the oesophagus is generally treated with definitive chemo-RT (like a head and neck primary). For SCC anywhere else in the oesophagus, chemo-RT appears to produce similar results to radical surgery.
  - For patients who have locally advanced tumours, so-called trimodality treatment is an option. Here chemo-RT is followed by surgery if the tumour is down-staged. This appears to offer a survival advantage over chemo-RT alone.
  - Clearly all these treatment options need to be discussed in a multidisciplinary team meeting and individualised according to the appropriate patient and disease-related factors.
- Surgical treatment of oesophageal cancer
  - Subtotal oesophagetomy in all patients with SCC/adenocarcinoma of middle and lower third as extensive submucosal spread.
  - The general principles of oesophagectomy for cancer requires abdominal and mediastinal lymphadenectomy. This provides superior staging and there is some evidence that it improves loco-regional control.

- Splenectomy may be performed in patients with junctional adenocarcinoma, although there is no evidence that this is of benefit.
- Reconstruction using the stomach as a conduit generally gives best functional outcomes and there is increased mortality associated with colonic or small bowel conduits.
- Generally, vagus-sparing oesophagectomy, without lymph node dissection, is used only with early tumours confined to mucosa (not reaching the muscularis mucosae) diagnosed by EMR. This is not standard and many of these tumours would now be treated by EMR.
- There is no evidence for benefit of routine three-field nodal dissection.
- Feeding jejunostomy is best option for post-oporative nutrition.
- There are four commonly used options in open oesophageal resection for cancer.
  1. The left thoracoabdominal (Sweet) approach involves an incision in the sixth intercostal space with division of diaphragm. It offers excellent exposure of GOJ but access to the proximal oesophagus is limited by the arch of aorta.
  2. The laparotomy and right thoracotomy (Ivor-Lewis) procedure is the most commonly used in Australia. Through the abdominal incision the stomach is mobilised, the cardia is resected (along with the left gastric artery). A gastric conduit is fashioned where the stomach survives on the right gastric and/or gastro-epiploic artery. The exposure of the GOJ from the chest is limited, but the exposure of rest of thoracic oesophagus is excellent. Generally the azygous vein is divided to allow access to oesophagus.
  3. The transhiatal (Grey-Turner) oesophagectomy (as popularised by Orringer) involves an incision in the abdomen and neck only. The oesophagus is mobilised by blunt dissection in posterior mediastinum from neck and abdomen. The nodes in the upper and middle third of mediastinum cannot be removed *en bloc*. There is an increased risk of damage to bronchus and azygous vein with tumour of the upper and middle third. Whilst this procedure does avoid a thoracotomy, and can be used in a patient with poor lung function, it probably achieves inferior oncological staging (if not results) due to the inability to dissect the mediastinal nodes *en bloc*.
  4. Finally the McKeown procedure is conducted as an Ivor-Lewis but includes an incision in the neck through which the anastomosis is fashioned. Although initially proposed as a means of circumventing an intra-thoracic leak (should one occur), the anastomosis usually falls back into the thoracic inlet and still causes mediastinitis if leak occurs.

- Palliative treatment of oesophageal cancer
  - Most patients either present with disease too advanced for surgery or are unfit for surgery. Therefore the main challenge in care of oesophagus cancer is effective palliative treatment.
  - A palliative pathway is indicated if the patient so desires after being fully informed or if they are not fit for surgery or definitive chemo/RT. Equally, palliation is required if they have clear evidence of systemic spread or non-resectability.
  - Both localised disease and metastatic symptoms may require attention. Localised symptoms include dysphagia, odynophagia, haematemesis, cough, chest pains, reflux hoarseness and chronic bleeding leading to anaemia. Metastatic symptoms include anorexia, weight loss, fatigue, upper abdominal pain and constipation. The options for treatments are set out below.
    - Palliative chemotherapy: there is little evidence to suggest that this is superior to best supportive care.

- Palliative external beam radiotherapy: achieves palliation of dysphagia in < 40% of patients and has largely been superseded by brachytherapy or multi-modality treatment.
- Palliative brachytherapy: this treatment consists of a single dose intracavity radiation (12Gy). Brachytherapy has been shown to offer similar palliation to metal stents with fewer complications (bleeding, perforation) and should be considered as a primary mode of palliation for patients with a life expectancy greater than 3 months.
- Self expanding metallic stents (SEMS): SEMS have superseded intubation with rigid prostheses because of greater efficacy and fewer complications.
- Neodymium — yttrium aluminium garnet (YAG) laser: YAG laser is useful for temporary relief of dysphagia before surgery or definitive palliation with SEMS or brachytherapy. It is useful for tumour ingrowth or overgrowth over a SEMS. It is useful for the cervical oesophagus where stent placement is impossible, but may require multiple treatments. Argon coagulation has same advantages as laser but is cheaper and more available.

3.3.6 Chronic liver disease

In the fellowship examination, patients with chronic liver disease have usually had an operation for another indication and the background history of chronic liver disease is an issue in the peri-operative setting. In this example we will describe a patient who has had surgery for a strangulated umbilical hernia.

The evaluation of a patient with suspected chronic liver disease should include:

- diagnosis of the cause of liver disease
- determination of the functional hepatic reserve
- definition of the portal venous anatomy and hepatic haemodynamic evaluation, and
- localisation of the site of upper gastrointestinal haemorrhage, if present.

The history

- Introduce yourself and ask the patient what has been going on. The patient will indicate that he needed an emergency operation for a lump at the umbilicus.
- Try to maintain a structure to your history, using the framework above. Begin by orientating yourself.
- The presenting symptoms and history of presenting complaint:
  - *presentation of lump*: when first appeared, how noticed, changes since then (bigger?), any other lumps, does/did it disappear when laying flat
  - *symptoms of complications*: incarceration — irreducible; strangulation — pain, skin changes, unwell; obstruction — nausea, vomiting, abdominal pain/distension
  - *associated symptoms of liver disease*: weight loss; anorexia; malaise; jaundice (painful/painless), pale stools, dark urine, bruising, bleeding (haematemesis, melaena, per rectum), abdominal distension, leg oedema
  - *previous investigations/interventions/treatments.*
- Risk factor assessment:
  - chronic alcoholism, hepatitis, complicated biliary disease
  - tattoos, IVDU, blood transfusion, contact with rats (Farm)
  - exposure to hepatotoxins.
- Past medical history.
- Surgical history.

- Drug history and allergies.
- Family history.
- Social history: occupation, home circumstances, smoking tobacco and alcohol consumption.

The examination

- Preparation — see above:
  - position the patient flat with one pillow under the head
  - expose the abdomen from nipples to pubic symphysis but state that ideally you would like to expose the patient to mid-thigh.
- General examination from the end of the bed:
  - overall condition
  - drains, tubes, infusions, TPN, IDC, oxygen etc.
- Assessment for peripheral stigmata of chronic liver disease, unless instructed otherwise:
  - vital signs
  - hands: anaemia, clubbing, malnutrition, leukonychia, palmar erythema, bruising, asterixis (liver flap)
  - head and neck: cachexia (wasting of temporalis)/jaundice/pallor/lymphadenopathy, fetor hepaticus
  - chest: gynaecomastia, loss of body hair, spider naevi, bruising, pectoral muscle wasting, scratch marks.
- Examination of the abdomen:
  - check the surgical site for healing, infection, recurrence of hernia
  - hepatosplenomegaly, ascites, testicular atrophy, signs of portal hypertension, dilated abdominal wall veins (Caput medusae).
- Conclusion:
  - say that you would do a digital rectal examination
  - cover the patient
  - reposition the patient
  - thank the patient
  - clean your hands again
  - only now turn to face the examiners.

The discussion

- Relevant investigation of a patient with chronic liver disease:
  - FBC — look for anaemia, low platelet count, low WCC. Cirrhosis is often accompanied by anaemia, leukopoenia and thrombocytopenia
  - coagulation studies — look for elevated INR, prolonged PT due to deficiency of the fat-soluble Vitamin K dependent clotting factors 2, 7, 9, 10 (the original terrestrial TV channels in Australia)
  - EUC — look for low Na, low K, metabolic alkalosis from recurrent vomiting, diarrhoea and hyperaldosteronism that accompanies cirrhosis
  - LFTs to differentiate cholestasis from hepatocellular injury and to assess level of hepatic decompensation
  - albumin — hypoalbuminaemia
  - hepatitis Serology — HCV, HBV
  - α-fetoprotein — HCC
  - liver biopsy — percutaneous liver biopsy is a useful in establishing the cause of cirrhosis and for assessing activity of the liver disease. Percutaneous liver biopsy is

not done when either coagulopathy or moderate ascites is present. In these situations, liver tissue can be obtained by means of a transjugular venous approach or at laparoscopy.

- Assessment of functional hepatic reserve in chronic liver disease:
  - this can be measured by using the Child-Pugh or MELD scoring system. These scoring systems give a risk assessment of morbidity and mortality.

Table 3.3.6 Child-Pugh criteria for chronic liver disease

MEASURE	1 POINT	2 POINTS	3 POINTS
Encephalopathy (grade)	None	1 or 2	3 or 4
Ascites	None	Mild	Moderate
Bilirubin (mg/dl)	< 2.0	2.0–3.0	≥ 3.0
Albumin (g/dl)	> 3.5	2.8–3.5	< 2.8
Prothrombin time prologation (s) (INR)	< 4 (< 1.7)	4–6 (1.7–2.3)	>6 (> 2.3)

  - Results in a score ranging from 5 to 15 points:
    - Class A = 5–6
    - Class B = 7–9
    - Class C = 10–15.
  - Operative mortality risk according to Child-Pugh Class is:
    - A = 0–5% mortality
    - B = 10–15% mortality
    - C = >25% mortality.
  - The overall 1-year survival rates for patients with Child-Pugh Class A, B, and C cirrhosis are approximately 100%, 80%, and 45% respectively.
  - MELD score (Model of End stage Liver Disease) has been found to be as predictive of mortality as Child-Pugh. It is derived from a complex formula incorporating bilirubin, INR and creatinine. It has been suggested that patients with a MELD score below 10 can undergo elective surgery, those with a MELD score of 10 to 15 may undergo elective surgery with caution, and those with a MELD score >15 should not undergo elective surgery.
- Assessment of the porto-systemic anatomy:
  - CT angiography is the investigation of choice for assessing the porto-systemic circulation and locating the presence of varices
  - doppler ultrasonography is a non-invasive technique for assessment of portal venous patency, direction of portal flow, and shunt patency status
  - ultrasound is also useful for assessing liver size, spleen size, and the presence of liver masses. It can also detect ascites in its earliest stages (≥100 mL)
  - visceral angiography, but is not as popular as before because it is invasive.
- How do you treat an umbilical hernia in a patient with chronic liver disease?
  - It depends on the degree of liver disease and the nature of the presentation of the hernia and whether it is symptomatic and there is evidence of complication (strangulation/obstruction).
  - Patients with Child-Pugh class B and C should be managed conservatively unless there is a clear emergency surgical indication for surgery (e.g. strangulation/obstruction) due to the high risk of morbidity and mortality.
  - Patients with asymptomatic hernias should be managed conservatively, with surgical correction of the hernia performed at the time of liver transplantation. The

cornerstone of conservative management in asymptomatic patients with umbilical hernias is aggressive management of ascites. Elastic/velcro abdominal binders can also help reduce pain and minimise further enlargement of the hernia.

- All patients should be managed in a multidisciplinary team environment (hepatologist, surgeons, nursing and allied health staff capable of looking after such patients).
- Patients should be optimised medically if surgery is being contemplated with:
  - reduction in ascites (salt restriction, spironolactone ± Furosemide)
  - nutritional optimisation (high protein high calorie supplements)
  - treatment of portal hypertension (propanolol/TIPPS).

3.3.7 Liver metastases

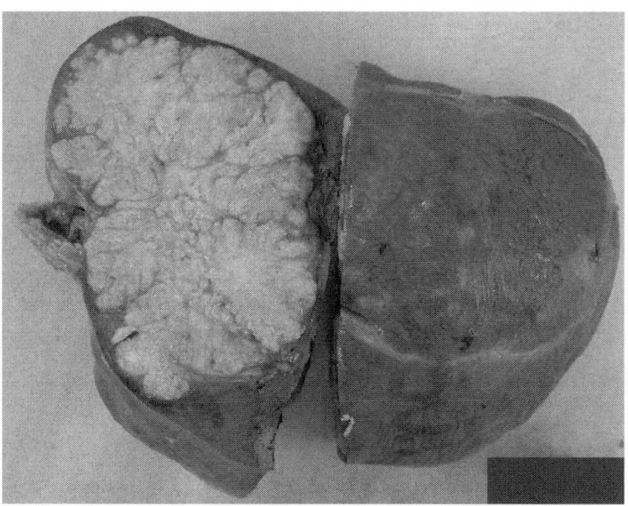

Figure 3.3.7
Right hemi-hepatectomy for colorectal liver metastasis

The history

- Introduce yourself and ask the patient what has been going on. The patient may indicate that he had bowel cancer that spread to the liver.
- Try to maintain a structure to your history, using the framework above. Begin by orientating yourself.
  - Has the liver metastasis been removed?
  - Has the bowel cancer been removed?
  - Was the liver metastasis removed before or after the bowel cancer?
- The detail relating to the bowel cancer:
  - Was the spread to his liver discovered at the same time as the bowel cancer or afterwards?
  - Did he have any treatment before the bowel surgery (particularly chemotherapy)?
  - What bowel surgery did he have done? Laparoscopic or open procedure? Which bowel operation? Patients will usually know if the left, right or most of the colon was removed.

  - Did he have a stoma or peri-operative complication?
  - Did he have chemotherapy post-operatively?
  - What follow-up imaging/colonoscopy has he had?
- The detail relating to the liver metastasis:
  - When was the liver metastasis discovered?
  - How were they picked up, on a CT scan or PET or MRI?
  - Has he had surgery yet?
  - If he has had surgery, what type?
  - Was it a major liver resection?
  - Did he require pre-operative portal vein embolisation?
  - Did he have a post-operative complication such as bile leak or return to theatre?
- Current functional status (diet, mobility, bowel function, expected date of discharge).
- Risk factor assessment:
  - personal or family history of polyps/colorectal cancer/inflammatory bowel disease.
- Past medical history.
- Surgical history.
- Drug history and allergies.
- Family history — particularly of endometrial/gastric/ovary/urothelium (HNPCC).
- Social history: occupation, home circumstances, smoking tobacco and alcohol consumption.

The examination

- Preparation (see above):
  - position the patient flat with one pillow under the head
  - expose the abdomen from nipples to pubic symphysis but state that ideally you would like to expose the patient to mid-thigh.
- General examination from the end of the bed:
  - overall condition
  - if post-operative: drains, tubes, infusions, TPN, IDC, oxygen etc.
- Assessment for peripheral signs, unless instructed otherwise:
  - vital signs.
- Examination of the abdomen:
  - inspection: look for previous scars and presence of a portacath — get the patient to point out scars. (Note: unless the patient has had laparoscopic liver surgery they will have a subcostal or upper midline incision. There may be a diverting ileostomy from an ultra-low rectal resection. The colonic surgery is often laparoscopic and so the incisions may be hard to see. Look for a portacath. Inspect drains, dressings, bruising. Inspect wounds for signs of infection
  - palpation: soft; tender; organomegaly (liver edge); ascites. Assess groin and incision for evidence of a cough impulse. Palpate the testicles
  - percussion: not usually relevant post-operatively unless distended and you want to determine if it is gas or fluid (ascites/ileus). Percussion for shifting dullness/fluid thrill
  - auscultation: listen in four quadrants for the character of borborygmi, bruits over the renal arteries, aorta and liver.
- Conclusion:
  - say that you would do a digital rectal examination in the pre-operative setting
  - cover the patient
  - reposition the patient

- thank the patient
- clean your hands again
- only now turn to face the examiners.

The discussion

- The examiners may ask you to tell them what you found. An example of a succinct summary for this case would be as follows. 'Mr Y is a 59-year-old man who had a right hemicolectomy 3 years ago for a colonic cancer. He received adjuvant chemotherapy after his colonic resection. Six months ago he was discovered to have a liver metastasis because of a rising CEA noted by his GP. The tumour was in the right side of the liver and was large. He had what sounds like a portal vein embolisation and then an extended hepatectomy. He was in hospital for 4 weeks after his liver surgery. It sounds like he may have had a bile leak and liver failure post-operatively, but he made a complete recovery.'
- Detection and assessment of liver metastases after surgery for colorectal cancer
  - All patients who have undergone curative surgery and are fit for further intervention should be offered surveillance to detect metachronous colorectal cancers and liver metastases.
  - This follow-up involves CEA measurement, CT scanning of the chest/abdomen/pelvis and colonoscopy; the former two investigations are integral to the early detection of (liver) metastases.
  - CEA measurement and CT scanning is usually arranged 3–6 monthly in conjunction with the clinical review of the patient. There is evidence of survival benefit to this practice when compared with no surveillance at all. RCTs comparing intensive (including CEA/CT) vs less intensive surveillance show an overall survival benefit to intensive follow-up. Follow-up should be 3–6 monthly for 2 years and 6 monthly thereafter.
  - Once a liver metastasis is diagnosed, search for extra-hepatic disease using PET-CT scanning should be considered in high-risk patients. PET-CT will detect occult metastasis (not revealed by other investigations) and change clinical management in about 25% of cases. However, after commencement of chemotherapy, PET-CT has a significant false-negative rate because of altered metabolic activity within the lesions.
  - Non-therapeutic laparotomy can be avoided using laparoscopy and intra-operative ultrasound. This allows the evaluation of visceral and parietal surfaces of the abdomen (and biopsy of suspicious lesions) and the porta hepatis for occult nodal disease. Intra-operative ultrasound can be used to detect unexpected lesions in the liver remnant that will persist following resection.
  - Portal hypertension can also be evaluated and the normal liver biopsied.
  - The Clinical Risk Score (CRS) can be used to predict which patients are most likely to be non-resectable at laparoscopy.
  - Within the CRS a point is given for each of:
    - >1 liver tumour
    - liver tumour >5 cm
    - node-positive colorectal primary
    - disease free interval <1 yr and
    - CEA >200.
  - If the score is 0, patients are likely to remain resectable at laparoscopy. If the score is 4–5, 25% of patients will be non-resectable at laparoscopy. Laparoscopy should be restricted to those with high CRS.

- What are the principles of treatment of liver metastases after surgery for colorectal cancer?
  - About 20% of patients have liver metastasis at initial presentation of a colorectal cancer (synchronous).
  - About 30% of patients develop metastases after resection of a colorectal cancer (metachronous).
  - Approximately one-quarter of the liver metastasis are resectable, although liver surgeons continue to push the boundaries with safe liver resection.
  - In appropriately selected patients, liver resection offers 5-year relapse-free survival rates of 30% and 5-year overall survival rates of approximately 58%.
  - The optimal selection of patients for resection continues to evolve. However, resection should *not* be considered in the following situations:
    - non-resectable extrahepatic disease detected by CT, PET-CT or laparoscopy
    - involvement of the common hepatic artery or main portal vein
    - inadequate liver remnant after resection
    - unfit for surgery.
  - Modern multidisciplinary consensus defines resectable CRC liver metastases as tumours that can be resected completely, leaving an adequate liver remnant.
  - The liver remnant must retain adequate hepatic arterial and portal venous inflow and venous and biliary drainage. Future liver remnant (FLR) is calculated by CT volumetric study. The normal liver constitutes approximately 2% of body weight. For a successful liver resection FLR needs to be:
    - normal liver: 20% or > if pre-operative chemo
    - cirrhosis/diabetics: >40%.
  - Consider portal vein embolisation if:
    - FLR <20% in normal patients or
    - FLR <40% in cirrhotics/diabetics.
- What are the main approaches for the treatment of resectable liver metastases after surgery for colorectal cancer?
  - *Liver first approach*:
    - this option is usually favoured if the primary is under control (non-obstructing/no bleeding) and there is large volume liver disease. Most liver surgeons believe that the liver is the determining factor for survival and therefore argue that the liver resection should be done first. Also, in the case of rectal cancer, liver surgeons argue that a complication post-pelvic surgery can delay liver surgery to the point where the patient may become inoperable.
  - *Synchronous resection approach*:
    - this approach should be considered for patients with low volume uncomplicated liver lesions; for example, single solitary peripheral metastasis or planned segment 2 or 3 liver resection where there is a lesser risk of peri-operative and post-operative morbidity and mortality.
  - *Colorectal primary first approach*:
    - this is the preferred pathway in most institutions, as the primary tumour is believed to be the source of the metastatic cells. Liver resection occurs 6–8/52 after bowel resection.
  - *Chemotherapy first approach*:
    - chemotherapy/re-evaluate/ ±liver resection. This approach is preferred in patients with high volume liver disease, as if there is disease progression on chemotherapy then resection is not suitable. This can avoid unnecessary liver resection. If, on the other hand, the disease has responded or is stable, resection

of the metastatic disease should be attempted. No more than two to three courses of pre-operative chemotherapy are recommended before liver resection as it causes CASH (chemotherapy-associated steatohepatitis). Chemotherapy treatment is not standardised and varies between institutions and countries. The optimal chemotherapy regimen is not established, but FOLFOX/ FOLFIRI are considered to be reasonable choices. For non-resectable disease, 'up front' chemotherapy is an appropriate option in an attempt to down-stage a patient to the point of resectability. This occurs in approximately 10–15% of patients. Note, longer durations of pre-operative chemotherapy increase the potential for liver toxicity and post-operative complications.
- Non-resectable liver metastases should be considered for RFA/TACE.
- Following complete resection of liver metastases, the best post-operative strategy is uncertain. In the absence of published randomised trials to guide clinical practice following metastasectomy, completion of a full 6 month course of systemic chemotherapy containing oxaliplatin is recommended.

3.3.8 Abdominal mass

You are asked to take a history and examine a patient who has presented with an abdominal mass. Outlined below are the pertinent aspects of history, examination and presentation of the differential diagnosis and treatment plan.

Consider the classification of abdominal masses. They can be classified by location, region or aetiology.

- Location — a good idea to keep this classification in mind during the history and examination:
  - anterior abdominal wall
  - intraperitoneal
  - retroperitoneal.
- Region:
  - right upper/lower quadrant
  - left upper/lower quadrant
  - midline masses may be supraumbilical or infraumbilical.
- Aetiology:
  - neoplastic (benign or malignant)
  - infective (e.g. hydatid cyst, liver abscess)
  - inflammatory (e.g. phlegmon secondary to appendicitis or Crohn's disease)
  - vascular (aneurysm, rectus sheath haematoma).

The history

- Introduce yourself and ask the patient what has been going on.
- Try to maintain a structure to your history, using the framework above. Begin by orientating yourself (see above).
  - Be aware that the lump may have been an incidental finding and not associated with any clinical symptoms. Even if this is the case, you should run through the list of questions below to demonstrate to the examiners that you know what you should ask about.
- The presenting symptoms and history of presenting complaint:
  - *the lump*: when it first appeared, how noticed, progression since then (bigger?), any other lumps

- *associated symptoms*: pain (SOCRATES) or distension
- *GI symptoms (from upper to lower GI tract)*: dysphagia, dyspepsia, early satiety, postprandial vomiting, reflux, haematemesis, jaundice, abdominal distension, altered bowel habit (constipation/ diarrhoea/ both), bleeding per rectum etc.
- *other associated symptoms — systemic*: fevers, weight loss; anorexia; malaise; shortness of breath
- *other associated symptoms — urinary*: frequency, dysuria, haematuria, pneumaturia, UTI
- *other associated symptoms — gynaecological in females*: menstrual cycle, menorrhagia, dysmenorrhoea, intermenstrual bleeding, last Pap smear, obstetric history
- *other associated symptoms — vascular*: claudication, risk factors for cardiovascular disease, aneurysms
- *investigations:*
    - details of those performed to date
    - results
    - presumed diagnosis
- *treatment:*
    - Was the patient admitted electively or acutely?
    - What procedure was performed?
    - Was neo-adjuvant treatment required or discussed?
    - Were there any complications after the operation?
    - Current status of the patient (diet, mobility, bowel function, expected date of discharge).
    - Will adjuvant treatment be required (radiotherapy or chemotherapy)?

- Risk factor assessment:
    - personal or family history of cancer.
- Past medical history:
    - history of malignancy (including GIT, breast and melanoma) and/or prior surgery including non-abdominal surgery (including skin excisions)
    - previous gastroscopy/colonoscopy (when/where/findings)
    - pancreatitis
    - IBD.
- Surgical history.
- Drug history and allergies.
- Family history — history of malignancy within family members and other diseases within the family including AAA.
- Social history: occupation, home circumstances, smoking tobacco and alcohol consumption, travel/migration.

The examination

- Preparation (see above):
    - position the patient flat with one pillow under the head
    - expose the abdomen from nipples to pubic symphysis but state that ideally you would like to expose the patient to mid-thigh.
- General examination from the end of the bed:
    - overall condition
    - drains, tubes, infusions, TPN, IDC, oxygen etc if post-operative.
- Assessment for peripheral signs, unless instructed otherwise:
    - vital signs

- hands: stigmata of gastrointestinal disease — Dupuytren's contractures, nail changes (leukonychia, clubbing), pallor of the palmer creases (anaemia). Ask the patient to squeeze your hand as poor grip strength is a marker of inadequate nutrition
- examine the head and neck: cachexia (wasting of temporalis; assess the eyes looking at the sclera for icterus and the conjunctiva for pallor; assess the mouth for angular stomatitis and glossitis
- examine the supraclavicular fossa for nodal metastases
- examine the chest for gynaecomastia, skin changes; auscultate for pleural effusions.

- Examination of the abdomen:
  - inspection: careful inspection as often the mass will be obvious by kneeling beside the patient with your eyes level with the abdomen. Observe movement with respiration; distension; scars; stomas; dressings; bruising. Inspect wounds for signs of infection. Look at drains, stomas and urine bag if present
  - palpation: soft; tender; organomegaly; ascites
  - percussion: not usually relevant post-operatively unless distended and you want to determine if it is gas or fluid (ascites/ileus). Percussion for shifting dullness; fluid thrill
  - auscultation: listen in four quadrants for the character of borborygmi, bruits over the renal arteries, aorta and liver.

For any mass it is important to describe it according to the mnemonic 'Should The Children Ever Find Lumps Readily' (see below, and Chapter 3.4, exam technique). In addition, it is crucial to assess the following to help distinguish the aetiology of an abdominal mass. Use the acronym **SPRUE** as an aide-memoire:

- **s**ite of enlargement
- **p**ercussion note
- **r**espiratory movement
- **u**nable to get above it
- **e**dge characteristics.

- Conclusion:
  - say that you would do a digital rectal examination in the pre-operative setting.
  - cover the patient
  - reposition the patient
  - thank the patient
  - clean your hands again
  - only now turn to face the examiners.

The discussion

- Having completed a history and examination the differential diagnosis needs to be considered. Refer to Chapter 3.5, Figure 3.5.13 and Table 3.3.8A, for a full list of differentials.
- Differential diagnosis of causes of intra-abdominal masses by location and organ of origin in the abdomen.
- Present a list of the differential diagnoses that you consider are most likely in the patient you have seen. They could be ordered from most common to least common or you could start with those that are most important to exclude (e.g. malignancy).

- Present a management strategy for the patient. Your management should include whether the patient needs admission to hospital or can be managed as an out-patient (i.e. is the patient sick?). Further investigation involves blood tests, imaging and endoscopy as appropriate.
  - Blood tests:
    - FBC — anaemia, leucocytosis
    - coagulation profile — INR raised in liver synthetic dysfunction, pre-operative
    - EUC — electrolytes, renal impairment
    - LFTs — hepatic dysfunction, raised bilirubin
    - amylase/lipase if indicated
    - tumour markers if indicated (CEA — colon; Ca19.9 — pancreas, gastric, biliary; AFP — HCC, testicular; Ca125 — ovarian)
    - HBV/HCV/Hydatid/amoebic serology if indicated.
  - Imaging:
    - a CT abdomen/pelvis with iv and oral contrast is the best initial test for an undifferentiated abdominal mass
    - other imaging modalities that may be useful — vascular duplex ultrasound (AAA); pelvic ultrasound
    - CXR should be obtained routinely if surgery is considered and as a screening test for thoracic pathology)
    - in certain instances further imaging may be required (e.g. 4 phase CT scan for characterisation of liver or pancreatic tumours or MRI).
  - Endoscopy:
    - upper GI endoscopy if the origin is thought to be UGIT
    - ERCP may be indicated in the setting of a RUQ mass and biliary obstruction
    - endoscopic ultrasound and FNA is valuable in the assessment of pancreatic masses
    - colonoscopy if suspected colonic malignancy to confirm diagnosis and exclude synchronous lesions.
- After presenting the differential diagnoses and a management plan, list the issues that need to be addressed. The list may include:
  - confirmation of diagnosis
  - staging in the setting of malignancy
  - MDT discussion of patients with malignancies with consideration of surgical or non-surgical management and any indications for neo-adjuvant or adjuvant treatment
  - management of sepsis (if present)
  - disease specific management or appropriate referral
  - nutrition
  - immediate and longer term treatment goals.
- The clinical profile, examination, investigations, aetiology and discussion points for intra-abdominal masses are detailed in Tables 3.3.8A, B, C and D.

Table 3.3.8A Clinical profile, examination, investigations, aetiology and discussion points for intra-abdominal masses (splenomegaly, gall bladder mass, liver mass)

	SPLENOMEGALY	GALL BLADDER MASS	LIVER MASS
Mass symptoms	Asymptomatic Progressive enlargement	Asymptomatic Acute hx if infective cause Chronic hx if malignant	Asymptomatic Progressive enlargement Generalised if ascites

Table 3.3.8A Continued

	SPLENOMEGALY	GALL BLADDER MASS	LIVER MASS
Painful mass	Discomfort or acute pain if infarction or infection Can radiate to left shoulder	Yes (infective) Radiates back, epigastrium or right shoulder	Pain associated with acute causes, bleeding from lesion, congestion
Appetite	Can be reduced	Reduced	Can be reduced
Nausea/vomiting	No	Yes (infection, jaundice)	Not usually
Haematemesis	Low platelets or portal HT	No	Low platelets or portal HT
Fullness/bloating	Yes (massive spleen)	No	Some liver conditions
Dyspepsia	Yes (massive spleen)	Can occur with gall stones	Some liver conditions
Weight loss	Yes	Can occur with malignancy	Yes
Altered bowel habit	No	No	No unless colorectal cancer metastases
Jaundice etc	Assoc with liver disease, haemolytic anaemia	Yes — stones, malignancy	Yes
Fevers etc	Yes	Yes — infection	Can occur
Past history	Immunological disorders Abnormal FBC Hepatitis Risk factors (RF) for hepatitis/chronic liver disease (IVDU/ alcohol) FHx anaemia, RA, SLE	Known gall stones Previous cholecystitis	Malignancy Hepatitis and RF for hepatitis/chronic liver disease (IVDU/ alcohol) Haematological disorders Cardiovascular disease FHx: polycystic disease
Examination	Spleen enlarges infero-medially; moves down with respiration Splenic notch Bimanual palpation Signs rheumatological disease, chronic liver disease, lymphadenopathy	Tender poorly defined mass that cannot get above in the midclavicular line on the right (infective causes) Non tender mass associated with jaundice in this location suggests malignancy of distal CBD	Tender diffuse liver enlargement with acute infective hepatitis Non-tender hard, irregular liver indicates malignancy Cystic lesions — smooth Signs of chronic liver and rheumatological disease
Investigations	FBC, LFTS, EUC, CRP	FBC, LFTS, EUC, CRP	FBC, LFTS, EUC, CRP
	Blood film examination	Coagulation studies	Coagulation studies
	Coagulation studies	CA 19.9, CEA	CA 19.9, CEA, AFP, CA 15.3
	Blood cultures	Ultrasound	Ultrasound (cystic vs solid)
	Viral serology (EBV, CMV) Echinococcus serology	CT Abdomen/Pelvis	Viral serology (EBV, CMV) Echinococcus, hepatitis
	CT Abdomen/Pelvis	Blood cultures	CT Abdomen/Pelvis
	CT Chest/neck	EUS	PET scan
	PET scan	ERCP/MRCP	MRI liver
	Bone marrow bx		Gastroscopy/colonoscopy (GIT primary)
	Excisional lymph node bx		

Table 3.3.8A Continued

	SPLENOMEGALY	GALL BLADDER MASS	LIVER MASS
Aetiology	Haematological malignancy	Mucocoele	HCC, cholangiocarcinoma
	Myeloproliferative disease	Acute cholecystitis	Metastases (colorectal)
	Infections (EBV, CMV, malaria, infective endocarditis)	Empyema	Infections (acute hepatitis, EBV, CMV, hydatid cyst)
	Portal hypertension	Biliary obstruction	Hepatic adenoma, FNH
	Immunological (RA, SLE)	Gall bladder carcinoma	Polycystic disease
	Infiltrative (e.g. sarcoidosis)		Right heart failure
	Splenic cysts		Haematological diseases
	Metastases (lung, pancreas, stomach)		Riedel's lobe
			Simple cyst, cystadenoma
Discussion points	Indications for splenectomy	Management of obstructive jaundice	Management of hepatic colorectal metastases
	Post-operative complications of splenectomy	Management of gall bladder carcinoma	Management of HCC
	OPSI and its prevention	Management of acute cholecystitis	Management of hydatid disease

Table 3.3.8B Clinical profile, examination, investigations, aetiology and discussion points for intra-abdominal masses (pancreas, stomach, colon)

	PANCREAS	STOMACH	COLON
Mass symptoms	Progression over time	Progression over time	Progression over time May not generalised distension due to LBO
Painful mass	Yes — radiating to back	Often non-tender	If associated perforation or obstruction
Appetite	Reduced	Reduced	Reduced
Nausea/vomiting	Present	Present	Associated with LBO
Haematemesis	Can occur if tumour erodes into duodenum/ stomach.	Can be present	No
Fullness/bloating	Present	Present	Yes
Dyspepsia	Can occur	Present	Associated with LBO
Weight loss	Yes	Yes	Yes
Altered bowel habit	Neuroendocrine tumours can cause diarrhoea	No	Constipation or diarrhoea, bleeding (fresh or dark), mucous Thin stools
Jaundice etc	Can occur	No	No

Table 3.3.8B Continued

	PANCREAS	STOMACH	COLON
Fevers etc	Can occur	No	Associated with infective causes/complications
Urinary symptoms	No	No	Can occur
Past history	Pancreatitis Diabetes Alcoholism FHx: pancreatic cancer	Peptic ulcer/H. pylori Previous gastrectomy/ ulcer surgery. FHx: stomach cancer	Hx previous colonoscopy and polyps IBD FHx — colon cancer
Examination	Carcinoma: cachexia and a firm poorly defined fixed mass deep in epigastrium Pseudocyst: smooth poorly defined epigastric mass	Cachexia Usually a poorly defined mass in epigastrium Gastric distension can be present (succussion splash)	Usually a poorly defined mass Maybe associated with LBO
Investigations	FBC, LFTS, EUC, lipase, CRP	FBC, LFTS, EUC, CRP	FBC, LFTS, EUC, CRP
	Coagulation studies	CEA, CA 72.4, CA 19.9	CEA
	CA 19.9, CEA	Endoscopy + biopsy	Colonoscopy + bx
	EUS/ERCP/MRCP	CT Chest/Abdomen/Pelvis	Blood cultures, MSU
	CT Chest/Abdomen/Pelvis		CT Chest/Abdomen/Pelvis
Aetiology	Carcinoma pancreas	Carcinoma stomach	Colorectal cancer
	Pancreatic pseudocyst	GIST stomach	Diverticular abscess/ phlegmon/fistula
	Neuroendocrine tumour	Neuroendocrine tumour	
Discussion points	Management of pancreatic pseudocysts	Management of adenocarcinoma of stomach	Management of colorectal cancer
	Management of pancreatitic cancer	Management of GIST tumours	Management of diverticular abscess

Table 3.3.8C Clinical profile, examination, investigations, aetiology and discussion points for intra-abdominal masses (omentum, ovarian, uterine)

	OMENTAL MASS	OVARIAN MASS	UTERINE MASS
Mass symptoms	Generalised distension if ascites present	Acute onset if due to ectopic/torsion	Suprapubic fullness/ sensation of heaviness
Painful mass	Discomfort more common	Ectopic, torsion, endometrioma associated with acute pain	Can cause discomfort and pain Cramping can occur with bleeding
Appetite	Reduced	Usually normal	Usually normal
Nausea/vomiting	Can be present	Can occur with acute pathologies	No
Haematemesis	No	No	No
Fullness/bloating	Yes	Associated with malignancy	No

Table 3.3.8C Continued			
	OMENTAL MASS	OVARIAN MASS	UTERINE MASS
Dyspepsia	Can be present	No	No
Weight loss	Yes	Yes if malignancy	Yes if malignancy
Altered bowel habit	Constipation	No	Uncommon
Jaundice etc	Can be present	No	No
Fevers etc	Often absent	No	No
Urinary symptoms	Bladder compression can cause frequency	Bladder compression can cause frequency	Bladder compression and fistulae can cause irritative symptoms
Gynaecological symptoms	If associated with gynaecological primary	Symptoms associated with menstrual cycle Possible pregnancy Dysfunctional uterine bleeding Post-menopausal bleeding	Symptoms associated with menstrual cycle Possible pregnancy Dysfunctional uterine bleeding Post-menopausal bleeding
Past history	Malignancy Appendicectomy Ovarian pathology FHx: malignancy (colorectal, gynaecological)	Malignancy (breast) Parity PCOS Endometriosis FHX: malignancy (breast, gynaecological)	Malignancy (breast) Parity OCP/HRT FHX: malignancy (breast, gynaecological)
Examination	Cachexia Ascites Often multiple small hard non-tender masses with fixation to anterior abdominal wall PR — Blummers shelf	Ovarian masses can be felt deep in iliac fossae but are better assessed with PV / bimanual palpation Determine fixation Examine cervix PR — Blummers shelf	Uterine masses can be felt suprapubically Unable to get below PV and bimanual examination PR
Investigations	FBC, EUC, LFT, CRP	FBC, EUC, LFT, CRP	FBC, EUC, LFT, CRP
	CA 125, CEA, CA 72.4, CA 19.9	CA 125, AFP, β-HCG	CA 125, CA
	CT abdomen/pelvis	Pelvic ultrasound	Pelvic ultrasound
	Ascitic tap for cytology	CT abdomen/pelvis	CT abdomen/pelvis
	Gastroscopy/colonoscopy	Diagnostic laparoscopy	Hysteroscopy + bx
Aetiology	Peritoneal mesothelioma	Malignant tumour	Carcinoma
	Pseudomyxoma peritonei	Torsion	Fibroids
	Metastases — ovarian, stomach, pancreas, colorectal	Cysts	
		Ectopic pregnancy	
		Dermoid	
		Endometrioma	
Discussion points	Pathophysiology of pseudomyxoma peritonei		
	Management of unknown primary with omental metastases		

Table 3.3.8D Clinical profile, examination, investigations, aetiology and discussion points for intra-abdominal masses (renal, bladder, small intestine)

	RENAL MASS	BLADDER MASS	SMALL INTESTINE
Mass symptoms			
Painful mass	Back or loin pain	Suprapubic pain, flank pain due to ureteric obstruction	Periumbililcal discomfort or colicky pain if SBO
Appetite	Usually normal	Usually normal	Can be reduced
Nausea/vomiting	No	No	Yes
Haematemesis	No	No	Usually no
Fullness/bloating	No	Suprapubic swelling	Yes
Dyspepsia	No	No	Yes
Weight loss	Yes if malignancy	Yes if malignancy	Yes if malignancy
Altered bowel habit	No	No	Yes — constipation, diarrhoea (carcinoid)
Jaundice etc	No	No	No
Fevers etc	Yes (paraneoplastic)	No	Yes — carcinoid
Urinary symptoms	Haematuria Frequency	Irritative or obstructive symptoms	No
Past history	Occupation — carcinogen exposure Smoking Obesity Analgesic abuse HTN, DM FHx: polycystic disease, renal failure	Occupation — carcinogen exposure Smoking Recurrent UTI	Malignancy IBD or FHX IBD Abdominal surgery
Examination	Cachexia Flank mass that may be balloted Scrotal varices Polycystic liver	Distended fluid filled mass unable to get below PR to examine prostate	Generalised abdominal distension (SBO) Discrete mass uncommon Examine hernia orifices and for incisional hernia
Investigations	FBC, EUC, LFTs, CMP	FBC, EUC, LFTs, CMP	FBC, EUC, LFTs, CMP
	MSU	PSA	Chromogranin A
	Renal tract ultrasound	MSU	CT abdomen/pelvis
	CT Abdomen/Pelvis	CT abdomen/pelvis/IVP	Octreotide SPECT/CT
		Urine cytology	Colonoscopy with TI intubation
		Cystoscopy + bx	
		TRUS prostate + bx	

Table 3.3.8D Continued

	RENAL MASS	BLADDER MASS	SMALL INTESTINE
Aetiology	Carcinoma	Bladder neck obstruction — prostate cancer/BPH	Adenocarcinoma
	Polycystic disease/ simple cysts	Bladder tumour	GIST
	Hydronephrosis		Carcinoid tumour
	Pyonephrosis		Lymphoma
			Small bowel obstruction
			Terminal ileitis
Discussion points			Management of carcinoid tumour and carcinoid syndrome
			Management of SBO

3.3.9 Malignant melanoma

The possible scenarios that you will encounter include a patient with either:

- stage I/II disease: localised melanoma, further investigation and treatment depends on pathology of primary lesion
- stage III disease: nodal metastases. Includes nodal recurrence and in-transit disease, or
- stage IV disease: systemic metastases.

The history

- Introduce yourself and ask the patient what has been going on. The patient may indicate that he or she had an operation for a melanoma on their back 1 month ago and now has had an operation on their axilla.
- Try to maintain a structure to your history, using the framework above. Begin by orientating yourself.
- The presenting symptoms and history of the primary melanoma:
  - suspicious features (ABCDE of melanoma)
  - excision or partial/punch biopsy
  - pathology of the melanoma — Breslow, ulceration, mitoses, margins.
- History of lymph node(s) assessment:
  - Is there a palpable nodal mass/lymphoedema?
  - Was sentinel lymph node biopsy (SLNB) performed?
  - How many nodes were removed, presence of metastases?
  - Lymph node (LN) dissection — for clinically evident disease or positive SLN or for nodal relapse?
  - Were there complications from surgery?
- History of systemic metastases:
  - where, how many, symptomatic versus non-symptomatic
  - weight loss, anaemia, neurological symptoms

- history of resection versus non-operative management (e.g. Radiotherapy [RTx], BRAF inhibitors, chemotherapy).
- Adjuvant treatment:
  - RTx, IFN, chemotherapy, ipilumimab, BRAF inhibitors, trials, isolated limb infusion.
- Risk factor assessment:
  - personal or family history of previous melanoma/non-melanoma skin cancers
  - history of sun exposure (e.g. occupation).
- Past medical history.
- Surgical history.
- Drug history and allergies.
- Family history.
- Social history: home circumstances, smoking tobacco and alcohol consumption.

The examination

- Preparation (see above):
  - position the patient comfortably
  - expose the patient completely, while preserving his/her dignity as much as possible.
- Inspection:
  - comment on general appearance and then general features of skin damage (e.g. fair skin with solar keratoses/BCC/SCC/multiple previous excision sites)
  - look for evidence of RTx changes
  - evidence of recent/previous surgery: where, drains and output
  - look for other suspicious lesions, presence of other dysplastic naevi.
- Examination for locoregional disease:
  - examine excision site for evidence of local recurrence/residual tumour/satellite lesions
  - examine draining LN basin (may need to examine multiple areas e.g. both groins for lower mid back primary site, bilateral neck for central scalp)
  - assess for clinically palpable masses and characterise
  - if previous dissection evident, examine that area then examine for recurrence
  - comment on presence/absence of lymphoedema if previous lymph node dissection
  - complications of previous surgery; for example, nerve damage with lymph node dissection.
- Complete the systemic examination:
  - start with hands if you have time
  - examine major nodal groups (bilateral axillae/groin/cervical/supraclavicular) especially if stage III/IV disease
  - percussion and auscultation of chest to exclude pleural effusion or other features associated with lung metastases
  - palpate the abdomen for liver metastases and other intra-abdominal masses; for example, LN/retroperitoneal/bowel metastasis.
- Conclusion:
  - cover the patient
  - reposition the patient
  - thank the patient
  - clean your hands again
  - only now turn to face the examiners.

The discussion

- How do you stage melanoma?
  - Use The American Joint Committee on Cancer (AJCC) TNM system.
  - Stage I/II (Localised melanoma):
    - T1–4 N0 M0 disease
    - T stage melanoma thickness
    - Tis: melanoma in situ (tumour remains in the epidermis)
    - T1: ≤1.0 mm thick
    - T2: 1.01 to 2.0 mm
    - T3: 2.01 to 4.0 mm
    - T4: >4.0 mm
    - each is subdivided according to absence (substage a)/presence (substage b) of ulceration
    - Breslow thickness, mitotic rate and the presence of ulceration are significant independent prognostic predictors of survival in this group of patients:
    - stage I (T1, T2a): 85–99% 5 year survival
    - stage II (T2b, T3, T4): 40–85% 5 year survival.
  - Stage III (Nodal disease):
    - the number of regional LNs involved, regional node tumour burden (micro vs macro) and ulceration of the primary tumour are independent predictors of survival in this group
    - the number of involved LNs is the most important predictor of survival
    - in-transit disease (in lymphatics) and satellite lesions (of skin) are included in stage III
    - 25–60% 5-year survival.
  - Stage IV (distant metastases)
    - 15% 5-year survival.
- What is the management strategy of patients with malignant melanoma?
  - Stage I/II patients:
    - staging for metastatic disease is not indicated in asymptomatic patients due to low yield (as per NHMRC guidelines)
    - SLNB should be performed for patients with primary melanoma >1 mm in thickness. Lymphoscintigraphy with Tc99 labelled sulphur colloid and intra-operative patent blue dye
    - any palpable lymphadenopathy should be investigated with an ultrasound guided FNA of any suspicious nodes
    - all patients with stage II or greater disease should be referred to a melanoma centre.
  - Stage III patients:
    - FDG PET scan with CT Brain or CT brain/chest/abdomen/pelvis to stage if the detection of occult metastatic disease would influence management
    - in-transit/locally recurrent disease should be confirmed histologically by excision/FNA biopsy of a nodule.
  - Stage IV or suspected stage IV disease:
    - FDG PET scan with CT Brain or CT brain/chest/abdo/pelvis
    - MRI brain to further characterise brain metastases may be indicated
    - tumour tissue can be tested for specific tumour mutations for consideration of targeted therapies which are available on trials for metastatic disease; for example, BRAF inhibitors for V600 mutations. BRAF and NRAS mutation testing.

- What are the principles of surgical management of malignant melanoma?
  - Wide excision of the primary cutaneous melanoma and management of the regional lymph nodes.
  - The prognosis is most closely associated with Breslow thickness (depth measured in millimetres (mm) from the granular layer of the epidermis to the point of deepest invasion using an ocular micrometre), ulceration and mitoses.
  - Treatment of the primary melanoma:
    - margins (NCCN guidelines):
      - melanoma in situ (Tis): 5 mm margin
      - <1 mm (T1): 1 cm margin
      - 1–2 mm (T2): 1–2 cm margin
      - >2 mm (T3,4): 2 cm margin
    - meta-analysis of WHO Trial, the Intergroup Melanoma Trial, the Swedish Melanoma Study Group Trial and the French Cooperative Group trial concluded that wide (3–5 cm) margins did not improve the overall mortality compared with narrow margins in the surgical treatment of primary cutaneous melanoma (Lens et al. Excision margins for primary cutaneous melanoma: updated pooled analysis of RCTs. *Arch of Surg* 2007).
  - Management of regional lymph nodes:
    - risk of LN metastases:
      - <0.75 mm: rare
      - 0.75–1 mm: 5%
      - 1–4 mm: 8–30%
      - >4 mm: 40% or higher
    - 20% of newly diagnosed stage I and II melanoma patients are considered to have an intermediate or high risk of harbouring occult regional nodal disease, whereby elective lymph node dissection (ELND) is not justified
    - SLN identification rate with lymphoscintigraphy and blue dye is >99%
    - Breslow thickness and ulceration are the strongest independent predictors of SLN involvement
    - important prognostic indicator: 5-year survival is 56% if SLN positive vs 90% if SLN negative. Allows for staging of patient, predicts prognosis, and assists with selection for adjuvant therapies
    - indications for SLN biopsy if clinically negative nodes:
      - Breslow >1 mm, need to discuss SLNB
      - patients with melanomas 0.75–1.2 mm with primary tumour demonstrating ulceration
      - Clark level IV or V or high mitotic rate should have discussion of SLNB (12% risk of metastases)
    - MSLT-1: Multicentre Selective Lymphadenectomy Trial 1 for primary melanomas 1.2–3.5 mm were randomised to:
      - (1) wide excision (WE) followed by nodal observation and therapeutic TLND when developed clinical nodal disease or
      - (2) WE plus SLNB followed by complete CLND if SLN positive
      - 5-year disease free survival was 73% in group 1 and 78% group 2. Five-year survival was significantly higher in group 2 compared with group 1 (71% vs 55%). Preliminary follow up information shows a significantly lower rate of distant metastasis in group 2 compared with group 1 (18% vs 21%). No overall survival advantage has been demonstrated yet

        - only 10–20% of patients with a positive SLN are found to have additional microscopic nodal disease within non sentinel LN, so it is unclear whether CLND is indicated. MSLT-2 is addressing this question and is currently recruiting to assess the incidence of nodal failure after removal of a positive SLND in the absence of a completion dissection, the incidence and predictors of additional positive non-SLNDs in the same basin and the survival impact.
    - Clinical nodal disease (confirmed on FNA) requires therapeutic lymph node dissection.
    - Lymph node dissection for melanoma:
        - axilla: level III dissection with resection of pectoralis minor
        - groin: complete clearance of subinguinal LNs in the femoral triangle including Cloquet's node. May be extended to an ilio-inguinal dissection of nodes in the pelvis if evidence of involvement of pelvic (obturator, internal/external iliac) nodes on imaging, gross clinical involvement of >3 groin LNs or clinically suspicious nodes high in the groin
        - neck: modified radical neck dissection, may need to add superficial parotidectomy
        - patients with LN metastases need discussion in a multidisciplinary team with a view to enrolment in clinical trials
        - an alternative to SLNB in older patients is to mark the SLN with lymphoscintigraphy and tattoo and undergo ultrasound follow-up. This may be appropriate as increasing morbidity of SLNB especially of the groin in older patients and even mild lymphoedema may affect the quality of life significantly.
- Treatment of locoregional recurrence:
    - persistent melanoma or melanoma with close margins should be re-excised
    - adjuvant radiotherapy should be considered for close or positive margins unsuitable for repeat resection
    - in-transit metastases and satellitosis:
        - low volume disease can be re-excised
        - local treatments include radiotherapy, cryotherapy, rose Bengal injection, laser
        - rapidly progressive limb disease can be managed with isolated limb infusion, which involves percutaneous cannulation of an artery and vein, proximal occlusion of the blood supply and delivery of local chemotherapy using melphalan under hyperthermic conditions It can achieve 90% response rates and 60–70% complete response rates. Systemic therapies and immuno-modulators may be necessary.
- Regional lymph nodes:
    - SLNB should be considered if recurrence occurs and the nodal basin has not been dissected and no clinical evidence of nodal involvement
    - lymph node dissection for clinically involved nodes following pathological confirmation
    - post-operative radiation therapy should be considered for adverse pathological findings
    - clinical recurrence in a previously dissected nodal basin should be managed by excision followed by RTx.
- The role of radiotherapy (RTx) in melanoma:
    - RTx to primary site for:
        - inoperable disease

    - involved or close margins that cannot have further excision due to anatomical constraints
    - high risk for local recurrence (e.g. Breslow >4 mm, ulceration, satellitosis, lymphovascular invasion).
  - RTx to regional LN basin after LN dissection:
    - >3 LNs involved
    - LN >3 cm
    - extracapsular extension of clinically palpable disease
    - regionally recurrent disease.
  - Palliative radiotherapy for symptomatic bone and brain metastases: brain metastases confer the worst prognosis for stage IV disease (1 year survival 10–15%). Most patients die from complications of CNS metastases. Options for brain metastases include: surgical resection, whole brain radiotherapy (WBRT), stereotactic radiosurgery and chemotherapy. WBRT is standard treatment for melanoma brain metastases. Resection followed by WBRT is superior to WBRT alone for single metastasis.
- The role of surgery in stage IV disease:
  - staging: M1a (skin, soft tissue, LN metastases), M1b (lung metastases), M1c (visceral, brain metastases, raised LDH). Site of metastases affects prognosis
  - metastasectomy: (a) patient selection is crucial; (b) surgical resection of selected patients with metastatic melanoma in up to five sites leads to a 5-year survival of 42.5%; (c) most important prognostic factor for survival is the presence of a solitary metastasis; (d) patients with surgically operable metastasis should be considered for resection.
- Adjuvant therapies for melanoma
  - Immunotherapy:
    - high dose Interferon (IFN) alpha. Only adjuvant regimen approved by FDA for stage IIB, IIC and III patients. Improves relapse-free survival by 10% at 5 years but no overall survival advantage. Substantial toxicity but should be considered in patients at high risk for recurrence
    - interleukin (IL)-2. Proleukin — response in 16% of patients (not used in Australia).
  - Chemotherapy:
    - darcarbazine, temozolomide, fotemustine — complete response rates in < 5%.
  - BRAF inhibitors:
    - 60% of melanomas contain a B-Raf gene mutation. The B-Raf inhibitor, Vemurafenib, acts against V600E mutation in melanoma, and causes apoptosis in melanoma cell lines which carry the mutation. Currently, subject to trial in disseminated disease.
  - Ipilimumab:
    - monoclonal antibody that binds CTLA-4 on cytotoxic T lymphocytes. Approved for use in stage IV melanoma; it causes hepatic toxicity.
- Follow-up of melanoma patients:
  - stage I: 6 monthly for 5 years then yearly thereafter
  - stage II/III/IV: 3–4 monthly for 2 years, 6 monthly until 5 years, yearly thereafter.

Chapter 3.4

The short case clinical examination

A person's way of doing things is the direct result of the way he [she] thinks about things. (Wallace D Wattles, 1860–1911)

The examination format

The short case clinical examination comprises six shorts cases in 40 minutes. Certain patients and cases are suited to the short cases. Organising short cases is a difficult task. Nearly all surgical patients in hospital have been operated on. This means that lumps and bumps and surgical conditions tend to be found coincidentally in patients on the general surgical, medical or vascular wards. Many other patients that are used in the short cases are out-patients with chronic conditions. Accordingly, prediction of the likely cases that you will encounter is possible.

After the bell rings, the examiners take you through each case. The examiners make focused examination statements, such as 'can you examine this man's groin?', 'can you examine this woman's abdomen?', 'can you examine this woman's breast?' or 'can you examine this young lady's thyroid?'. The examiners keep careful track of time and limit you to 6.5 minutes per short case to keep you moving along. For each case, the examiners will let you know whether you can or should ask the patient questions before, during or after the examination. They will usually also let you know if they just want you to examine the patient and not ask any questions.

Exam technique

After introducing yourself to the patient, ask focused questions pertinent to the region being examined (if instructed to ask questions) or just start examining if requested to do so. If you are instructed to ask the patient some questions first, make sure that you leave enough time to complete your examination. Obviously you will need to speak with the patient to gain their cooperation to complete the examination.

To avoid repetition in the description of short cases that follow in Chapter 3.5, a complete structure will not be reiterated for every case described. However, it is imperative that you adhere to the following structure for *every* short case.

1. Listen *carefully* to the examiner's *instruction*.
2. *Approach* and preparation — the 5Ps:
   - **p**lace your hands in the sink or under the hand sanitiser
   - **p**ermission to perform the examination
   - **p**osition the patient
   - **p**reserve the patient's dignity during exposure
   - **p**rogress to the foot of the bed.
3. For most short cases, it is appropriate to divide your examination into three parts, although most time should be spent on part (b) below:
   a. general inspection from the foot of the bed
   b. examination of the system and/or area of interest:
      i. inspection
      ii. palpation
      iii. percussion
      iv. auscultation
      or
      v. look
      vi. feel
      vii. move
   c. examination of associated/allied systems (e.g. for thyroid status following thyroid examination).
4. Conclusion:
   a. say that you would do the things that form part of the examination but that are inappropriate in the exam setting (e.g. digital rectal examination etc.)
   b. cover the patient
   c. reposition the patient
   d. thank the patient
   e. clean your hands again
   f. only now turn to face the examiners.

Avoid causing the patient pain during examination, and only expose what parts need to be accessed during the examination. Kindness, respect and consideration towards the patient are just as important here in the examination as they are in clinical practice.

One common area of contention is whether to report your findings to the examiners as you progress with your examination. This is a stylistic issue and there is no absolute answer. However, reporting your findings as you go along offers two potential advantages. Firstly, you can accumulate points as you examine and emphasise manoeuvres that the examiners may have otherwise missed. Secondly, it is a more efficient use of the time (6.5 mins/case). If you have finished the examination just start talking to the examiners.

Remember to have well-rehearsed routines for all common examinations. In particular, you must be ready and able to comprehensively examine (and describe) any lumps that you detect. We recommend using the following mnemonic 'Should The Children Ever Find Lumps Readily':

S site/size/shape/surface/skin/scars/symmetry
T temperature/tenderness/transilluminability
C colour/consistency/compressibility

E edge/expansility
F fluctuation/fluid thrill/fixation
L lymph nodes
R resonance/relations to surrounding structures.

A standard format for each short case would involve 3 minutes to examine and a further 3 minutes for discussion. You may lead the discussion but sometimes you will be asked questions. If the examiners speak first after the examination, they often ask 'what did you find?', 'can you tell me what you found?' or 'what do you think?'. Summarise concisely and precisely. Sometimes an obvious diagnosis should be stated first, such as 'this woman has a large multinodular goitre causing tracheal compression', 'this man has a large reducible incisional hernia in a midline abdominal incision, on a background of an abdominoperineal excision for rectal cancer. There is a colostomy in the left lower quadrant of the abdomen'. Then continue with a more detailed explanation of the examination findings. Be prepared to be interrupted and do not be put off by the 'stop-start' nature during the physical examination or the discussion. Being stopped does not mean failure. By the contrary, it usually means that you are doing well and the examination needs to move on.

The discussion of the short case will often involve:

- a summary of the physical findings (if not already described during the examination)
- a provisional diagnosis and differential diagnosis
- a discussion of disease factors, patient factors, investigations and treatment as in the medium case in Chapter 3.2
- you will commonly be shown relevant imaging such as CT scans and be asked to discuss and comment on them.

Many of these techniques will be demonstrated in the model answers in Chapter 3.5.

Preparation and practising

Look at the list of common short cases in Chapter 1.3 and make sure that you can perform a perfect examination for each of these cases. You absolutely *must* have a methodical and deliberate structure for examination of each of the common surgical systems. The examination must be well rehearsed and you need to be fluent. In Chapter 3.5, examples of common short cases will be provided. However, you must be competent performing examination of superficial lumps and ulcers; the neck and thyroid gland; the abdomen and trunk, including ventral and groin hernia and scrotal contents; the breast; the musculoskeletal system for peripheral nerve injuries; the circulation and lymphatics, including arterial and venous system assessment, as well as the diabetic foot, as a minimum. The use of a dedicated clinical examination book is mandatory (see the suggested reading list in Chapter 1.4).

As with many other parts of the fellowship examination, repeated practise is imperative so that you can deliver a faultless, flowing performance in front of the examiners. This section of the examination offers the opportunity to really 'hit home-runs' with straightforward surgical cases, such as hernia, abdominal examination etc. However, the ability to conduct clinical examinations of such common cases is fully expected of surgical trainees and this brings with it a unique pressure that adversely affects many candidates in this part of the examination. During the examination it is important that you demonstrate to the examiners that you have sound clinical examination skills and that you are capable of detecting clinical signs with your technique. Your examinations must be smooth and confident. You can only achieve this level of performance if you have practised many times with your colleagues and in front of your mentors. The examiners will be fully able to judge how experienced you are. You must be able to perform the examination automatically without thinking about what comes next so that you can focus your attention on the detection of clinical signs and their assimilation to create meaningful, accurate differential diagnoses.

Chapter 3.5

Common short cases

3.5.1 Inguinal hernia

See also 4.2.1 Laparoscopic preperitoneal anatomy, 4.4.1 Inguinal hernia repair and 4.4.2 obstructed femoral hernia.

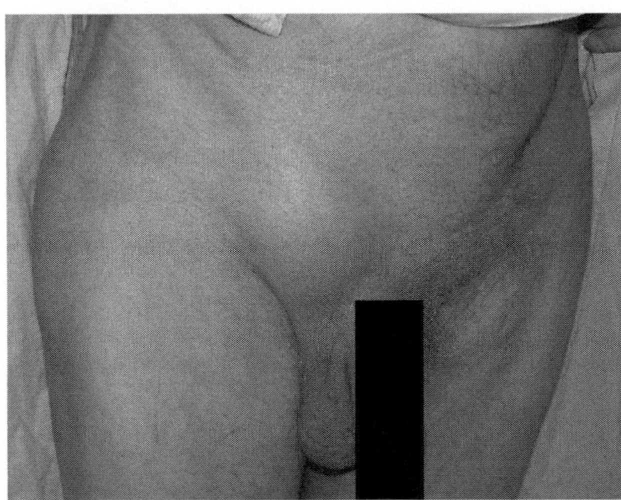

Figure 3.5.1
Right inguinal hernia

Instruction

'Please examine this man's groin.'

Approach

- Wash your hands or use the hand sanitiser.
- Introduce yourself and ask permission to perform the examination.
- Expose the patient from umbilicus to knees.
- Ask the patient if there is any pain anywhere.
- Often an obvious lump is visible.

- It doesn't matter if the hernia is examined with the patient lying down or standing up. It is generally considered to be easier to define the anatomy with the patient supine, and if the hernia can be detected with the patient on the couch, then examine there. If no lump can be felt, or if no couch is available, then stand the patient up first.

- The three objectives of the examination are to:
  - confirm that the lump is a hernia
  - differentiate an inguinal from a femoral hernia
  - if it is an inguinal hernia, establish whether it is direct or indirect.

Inspection

1. Scars (is it a recurrent hernia?).
2. Look for lump/swelling — describe its relation to the pubic tubercle. Is it above or below the inguinal ligament. Does it extend into the scrotum?
3. If the hernia is obvious, then begin to examine it.
4. If it cannot be seen then ask the patient to cough and observe for a lump.
5. If it is still not obvious, ask 'Have you noticed a lump in your groin?' and get the patient to demonstrate it / stand up.

Palpation

1. Confirm the presence of a cough impulse. This fulfills objective 1 above.
2. Define the anatomy — location of the pubic tubercle and ASIS.
3. Demonstrate the inguinal ligament running between these two points.
4. Is the hernia arising above the ligament (inguinal) or below and lateral to pubic tubercle (femoral)? This fulfills objective 2 above.
5. What is the relation to the femoral artery (located 1–2 cm below the mid-inguinal point).
6. Does it extend into the scrotum?
7. If the hernia is persistently protruding out, ask the patient if the hernia is reducible.
8. Try not attempt to reduce the hernia in the standing position. Ask the patient to lie supine and reduce the hernia.
9. With the hernia reduced, place your finger over the deep ring (1 cm above the mid-point of the inguinal ligament), then stand the patient up and/or ask him or her to cough. If this stops the hernia from coming out, it is most likely an indirect hernia.
10. Also, if the hernia extends into the scrotum it is likely to be an indirect hernia.
11. Examine both groins.
12. Examine both testicles.

Auscultation

- If the lump is irreducible listen for bowel sounds.

Complete the examination if allowed by performing a full abdominal examination; tell the examiner that you would like to finish by doing a digital rectal examination to assess for rectal and prostatic pathology.

The discussion

1. Summarise the findings to the examiner.
2. What is the differential diagnosis of a lump in the groin?

- Skin and soft tissue:
  - sebaceous cyst
  - lipoma
  - lymph node.
- Urogenital:
  - undescended testes
  - hydrocoele of the cord/lipoma of cord
  - renal transplant.
- Vascular:
  - femoral artery aneurysm/pseudoaneurysm
  - saphenovarix.
- Hernia:
  - inguinal
  - femoral.

Acronym **L-SHAPE**:

Lymph node
Saphenovarix
Hernia
Aneurysm of femoral artery
Psoas abscess/pathology
Ectopic testicle.

3. When do you repair an inguinal hernia?
   - Repair of all symptomatic hernias should be considered (pain/incarceration/strangulation/obstruction/perforation).
   - Asymptomatic hernias in high risk patients can be observed. Recent randomised evidence has suggested that there is no increase in morbidity or mortality with observation. However, approximately 25% of these patients will become symptomatic within the next 2 years and will require repair.
   - Those patients who are at an increased risk for general anaesthesia can have the hernia repaired under local anaesthesia. This is especially beneficial in patients with severe respiratory disease.
   - All femoral hernia should be repaired in patients fit for surgery.
4. What are the complications of inguinal hernia repair?
   - General: bleeding, haematoma, wound infection, respiratory infection, DVT/PE.
   - Procedure specific:
     - urinary retention (1%)
     - ischaemic orchitis (0.5%) — due to traction injury/direct trauma to the testicular artery or pampiniform plexus of veins resulting in thrombosis
     - recurrence (0.5–1%) for open repair, 2% for laparoscopic repair
     - major vessel, bowel, or bladder injury with laparoscopic repair
     - mesh infection (1%)
     - chronic pain (0.5–5%) — pain is normal after hernia repair but should improve steadily over 4–6 weeks recovery. During this time heavy lifting, strenuous exercise, straining or any activity that causes increased intra-abdominal pressure should be avoided. Pain that persists beyond 6–8 weeks post-operatively should initially be managed conservatively as the majority will slowly resolve after 6–12 months. During this time patients should avoid activity that produces pain and be prescribed anti-inflammatory drugs such as ibuprofen for pain relief.

The aetiology of chronic pain is not clearly understood but believed to be due to either: inguinal nerve injury, pubic tubercle trauma or the presence of the mesh itself. If pain persists beyond 6–12 months after repair then investigate:

- ultrasound to exclude recurrence
- bone scan to rule out pubic osteitis
- CT or MRI to rule out pelvic pathology and spinal diseases.

If above investigations are normal, refer to a pain clinic for steroid injections with local anaesthetic into the painful area. If these injections are unsuccessful, then more intensive, specific medication or possible radiofrequency ablation (RFA) or cryoprobe should be considered to alleviate pain. If pain is still persistent after these endeavours, groin exploration with triple neurectomy and possible mesh removal may be warranted.

5. What are the contents of the spermatic cord?
    - Rule of 3s
        - **3** layers of fascia:
            - external spermatic; from the external oblique aponeurosis
            - cremasteric; from the internal oblique aponeurosis
            - internal spermatic; from the transversalis fascia.
        - **3** arteries:
            - testicular artery (from the aorta)
            - cremasteric artery (from the inferior epigastric artery)
            - artery of the vas (from the inferior vesical artery).
        - **3** veins:
            - the pampiniform plexus of veins (draining the right testis into the inferior vena cava and the left into the left renal vein)
            - the cremasteric vein
            - vein of the vas deferens.
        - **3** nerves:
            - the genital branch of the genitofemoral nerve which supplies the cremaster
            - sympathetic fibres from T10–11
            - ilioinguinal nerve (lies on the cord).
        - Vas deferens.
        - Lymphatics.
6. What pathogenic factors are involved in the development of groin hernias?
    - Congenital:
        - male — patent processus vaginalis
        - connective tissue disorders — Marfan's syndrome, Ehlers-Danlos syndrome, Down's syndrome.
    - Acquired — thought to be due to increased intra-abdominal pressure:
        - male
        - increasing age
        - obesity
        - smokers
        - malnutrition
        - steroids
        - chronic cough
        - prostatic obstruction
        - straining at defaecation
        - pregnancy
        - ascites.

7. What are the benefits of laparoscopic versus open repair?
    - The decision to perform an open 'tension-free' mesh repair versus laparoscopic mesh repair remains a controversial area. Current evidence favours laparoscopic repair over open repair for recurrent or bilateral hernias. On the other hand, there seems to be agreement that large inguinal scrotal hernias are better repaired by an open technique. The jury still remains undecided with regard to the ideal surgical approach for other inguinal or femoral hernia.
    - Systematic reviews have demonstrated that laparoscopic repair is associated with less post-operative pain, quicker return to normal activities and work. However, there is an increased risk of rare and serious complications. Also, laparoscopic repair is more costly.
    - A large multicentre trial performed in the USA (N Engl J Med. 2004; 350: 1819) included 1983 patients randomly assigned to an open tension-free mesh repair or laparoscopic mesh repair demonstrated that patients who underwent laparoscopic repair had:
        - less pain on day 1 and at 2 weeks
        - returned to work one day earlier
        - higher recurrence rates at 2 years (10.1% vs 4.9 %)
        - more complications (39% vs 33.4%)
        - more serious complications (1.1% vs 0.1%) (bowel/ bladder/ major vascular injury).
    - The pros and cons of both procedures need to be discussed carefully with patients. Laparoscopic repair may be advantageous in returning patients who perform heavy manual labour to work earlier and open repair may be particularly advantageous in an older, less healthy patient. Open repair, as with laparoscopic repair, generally does not require overnight hospital stay.
8. When is ultrasound used in the assessment of groin hernias?
    - Groin pain with clinically insignificant hernia.
    - Groin pain with no evidence of a hernia.
    - Post-hernia surgery groin pain to exclude recurrence/missed hernia /identify other pathology (e.g. neuroma).

3.5.2 Incisional hernia

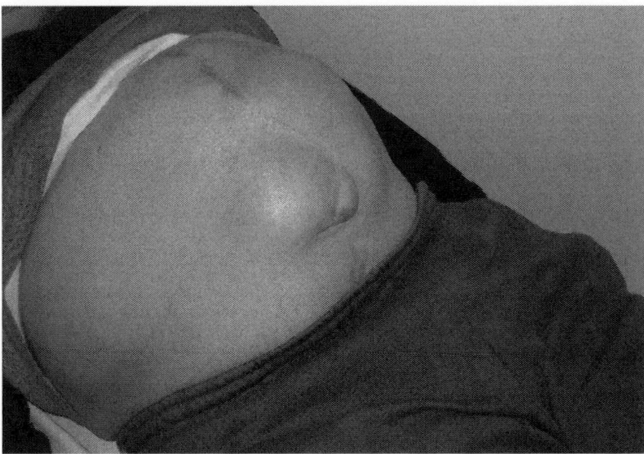

Figure 3.5.2
Incisional hernia

Instruction

'Please examine this patient's abdomen.'

Approach

- Wash your hands or use the hand sanitiser.
- Introduce yourself and ask permission to perform the examination.
- Lay the patient flat with one pillow beneath the head.
- Expose the patient from umbilicus to symphysis pubis.
- Ask the patient if there is any pain anywhere.

These notes should be read in conjunction with 3.3.8 and 3.5.13, abdominal mass medium and short case respectively.

Inspection

1. Look for and comment on obesity, striae, scars, swellings or lumps beneath the scar(s), distension or visible peristalsis.
2. Ask the patient to cough and look at scar(s) to see a cough impulse.
3. Ask patient to lift his/her head off the bed and see if the scar 'bulges'.

Palpation

1. Ask the patient if there is any pain or tenderness in the abdomen before palpating.
2. Palpate over the scar and ask the patient to cough to confirm your inspection findings.
3. Ask the patient to lift his/her head off the bed to help define the size and extent of the hernia.
4. Determine the width of the defect and whether the defect is the entire length of the scar.
5. If there are contents in the hernia sac, ask the patient if it is reducible. If yes gently reduce contents.
6. Complete the examination by palpating the abdomen for tenderness/masses/organomegaly/ascites. Examine both groins for herniae and the testicles in men.
7. Tell the examiner you would like to finish your examination by doing a digital rectal examination.

Percussion

Percussion of the abdomen may further characterise the hernia and associated masses or organs (liver/spleen/bladder). Check for ascites by shifting dullness/testing for a fluid thrill.

Auscultation

Auscultate for bowel sounds over a hernia to help determine whether there is bowel in the hernia.

The discussion

1. What factors predispose to incisional herniation?
   - Patient related factors:
     - advancing age, smoking, obesity, diabetes, medications (e.g. steroids, immunosuppressants, chemotherapy etc.), malignancy, renal failure, COPD, prostate enlargement, liver disease/ascites, gross intra-abdominal infection/contamination.

- Operative factors:
  - closure with too much tension on sutures, inadequate suture bites, wrong suture material.
- Post-operative factors:
  - wound infection, haematoma, respiratory infection, early intra-abdominal straining — going back to heavy work before 8 weeks post-operative recovery.

2. What are the complications of incisional hernia?
   - Pain, incarceration, strangulation, obstruction, skin excoriation.
3. What are the indications and contraindications for surgery?
   - Asymptomatic incisional hernias (with wide necks) can be managed conservatively in patients with multiple comorbidities or those who don't want surgery.
   - Surgical intervention is warranted in the following:
     - acute presentation with symptoms suggestive of complications (obstruction, strangulation, incarceration, perforation)
     - symptomatic hernias or those that complicate daily activities (e.g. dressing)
     - hernias with a high risk of complications (i.e. those with small necks/fascial defects).
   - Hernias that are less likely to become complicated include:
     - those in the upper abdomen
     - <1 cm in diameter, and >7–8 cm diameter (where bowel can move without restriction).
   - Contraindications to elective repair are those that preclude elective surgery (i.e. the unstable or high-risk patient due to comorbidities e.g. renal failure/chronic liver disease/severe cardiac or respiratory disease).
4. What are the surgical options?
   - Direct suture repair — the edges of the hernia sac are dissected out and defined, healthy fascia is exposed circumferentially. The fascial edges are sutured together with an appropriate non-absorbable suture (1 or 1/0 nylon or polypropylene) placing the sutures 1 cm from the fascia edge and 1 cm apart. This provides the optimal healing and reduces ischaemia. While outcome studies demonstrate a higher recurrence rate compared to mesh repair, it is still considered the appropriate repair for small hernias (<2 to 3 cm in greatest diameter). Suturing techniques such as Mayo/Keel repair may provide additional strength and reduce recurrence rates.
   - Mesh repair procedures.
     - Onlay — the mesh is placed above the fascia. Approximately 3 cm of healthy fascia is exposed beyond the margins of the hernia defect. If possible, the fascia is brought together and closed with sutures and a lightweight mesh is then placed over the repair and secured with sutures.
     - Inlay — the mesh is placed within the hernia defect as a bridge between the fascial edges. This provides a tension-free primary bridging of a large fascia defect. The mesh is fixed to the fascial edges by means of a running or interrupted sutures. Specific meshes have been designed (Gore Tex/Dual mesh/

PROCEED/PHYSIOMESH etc.) that permit placement in direct contact with peritoneal contents in the belief that there is reduced adherence to intraperitoneal structures.
  - Sublay — the mesh is placed beneath the fascia. The sublay technique has lower recurrence rates compared to both the onlay or inlay techniques. Sublay involves dissection of the hernia sac both above and beneath the fasica, ideally staying in the extraperitoneal plane. The mesh is then secured with sutures to the posterior surface of the sheath using non-absorbable sutures. The overlying anterior fascia is then closed to either itself or the mesh, depending on the degree of tension encountered.
  - The main complications of mesh repair are seroma formation and chronic mesh infection as a result of drainage procedures.
- Component separation — this involves, as the name suggests, the separation of the fasica and muscular components of the anterior abdominal wall to mobilise fascia to allow closure of the midline and abolition of the hernia defect. The hernia sac is dissected free and reduced into the abdomen. The subcutaneous tissue of abdominal wall is undermined to expose the external oblique aponeurosis all the way laterally beyond the mid-axillary line. The external oblique aponeurosis is incised 1–2 cm lateral to the lateral border of rectus abdominis muscle, from iliac crest to costal margin. This enables the fascial edges to be brought together in the midline without tension and without prosthetic material. Substantial hernia defects can be closed using this technique. The advantage of component separation is that it avoids the potential complications associated with the use of mesh (e.g. seroma formation, pain, chronic infection). This technique may also be employed laparoscopically.
- Laparoscopic mesh repairs — this technique involves placement of a large mesh intraperitoneally with a minimum of 3 cm overlap around the hernia defect. The technique of laparoscopic ventral hernia repair (LVHR) involves:
  - creation of a pneumoperitoneum
  - placement of laparoscopic ports
  - adhesiolysis to expose hernia defect
  - reduction of the hernia contents
  - measurement and placement of mesh sized to cover the defect with a 3 cm overlap
  - placement of sutures in four quadrants of the mesh to anchor it in place via small skin incisions. The suture ends are retrieved and tied loosely in a subcutaneous transfascial position
  - tacking of mesh into place with tacks (preferably absorbable)
  - drains are not usually used, unless the defect is large.

In LVHR, the mesh will almost always be in contact with bowel, and it is therefore important that the mesh be treated so that it does not provoke a high degree of adhesion (Gore-Tex/Dual Mesh/PROCEED etc.). Extreme care must be taken to avoid inadvertent and unrecognised bowel injury during adhesiolysis, as this can result in significant complications and potentially death.

3.5.3 Goitre

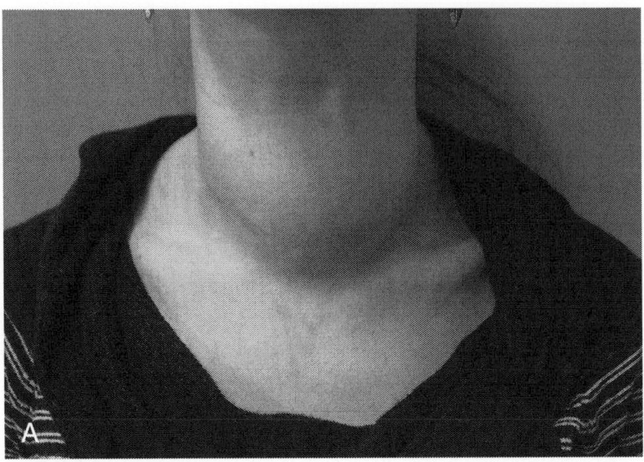

Figure 3.5.3A
Goitre from front

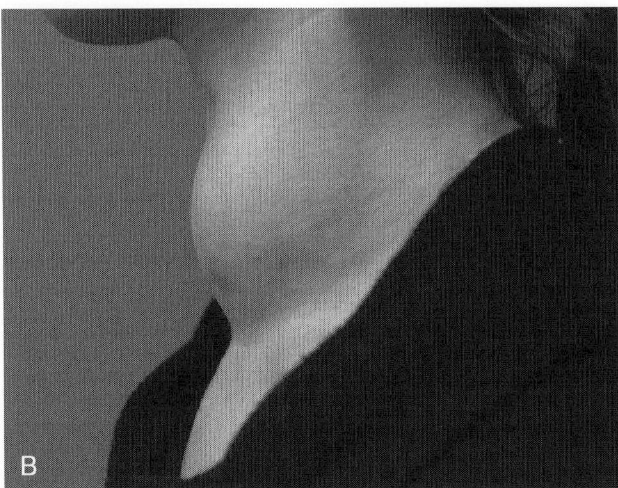

Figure 3.5.3B
Goitre from left side

This section should be read in conjunction with: 2.4.6, solitary thyroid nodules; 2.4.7 thyrotoxicosis; 4.2.3 thyroidectomy anatomy; 4.4.9 thyroglossal cysts; 4.6.8 thyroid cancer; and 4.6.9 multinodular goitre.

Instruction

'Please examine this woman's neck.'

Often the examiner will suggest that you ask the patient a 'few questions' (see below). Usually an obvious lump is visible. Focused history and inspection, will give you an indication whether you are dealing with a case of thyrotoxicosis or a thyroid nodule. Also listen to cues from the examiner. During the focused history, you can comment on whether the patient has a hoarse voice.

The history (if allowed or requested)

1. Symptoms related to the goitre:
   - duration/change in size
   - pain
   - mechanical symptoms:
     - discomfort during swallowing/dysphagia
     - dyspnoea/shortness of breath
   - hoarseness/change in voice
   - cosmetic symptoms.
2. Symptoms of thyroid dysfunction:

System	Hyperthyroidism	Hypothyroidism
Appetite	Increased	Decreased
Weight	Decreased	Increased
Thermoregulation	Heat intolerance	Cold intolerance
GI	Frequent, loose stools	Constipation
Neurological	Fine tremor	Carpal tunnel
Cardiovascular	Tachycardia/palpitations	Bradycardia
Neuropsychiatric	Nervous/irritable	Slow/depressed
Skin	Sweating	Dry skin/hair loss
Musculoskeletal	Proximal weakness	Fatigue

3. Associated symptoms — especially eye symptoms in thyrotoxicosis.
4. Associated symptoms of familial MEN syndromes: phaeochromocytoma (hypertension, sweats), hypercalcaemia (stones, bones, groans, psychic moans).
5. Past history of radiation increases index of suspicion, thyroid surgery, radioactive iodine.
6. Family History: Enquire specifically about familial thyroid cancer syndromes. These include medullary thyroid Cancer, MEN 2a, MEN 2b and Cowden's syndrome (PTEN).

Approach

- Wash your hands or use the hand sanitiser.
- Introduce yourself and ask permission to perform the examination.
- Expose the neck down to both clavicles.
- Ask the patient if there is any pain anywhere.

- Remember the objectives of the thyroid examination:
  - confirm that the abnormality is within the thyroid
  - determine if the enlargement is diffuse (smooth vs nodular) or due to a solitary nodule
  - examine the surrounding structures
  - assess the thyroid status of the patient.

Inspection

1. General inspection: looks well, frightened faces, sweating, anorexic (wasting).
2. Closer inspection focusing on the neck. Any scars? Jugular venous engorgement?
3. Determine if there is any swelling and confirm that it is in the midline.
4. Assess for thyroglossal cyst versus thyroid enlargement by initially extending the neck and then getting the patient to protrude the tongue.
5. Assess thyroid: ask for a glass of water for the patient and ask them to take a sip. The thyroid will rise with swallowing. Comment on it. Inspect lateral neck for any swelling.

Palpation

Approach from behind the patient.

1. Feel for the thyroid gland, which is lateral to trachea but anterior to SCM (within anterior triangle). Often deep palpation of both is necessary but be careful not to hurt the patient. Fix one lobe whilst examining the other.
2. Feel whether the enlargement is diffuse (smooth or nodular) or confined to a solitary nodule. Assess the consistency, characterise any nodules: fixed, texture, size, tender, solitary v multiple.
3. Again get patient to take sip of water. Can I get above it? Can I get below it? Retrosternal? Retroclavicular?
4. Lateral node exam: level 2 to 5 plus central level 6 (stratifying spread if thyroid cancer suspected).

Return to the front of the patient.

5. Check that the trachea is not deviated.

Percussion and auscultation

1. Percuss over the sternum for retrosternal extension and listen for a bruit from a high blood flow through the thyroid (pertinent to Graves' disease or a thyrotoxic patient).

Assess thyroid status and special tests

1. Hands: increased sweating, palmar erythema, thyroid acropachy (pseudo-clubbing), onycholysis (Plummer's nails — concave or ragged edge to nail bed), pulse, tremor.
2. Eyes: seven signs:
   - loss of hair, outer-third eyebrow
   - lid retraction
   - lid lag
   - ophthalmoplegia
   - exophthalmos
   - chemosis
   - proptosis.
3. Assess for Pemberton's sign. Ask the patient to lift the arms above their head for 1 minute. Pemberton's sign: facial flushing, distended head and neck superficial veins, raised JVP and inspiratory stridor with elevation of the arms, due to thoracic inlet obstruction (retrosternal goitre).
4. Finish by examining the lower limbs for:
   - proximal myopathy
   - pretibial myxoedema
   - slowly relaxing reflexes (hypothyroidism).

The discussion

1. Summarise findings to examiner.
2. Having performed a focused history and thorough examination, it will become evident whether the thyroid is diffusely enlarged (smooth/nodular) or contains a solitary nodule.
   - Diffuse enlargement — smooth or nodular:
     - multinodular goitre
     - toxic (i.e. hyperthyroid) = Grave's disease

- simple colloid goitre
- thyroiditis; for example, subacute (granulomatous) — de Quervain's; autoimmune (Hashimoto's); or Reidel's (invasive fibrous); in these cases the thyroid may be tender
- neoplastic goitre — benign/malignant.

- Solitary nodule:
  - degenerative cysts
  - neoplasms: benign (follicular adenoma), malignant — primary (papillary, follicular, medullary, anaplastic squamous cell carcinoma and malignant lymphoma) or secondary (metastatic from breast/kidney)
  - dominant nodule of a multinodular goitre masquerading as an 'apparently' solitary nodule.

3. At this point ask for results of supplementary investigations: TSH, ultrasound or nuclear medicine scan if thyrotoxic, fine needle aspiration cytology if performed.

3.5.4 Parotid mass

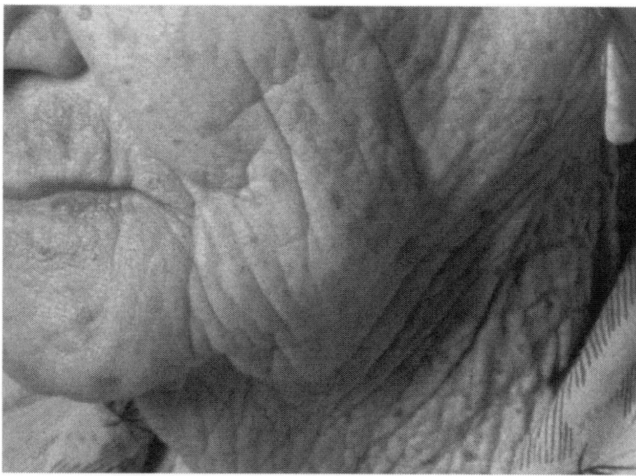

Figure 3.5.4
Left parotid mass

Instruction

'Please examine this woman's face and neck.'

Approach

- Wash your hands or use the hand sanitiser.
- Introduce yourself and ask permission to perform the examination.
- Expose the patient's neck down to the clavicles.
- Ask the patient if there is any pain anywhere.
- Explain to the patient that you will speak to the examiner as you examine.

- Things you *must not* forget in a parotid exam:
  - examination of the facial nerve
  - examination of the scalp for primary lesions
  - look inside the mouth/offer to perform bimanual examination and
  - examine the draining lymph nodes.

Inspection

1. Look at both sides of the face and neck.
2. Are there any scars?
3. Describe the mass that you find using the mnemonic 'Should The Children Ever Find Lumps Readily' (see above, and 'exam technique' in Chapter 3.4) to guide you.
4. Examine the entire scalp, face and neck for skin lesions/masses.
5. Ask the patient to open the mouth and inspect the opening of the parotid ducts (opposite 2nd upper molar).

A commentary to the examiner may go as follows: 'There is a mass in the right parotid region. The overlying skin is normal. I am looking for skin lesions or other masses in the region of the head and neck. I am looking over the scalp, behind the ear, over the face and the neck on both sides. I would like to have a look inside the mouth with a torch.'

Palpation

1. Continue the examination of the lump to ascertain all the characteristics of the mass by completing the mnemonic 'Should The Children Ever Find Lumps Readily'.
2. Establish which layer the mass lies in by drawing the skin over the top and checking relations to surrounding structures.
3. Offer to perform a bimanual examination, including assessment of the parotid duct. IF instructed to proceed, don a pair of gloves and examine inside the mouth bimanually.
4. Check for a facial nerve palsy by getting the patient to:
   - raise the eyebrows
   - screw the eyes tightly shut whilst you try to open them
   - whistle
   - blow out the cheeks whilst preventing you from 'popping' them
   - smile.
5. Move behind the patient (if possible) to palpate the nodal regions of the neck in a logical sequence (see 3.5.5 below).

The discussion

1. Summarise your findings. This may go something like, 'There is a solitary mass in the right parotid gland. The mass is not tender. It is 2 × 2 cm in size and discrete. It is ovoid and solid but not hard. The skin is mobile over the mass. The mass is not pulsatile or expansile. It does not transilluminate. There are no skin lesions in the head or neck, signs of previous surgery or lesions in the oral cavity. There are no masses in the lymph nodes of the neck. The facial nerve function is normal. This is likely to be a pleomorphic adenoma.'

2. What is the differential diagnosis for enlargement of the parotid gland?
   SIN:
   - **S**tones
   - **I**nfections/**i**nflammatory:
     - bacterial (staph, strep, E.coli, TB)
     - viral (mumps)
     - autoimmune (Sjogren's syndrome).
   - **N**eoplasia
     - benign:
       - pleomorphic adenoma
       - Warthin's tumour
       - monomorphic adenoma
       - oncocytoma.
     - malignant (primary/secondary):
       - adenocarcinoma
       - adenoid cystic carcinoma
       - mucoepidermoid carcinoma
       - acinar cell carcinoma
       - lymphoma
       - SCC.
3. How would you evaluate parotid lesions?
   - Clinical evaluation:
     - complete history and examination, including skin and scalp, ears (pneumatic otoscopy), mouth (lip, buccal mucosa, tongue including bimanual palpation), oropharynx and flexible nasendoscopic examination of nasopharynx, hypopharynx and larynx. Systematic cranial nerve examination. The chest and abdomen should also be examined.
   - Imaging:
     - (sialography); USS; CT scan; MRI
     - Consider complete imaging of head, neck and chest.
   - Fine needle aspiration cytology:
     - can be useful and influence decision to operate
     - concerns re: diagnostic accuracy in low-grade malignant lesions.
4. What is the treatment of parotid lesions?
   - If the FNA suggests a benign lesion or is non-diagnostic, I would recommend a superficial parotidectomy (for excision biopsy). Possibly enucleation for Warthin's tumour.
   - If the FNA shows malignancy, management would depend on what type:
     - total conservative parotidectomy for benign neoplasms within the deep lobe and for low-grade malignant tumours and occasionally high-grade malignant tumours without involvement of the facial nerve
     - radical parotidectomy for high-grade adenocarcinoma of the parotid.
   - If SCC is evident on FNA:
     - triple endoscopy under GA (oropharynx; nasopharynx; bronchial tree)
     - if no lesion is seen, blind biopsy of tonsillar fossa, piriform sinus (hypopharynx), nasopharynx and base of tongue
     - if still no primary is found, a modified radical neck dissection is performed on the ipsilateral side with post-operative RT to treat neck and likely occult primary sites.

3.5.5 Neck lymphadenopathy

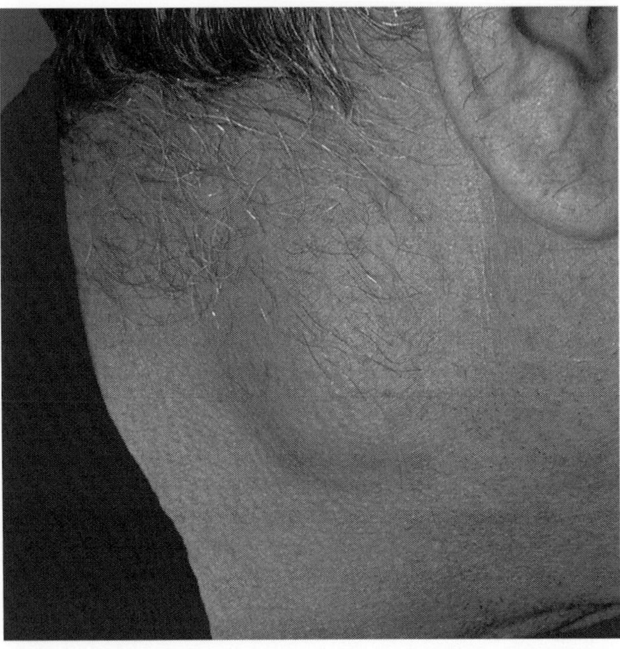

Figure 3.5.5
Mass in right side of neck

Instruction

'This patient has been complaining of a lump on the back of his neck for the past few months. Please examine this patient's neck.'

Approach

- Wash your hands or use the hand sanitiser.
- Introduce yourself and ask permission to perform the examination.
- Expose the patient down to the clavicles — you may need to expose the upper torso too.
- Ask the patient if there is any pain anywhere.
- Remember that the objective of this station is to identify the lymph nodes involved (describing their level) and determine the aetiology for enlargement. If you are doing well, there is an opportunity to discuss your treatment pathway.

Inspection

1. Are there any scars?
2. Examine the entire scalp, face and neck for skin lesions/masses.
3. If there is an obvious mass visible, describe it using the mnemonic 'Should The Children Ever Find Lumps Readily' (see above, and 'exam technique' in Chapter 3.4).
4. If no mass is evident, proceed to palpate all lymph nodes as described below.

Palpation

1. Move behind the patient (if possible) and palpate the nodal regions of the neck in a logical sequence:
   - begin at the chin — submental nodes
   - move along the jawline — submandibular nodes
   - at the ear — pre- and post-auricular nodes
   - move down the sternomastoid to the clavicles — upper/middle/lower jugular chain nodes
   - move laterally along the clavicles — supraclavicular nodes
   - move up towards the occiput — posterior triangle nodes
   - finish with the occipital nodes.
2. Systematically palpate all levels of lymph nodes bilaterally with the pads of your index and middle fingers. Report your findings as you go; for example, 'I am now feeling for level I lymph nodes, which appear normal' etc.
3. Examine the index node in detail. Report what you find. For example, the node is rubbery (hard/fixed/mobile), non-tender, approximately 2 cm in size with or without overlying skin changes.
4. Continue your examination to identify possible underlying aetiology.
5. Examine the scalp, behind the ear, the face and neck for any obvious skin lesion, especially melanomas.
6. Examine the oral cavity and thyroid gland for malignancy.

Conclusion

1. Say that you would like to go on and examine:
   - the nasopharynx
   - the rest of the lymphoproliferative system (other groups of lymph nodes, spleen and liver).

The discussion

1. What are the causes of cervical lymphadenopathy?
   - Use the acronym **LIST**:
     - **L**ymphoma
     - **I**nfection
     - **S**arcoidosis
     - **T**umour — primary or secondary
       - secondary: metastasis from other primary skin or aerodigestive system (e.g. nasopharyngeal cancer, tonsillar/tongue/laryngeal cancer, Virchow's node in left supraclavicular fossa may suggest gastric and other GIT cancers).
   - Infections can be sub-classified:
     - bacterial (strep/TB)
     - viral (CMV/Infectious mononucleosis/HIV)
     - protozoal
     - toxoplasmosis.
2. What further investigations would you perform in a patient with cervical lymphadenopathy?
   - Blood tests: haematological; viral serology, blood cultures.
   - Radiological: USS, CT scan, MRI.
   - Depending on the index of suspicion the patient will require either:
     - FNA aspiration for cytology of the node, preferably ultrasound guided or
     - excisional biopsy (if lymphoma suspected — ideally not SCC as spoils surgical field).

- If malignancy:
  - SCC: look for the primary cancer. The patient may require panendoscopy with biopsy of the primary lesion, ultrasound of the neck, CT scan of neck/thorax +/- abdomen and a PET scan
  - adenocarcinoma: look for thyroid/gastrointestinal/breast primary.
- Recruit the assistance of an oncologist or a haematologist to offer the patient comprehensive and multidisciplinary management.

3. Describe the various levels of cervical lymph nodes and tell me which sites drain to them.

LYMPH NODE LEVEL	ANATOMICAL LEVEL	SITES DRAINING
Level I	Submental and submandibular nodes	Floor of mouth, anterior tongue, lower lip, submandibular gland nasopharynx
Level II	Upper jugular chain of nodes	Oropharynx, nasopharynx, nasal cavity, larynx and parotid gland
Level III	Mid jugular nodes, bounded superiorly by the level of hyoid bone and inferiorly by the cricoid cartilage	Oral cavity, nasopharynx, hypopharynx, larynx
Level IV	Lower jugular behind lower border of SCM	Larynx, hypopharynx, thyroid and cervical oesophagus
Level V	Posterior triangle lymph nodes; nodes along spinal accessory nerve	Nasopharynx, oropharynx and skin of posterior scalp and neck. Virchow's node (GIT system related to thoracic duct drainage)
Level VI	Central compartment lymph nodes containing thyroid gland, bordered superiorly by hyoid bone and inferiorly innominate artery and laterally carotid sheath	Thyroid gland, subglottic larynx, cervical trachea, hypopharynx and cervical oesophagus

3.5.6 Dupuytren's contracture

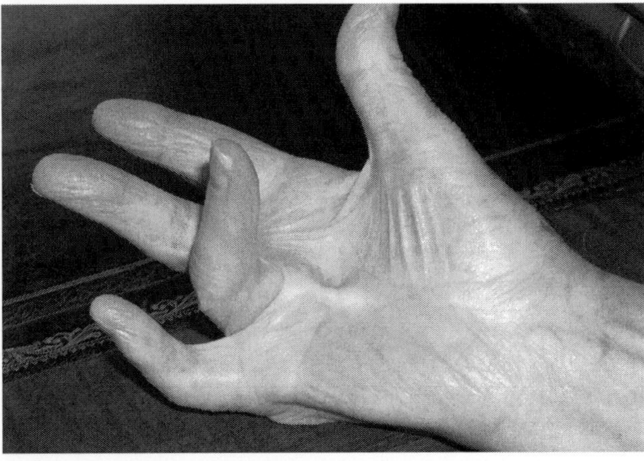

Figure 3.5.6
Dupuytren's contracture

Instruction

'Examine this patient's hands, but first ask him a few questions.'

Approach

- Wash your hands or use the hand sanitiser.
- Introduce yourself and ask permission to perform the examination.
- Ask the patient if there is any pain anywhere.
- Expose to elbows and ask the patient to place his hands palm upwards on a pillow (if available).

The history (if allowed or requested)

1. Ask the patient his age and which hand is his dominant hand.
2. Duration of symptoms and degree of functional impairment.
3. Past medical history; for example, diabetes.
4. Family history — patients less than 40–50 years of age usually have a family history and tend to have recurrence after surgery, including involvement of the non-dominant hand.
5. Occupational and social history — specifically assessing exposure to repetitive handling or vibration, and current cigarette smoking or alcohol consumption.

Look

1. Look at both hands; palmar and dorsal surfaces.
2. Describe any tethering or pitting of the skin on the palmar aspect of the hand and also note the appearance of any visible cords.
3. Look for fibrous nodules in the palm without significant deformity, which may signify early stages of the disease.
4. Look for scars from previous surgery.
5. Describe any flexion deformities at the metacarpophalangeal and proximal interphalangeal joints (MCPJ and PIPJ) of the involved fingers (ring and little fingers most commonly involved).
6. Look for involvement of the thumb and the first web space (a sign of more aggressive disease).
7. Ask the patient to turn his hands over to look for Garrod's pads (thickening of the subcutaneous tissues) over the PIPJ.
8. Joints should appear normal (no swelling/subluxation).
9. Exclude leukonychia, clubbing, palmar erythema, bruising, asterixis (peripheral stigmata of chronic liver disease).
10. Look for similar deformities on the other hand (Dupuytren diathesis has bilateral involvement and is familial).

Feel

1. Feel both palms, palpating the swelling, particularly noting its fixation to skin. Fibrous nodules in the palm along the flexor tendons, which may be mildly tender.
2. Palpate the muscle bulk of the thenar and hypothenar eminences.
3. Gently squeeze MCP joints to elicit tenderness, palpate each MCP, PIP and DIP joint. Inflammatory rheumatological signs are typically absent (erythema, joint swelling and pain).

Move

1. Assess the range of passive and active movement (flexion/extension) in the involved fingers.
2. Note the presence of fixed deformities by passively moving the involved joints.
3. Demonstrate movements to patient. Ask the patient to:
   - place the palms together to extend the wrists
   - place the backs of the hands together to flex the wrists
   - make two fists
   - fully extend the fingers
   - spread all the fingers apart, then back adduct together again
   - touch the thumb to the little finger.

Note the ability to extend MCP, PIP and DIP joints of affected digits.

4. Test passive extension of the affected joints, and measure or estimate the degree of flexion deformity, as this is used to stage the disease.
5. Assessment of functional status: assess grip strength, opposition strength, perform a practical task (e.g. undoing a shirt button).
6. Ask the patient to lay the involved hand flat against a hard surface, e.g. a table. This may facilitate assessment of the deformities and allow you to judge the extent to which they are fixed (table-top test).

Completing the examination

1. Say that you would like to examine:
   - the feet and the external genitalia as the disease can affect the soles of the feet and the penis
   - for signs of alcoholism and cirrhosis.

The discussion

1. Summarise findings to examiner. For example, 'This man has limited extension of the MCP joints of his little and ring fingers bilaterally. The flexion deformity is approximately 45 degrees at the MCP joints. There are associated visible cords and thickening of the palmar fascia, consistent with a diagnosis of Dupuytren's contracture. There appears to be minimal effect on function.'
2. What is Dupuytren's contracture?
   - It is a benign, slowly progressive thickening and shortening of the palmar fascia that may also affect the plantar fascia and penile corpus cavernosa (Peyronie's disease).
   - It involves a proliferation of fibroblasts (typically myofibroblasts which have contractile properties) and disordered deposition of collagen causing thickening of the palmar fascia, which progresses to cause contractures of the MCP and PIP joints of the affected fingers.
   - Nodules contain fibroblasts and type III collagen and are typical of the early proliferative phase of the disease. Increased fibrosis of the overlying skin cause it to become attached, puckered and tethered to the tendons below.
   - The tendons are normal. Progression is variable.
3. What is the aetiology of Dupuytren's contracture?
   - The exact aetiology is unknown.
   - There is an autosomal dominant hereditary form.
   - It is more common in males (5–10 : 1), most common in Caucasians, and increases with age (most over 50 years old). It is very common in Australia affecting 7% of the population over the age of 70.

- The following are associated with Dupuytren's contracture and can be remembered using the mnemonic '**deafest pail**':
  - **D**iabetes mellitus
  - **E**pilepsy
  - **A**ge (positive correlation)
  - **F**amily history (autosomal dominant)/**f**ibromatoses*
  - **E**pileptic medication (e.g. phenobarbitone)
  - **S**moking
  - **T**rauma and heavy manual labour
  - **P**eyronie's disease (fibrosis of the corpus cavernosum — seen in 3% of patients with Dupuytren's)
  - **AI**DS
  - **I**diopathic (most common)
  - **L**iver disease (secondary to alcohol).

4. What is Garrod's pad?
   - These pads are benign, well circumscribed, smooth, firm, skin- coloured papules, nodules or plaques, located in the skin (commonly) over the dorsal aspects of the interphalangeal joints.
   - They are four times more common in Dupuytren's contracture than the general population.
   - A history of repeated trauma related to sports or occupation is often present.
5. What are the differential diagnoses of Dupuytren's contracture?
   - Congenital:
     - contracture of the little finger — affects PIPJ.
   - Acquired:
     - skin contracture — look for scar from previous wounds
     - tendon contracture — thickened area, which moves on passive flexion of involved finger
       - trigger finger: typically causes flexion deformity of the fourth finger but can be extended with excessive force from the patient or by passive extension (with associated 'snap'). The finger and palmar skin will feel and look normal. The flexor tendon or tendon sheath maybe thickened over the metacarpal head and a snap may be felt as the finger is flexed and extended
     - ulnar nerve palsy — clawing of the fourth and fifth digits. The ring and little fingers are hyperextended at MCPJ and flexed at PIPJ. There is associated weakness of finger adduction/abduction and loss of sensation in the distribution of the ulnar nerve (fifth finger and ulnar aspect of the fourth). The finger and palmar skin will feel and look normal
     - palmar fibromatosis: rare condition associated with ovarian malignancy (also stomach, pancreas, lung). Progressive flexion deformities of all fingers of the hand. Thickening of the palmar skin and fascia is similar to Dupuytren's but is more diffuse.
6. What is the treatment of Dupuytren's contracture?
   - Non-operative:
     - physiotherapy — stretching exercises for early forms of the disease

*A group of disorders characterised by diffuse fibrosis, which include such diverse conditions as desmoid tumours, Reidel's thyroiditis, retroperitoneal fibrosis and Ledderhose disease (fibrosis of the plantar aponeurosis — seen in 5% of patients with Dupuytren's).

- local injections of triamcinolone acetonide into fibrous nodules may slow their progression and injections into synovial sheaths treat episodes of tenosynovitis. Main complication is tendon rupture
- other non-operative therapies in the literature: collagenase injections and external beam radiation. Most of these confer mild to moderate benefits in patients with early disease and all are associated with high rates of recurrence.

- Operative — surgical correction of deformities for advanced disease, causing significant functional impairment, is the most successful at correcting deformity:
  - fasciotomy — transection of fibrous bands
  - partial fasciectomy (with Z-plasty to lengthen wound) — in conjunction with post-operative physiotherapy (early active flexion range-of-motion exercises for grip strength) and night-time splintage in extension
  - complications: recurrence is common therefore patients are usually advised to defer surgery for as long as possible
  - dermofasciectomy (with full-thickness skin grafting) — associated with the lowest risk of recurrence
  - arthrodesis/amputation — for late presentations and repeated recurrences
  - percutaneous needle fasciotomy has been shown to improve MCP and PIP joint contractures but high rates of recurrence and poorer results compared to surgery.

3.5.7 Leg ulcers

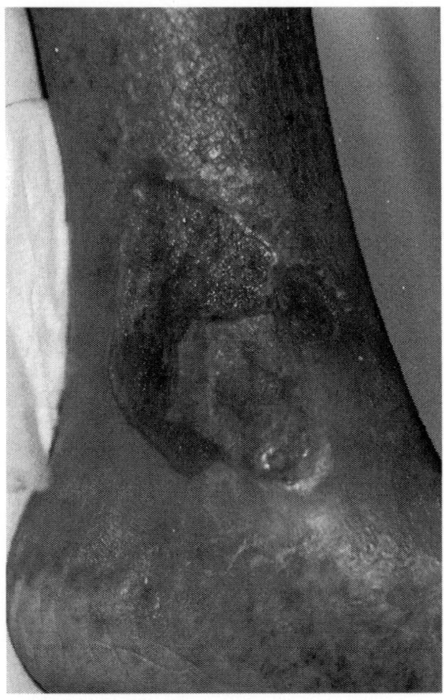

Figure 3.5.7
Venous ulcer left leg

Instruction

'Please examine this patient's legs.'

Approach

- Wash your hands or use the hand sanitiser.
- Introduce yourself and ask permission to perform the examination.
- Ask the patient if there is any pain anywhere.
- Expose both legs completely, whilst maintaining dignity by keeping the external genitalia covered.

> **TOP TIP**
>
> It is useful to examine the limbs using the following structured approach, focusing on the most obviously abnormal system:
>
> - arterial
> - venous
> - neurological
> - musculoskeletal/dermatological.

Inspection

1. Inspect both lower limbs.
2. Establish number and distribution of ulcers:
   - arterial: pressure areas — metatarsal heads/between toes/heel
   - venous: gaiter area — medial malleolus
   - neuropathic: pressure/exposed areas. Painless, associated with normal appearance of surrounding skin and sensory loss.
3. Describe the ulcer using the mnemonic 'Should The Children Ever Find Lumps Readily' (see above, and 'exam technique' in Chapter 3.4). For ulcers, also describe using the acronym BEDD:
   - **B**ase — granulation tissue/slough/malignant change/structures visible
   - **E**dge — sloping (healing); punched-out (ischaemic/neuropathic); undermined (pressure necrosis/TB); rolled (BCC); everted (SCC)
   - **D**epth
   - **D**ischarge — serous; sanguinous; serosanguinous; purulent.
4. Inspect for signs of chronic ischaemia (see 3.5.8 below):
   - pallor
   - loss of hair/shiny skin
   - gangrene/loss of toes
   - wasting of muscles
   - scars suggestive of surgical reconstruction.
5. Inspect for signs of chronic venous insufficiency — remembered using the acronym **LEGS**:
   - **L**ipodermatosclerosis
   - **E**czema
   - **G**aps in the skin (ulcers)/scarring from previous ulceration
   - **S**welling (ankle oedema)
   - look for evidence of varicose veins (see 3.5.10 below)/previous trauma precipitating DVT formation.
6. Inspect for Charcot arthropathy, claw toes (diabetic foot).
7. Look for the presence of cellulitis/infection and satellite lesions/other ulcers.

Palpation

1. Chronic ischaemia (comparing right to left; proximal to distal) (see 3.5.8 below):
   - skin temperature
   - capillary refill
   - systematic examination of pulses with comparison to contralateral side, exclude aneurysm (popliteal artery)
   - Buerger's angle.
2. Chronic venous insufficiency — if suspected you *must* stand the patient up to exam for varicose veins including (see 3.5.10):
   - oedema and thickness of skin
   - cough impulse in groin — saphena varix
   - Trendelenburg test (if varicose veins present).
3. Neurological assessment:
   - tone, power, sensation, reflexes, vibration:
     - monofilament examination (10 g) for light touch, joint proprioception, vibration — glove/stocking peripheral neuropathy.
4. Active/passive movement of all joints.
5. Draining lymph nodes.

Auscultation

1. For bruits.

Table 3.5.7 Clinical findings commonly seen in venous, arterial and neuropathic leg ulcers

	ARTERIAL	VENOUS	NEUROPATHIC
Location	Anterior shin Heel, over malleoli, over toe joints	Gaiter area Above malleoli	Pressure areas/bony prominences Metatarsal heads, over toe joints, heel, over malleoli
Surroundings	Signs of chronic ischaemia Atrophic skin changes, muscle wasting	Signs of chronic venous insufficiency Eczema	Can be normal (if not mixed disease) Callous indicating abnormal weight bearing Cellulitis due to concomitant infection
Edge	Demarcated, punched out	Sloping Purple in colour, epithelisation from margins	Demarcated
Base	Eschar may be present May expose underlying tendon/bone	Pink granulation tissue but if severe can expose tendon/bone	May expose underlying tendon/bone
Depth	Progressively deepen	Shallow	Progressively deepen
Exudate	Often minimal unless infected No bleeding	Excessive Seropurulent Bleed easily	Often minimal unless infected Infected ulcers with underlying osteomyelitis produce purulent discharge
Oedema	Usually absent unless infected	Present, can be significant	Usually absent unless infected
Pain	Severe	Mild to moderate	Absent
Pulses	Absent/weak Popliteal aneurysm may be present	Normal	Normal

The discussion

1. What are the causes of leg ulcers?
   - Remembered using the acronym **TIN CANS**:
     - **T**rauma
     - **I**nfection/**i**mmunological
       - TB/syphilis/rheumatoid arthritis
     - **N**eoplasia
       - SCC/BCC
     - **C**hronic venous insufficiency (including mixed arteriovenous disease).
     - **A**rterial insufficiency — atherosclerosis, embolism, Buerger's disease, diabetes.
     - **N**europathy — diabetes, nerve injuries
     - **S**kin conditions including, pyoderma gangrenosum, necrobiosis lipoidica etc.
2. What is the relative contribution of vascular disease in lower limb ulcers?
   - 60% chronic venous insufficiency
   - 15% arterial insufficiency
   - 15% mixed arterial and venous disease.
3. What is the aetiology of ischaemic ulcers?
   - Luminal:
     - emboli: atherosclerotic/cholesterol
     - thrombotic/ hyper coagulable states: anti-phospholipid syndrome.
   - Arterial wall — using the acronym SAD:
     - **S**pasm — Raynaud's phenomenon
     - **A**therosclerosis/**a**rteritis
       - Takayasu's
       - Buerger's disease
       - giant cell
       - polyarteritis nodosa
       - small vessel vasculitis — CTD, Behcet's etc.
     - **D**iabetes mellitus/**D**ilatation (aneurysm).
   - Outside the artery:
     - trauma
     - compression.
4. What is the aetiology of diabetic foot ulcers?
   - The 'diabetic foot syndrome' encompasses a number of pathologies including: diabetic neuropathy, peripheral occlusive arterial disease, Charcot neuroarthropathy, osteomyelitis, foot ulceration and the potentially preventable end-point of amputation.
   - Diabetic neuropathy and peripheral occlusive arterial disease are the major aetiological factors for the development of ulceration and may act alone, together or in combination with other factors such as microvascular disease, biomechanical abnormalities, limited joint mobility and increased susceptibility to infection.
   - Neuropathic (45–60% of ulcers).
   - Ischaemic due to peripheral occlusive arterial disease (10% of ulcers).
   - Mixed Neuroischaemic (25–45% of ulcers).
   - Opinion is divided as to whether diabetic neuropathy occurs due to (a) microvascular disease leading to nerve hypoxia or (b) direct effects of hyperglycaemia on neuronal metabolism or a combination of both.

- Atherosclerotic occlusive arterial disease is present (albeit in subclinical form in some) in virtually all long-term diabetics; vascular disease being responsible for 70% of diabetic deaths. The distribution of peripheral occlusive arterial disease is different in diabetics, predominantly affecting below-knee vessels.

5. How can you treat venous ulcers?
   - Non-surgical:
     - high success: 50–70% will heal at 3 months, 80–90% at 12 months
     - the patient should be warned to avoid trauma to the affected area
     - four-layer compression bandaging comprising:
       - non-adherent dressing over ulcer plus wool bandage
       - crepe bandage
       - blue-line bandage
       - adhesive bandage to prevent the other layers from slipping
     - encourage rest and elevation of leg
     - once healed, grade II compression stockings should be fitted and worn for life.
   - Surgical:
     - if the ulcer fails to heal, careful consideration should be given to excluding other causes (such as a malignant Marjolin ulcer) and the area may need to be biopsied (2% of chronic leg ulcers are malignant)
     - otherwise, a split skin graft should be considered with excision of the dead skin and the graft attached to healthy granulation tissue
     - if ulceration is due to primary varicose veins, surgery to the superficial veins is required.

3.5.8 Peripheral occlusive arterial disease

Please read in conjunction with 2.2.32, ischaemic leg.

Instruction

'Examine this patient's legs.'

Approach

- Wash your hands or use the hand sanitiser.
- Introduce yourself and ask permission to perform the examination.
- Ask the patient if there is any pain anywhere.
- Expose both legs completely, removing socks, whilst maintaining dignity by keeping the external genitalia covered.
- Remember:
  - as with examination of varicose veins (see 3.5.10), there are three main objectives for each of the inspection and palpation components of the examination
  - compare left and right; proximal and distal.

Inspection — three main objectives to assess

1. Colour changes:
   - the skin of the lower limb may be red (vasodilatation of the microcirculation due to tissue ischaemia), white (advanced ischaemia) or purple/blue (excess deoxygenated blood in the tissues).

2. Trophic changes:
   - loss of hair and small non-healing sores may be evident on the lower limbs/feet
   - wasting of muscles
   - gangrene (especially between and at the tips of the toes)
   - loss of digits, due to previous gangrene/amputation
   - arterial (ischaemic) ulcers are found typically in the least well-perfused areas and over the pressure points, such as lateral aspect of foot and malleoli:
     - the lesions are punched out (compromised ability to heal) and well circumscribed
     - they may be very tender and the surrounding skin is cold
     - they may vary considerably in size but are usually smaller than venous ulcers
     - there is no granulation tissue but there may be a thin layer of slough at the base. Otherwise the base is flat and pale
     - they may be very deep and penetrate surrounding tissue (including bone)
     - be sure to look between each of the toes on both feet
     - ask the patient for permission, then lift the foot up to observe the heel for ulcers (neuropathic ulcers are commonest here) and the sole of the foot for ulceration of the metatarsal heads.
3. Vascular (Buerger's) angle:
   - lift the leg until it becomes white as the perfusion drops
   - the angle between the horizontal and the leg when it becomes white is Buerger's angle
   - venous guttering can also be observed
   - a normal leg can be raised to 90° and still remain perfused; if the angle is less than 20°, this indicates severe ischaemia
   - assist the patient to 'drop their leg' over the side of the bed — this causes the diseased leg to become purple–red in colour due to reactive hyperaemia — this is the second part of Buerger's test. It represents dysfunction of the microcirculation (perhaps secondary to sympathetic dysfunction and loss of vasoconstrictive tone) and/or vasodilatation from accumulation of anaerobic (post-hypoxic) metabolites due to chronic ischaemia.

Palpation — three main objectives to assess

1. Temperature:
   - feel for skin temperature, using the back of the hand, comparing both sides simultaneously for any difference.
2. Capillary refill:
   - examine the toes for capillary refill
   - normally the toe blanches but then returns to the normal colour within 2 seconds. Any longer than this is abnormal.
3. Palpation of the peripheral pulses:
   - vascular surgeons palpate the peripheral pulses using the following technique:
     - use more than one finger to palpate the pulse if the artery is big enough
     - position your fingers in the direction of the artery to optimise your chances of feeling it
     - palpate both sides simultaneously to detect subtle differences
   - for the purposes of exams, peripheral pulses should be *confidently* reported to your examiner as: (a) present; (b) reduced; or (c) absent.

- Palpate the:
  - femorals (at the mid inguinal point, halfway between the anterior superior iliac spine and the pubic symphysis)
  - popliteals (by compressing it against the posterior aspect of the tibia)
  - foot pulses:
    - palpate from the bottom end of the examination couch
    - do not be tempted to palpate the dorsalis pedis (DPA) and posterior tibial (PTA) pulses simultaneously. Instead, examine each pulse in turn using two or three fingers, whilst simultaneously comparing it with the contralateral side
    - the DPA lies immediately lateral to the tendon of extensor hallucis longus this tendon
    - the PTA lies one finger's breadth below and behind the medial malleolus
    - remember that the foot pulses may be absent in 2% of normal subjects!

Auscultation

1. For bruits, especially over the femoral artery and in the subsartorial canal.

Completion

1. Tell the examiner you would:
   - examine the rest of the peripheral arterial system, including *all* peripheral pulses
   - examine the abdomen for aneurysmal dilatation of the aorta
   - measure the ankle brachial pressure indices (ABPI) on each side using a Doppler probe.

The discussion

1. How would you manage a patient who presents with claudication that impacts on his/her daily activities or QoL?
   - History:
     - intermittent claudication
     - critical ischaemia
     - cardiovascular history and risk factors.
   - Examination (as above):
     - lower limb
     - exercise challenge
     - ABPI
     - cardiovascular risk factors (BMI, BP, BSL).
   - Investigation:
     - urinalysis — glucose, micro spot for proteinuria
     - FBC (Hb, WCC)
     - EUC (renal function)
     - fasting BSL, HbA1C and glucose tolerance tests as required
     - coagulation studies and thrombophilia screens may be indicated in a small number of patient with family history
     - total cholesterol/TG/LDL/HDL
     - duplex imaging
     - radiological investigation:
       - diagnostic digital subtraction angiogram
       - CT angiography (if proximal disease is suspected)
       - MR angiography.

- Treatment: risk factor modification:
  - stop smoking
  - weight management
  - optimise lipid profile
  - aggressive treatment of hypertension/diabetes
  - antiplatelet therapy
  - exercise.
- Endovascular treatment:
  - angioplasty ± stenting (evidence for iliac stenoses and suboptimal flow after angioplasty, no place in femoro-popliteal disease).
- Surgical treatment:
  - indicated if failure of medical therapy or primary prevention
  - depends on level of obstruction and presence of comorbidities and patient's symptoms
  - aortoiliac disease:
    - unilateral disease:
      femoro-femoral cross over
      ilio-femoral bypass
      axillo-femoral
    - bilateral disease:
      aortobifemoral
      iliac angioplasty/stenting and femoro-femoral cross over
      axillo-bifemoral
    - infrainguinal disease:
      femoral (above knee or below knee)-popliteal bypass
      endarterectomy.

3.5.9 Lymphoedema

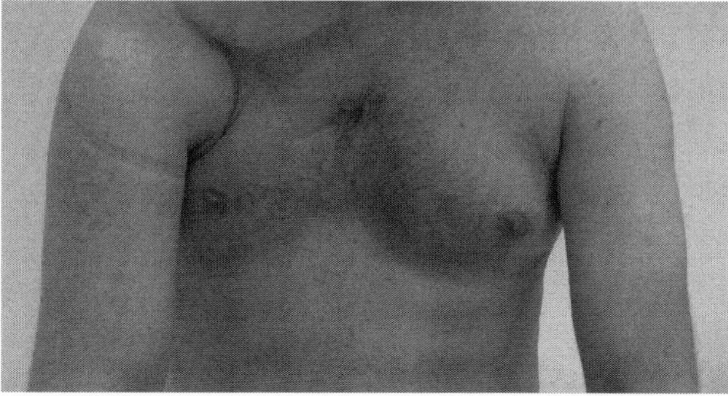

Figure 3.5.9
Lymphoedema right arm

Instruction

'Please examine this patient's arms' or 'Please examine this patient's legs.'

Approach

- Wash your hands or use the hand sanitiser.
- Introduce yourself and ask permission to perform the examination.
- Ask the patient if there is any pain anywhere.
- Expose the entire limb, whilst maintaining the patient's dignity.

Inspection

1. Limb girth. Compare right to left. Can be recorded and serial examinations are a measure of response to treatment.
2. The legs may be grossly swollen, with no particular distribution. The swelling tends to be bilateral.
3. Note the loss of contour at the ankle/wrist, which causes a 'buffalo hump' appearance on the dorsum of the foot/hand. This does not occur in venous disease.
4. There may be lichenified fronds on the toes and the skin looks thick and indurated (hyperkeratosis, lichenification and peau d'orange).
5. Yellow discolouration of nails.
6. Stemmer's sign: squaring of the toes.

Palpation

1. Pitting oedema (early disease), non-pitting late.
2. Thickened skin and dermal layers (fibrosis).
3. Stemmers test: unable to pinch the interdigital skin at the second toe or finger.
4. Examine draining lymph nodes (?enlarged from tumour infiltration).
5. Functional assessment of the affected limb.
6. Check all limb pulses.

The discussion

1. Which investigations would you do?
   - Blood tests:
     - WCC: eosinophilia (parasitic infection), neutrophilia (cellulitis)
     - albumin
     - creatinine (renal function).
   - Imaging:
     - CT: look for primary/recurrent malignancy, visualise dilated lymphatics
     - venous duplex ultrasound — exclude venous disease
     - arterial duplex ultrasound — exclude underlying arterial disease especially if compression therapy to be used
     - lymphangioscintography — technetium colloid injected intradermally in limb to be tested (interdigital space) and a gamma camera takes images at 5 minute intervals to monitor the uptake of the colloid. Time to inguinal lymph nodes when testing the foot is 15–60 min.
2. What is lymphoedema?
   - Progressive limb swelling due to accumulation of protein rich interstitial fluid due to inadequate lymphatic drainage.

3. What is the aetiology of lymphoedema?
    - Primary:
        - congenital: familial (Milroy's disease), non-familial
        - lymphoedema praecox (onset up to 35 yrs)
        - lymphoedema tarda (onset after 35 yrs).
    - Secondary:
        - malignancy: due to extrinsic compression of lymphatics or invasion by tumour
        - surgery — lymphadenectomy, vascular surgery
        - radiotherapy
        - infection, either parasitic — filariasis (from nematodes) is the most common cause in developing world, or bacterial — β-haemolytic streptococci, S. aureus, tuberculosis
        - trauma: circumferential trauma to limb/severe burns.
4. How do you treat lymphoedema?
    - Clinical staging:
        - 0: latent disease, swelling not evident
        - I: pitting oedema that reduces on limb elevation
        - II: pitting oedema and limb swelling that does not improve with elevation
        - III: non-pitting oedema, extensive limb swelling, skin changes.
    - Non-operative:
        - patient education is crucial
        - early intervention better than late
        - physical activity, elevation, manual lymphatic drainage (massage)
        - skin hygiene, protect skin integrity (cleanse, emollient moisturiser, avoid synthetic fabrics, good fitting footwear)
        - grade III compression bandages (to apply 40 mmHg pressure at the ankles)
        - treatment of infection (exacerbate swelling, cause pain)
        - topical anti-fungals (Clotrimazole 1% cream). Systemic therapy may be required.
    - Operative:
        - debulking or bypass:
            - indicated for severe disease, failure of conservative measures, recurrent infective complications:
                - debulking surgery — better for disease due to obliteration of lymphatics:
                    - removal of skin and subcutaneous tissue with primary closure or skin grafting (e.g. Homan's procedure)
                    - complications: wound infection and dehiscence, recurrence, poor cosmesis
                - bypass surgery — better for disease due to obstructed lymphatics:
                    - skin and muscle flaps — poor results
                    - omental bridges — poor results
                    - enteromesenteric bridges
                    - lymphatico-lymphatic bypass/transplant (normal lymphatics from contralateral limb)
                    - lymphatico-venous bypass.

3.5.10 Varicose veins

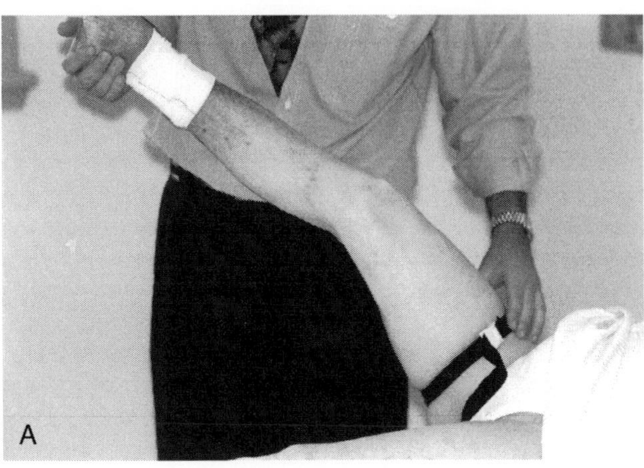

Figure 3.5.10A
Tourniquet test right leg

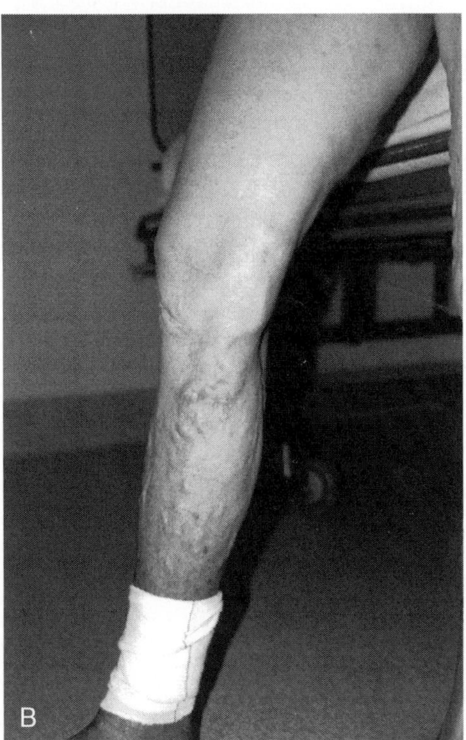

Figure 3.5.10B
Tourniquet test right leg after standing

Instruction

'Examine this patient's legs.'

Approach

- Wash your hands or use the hand sanitiser.
- Introduce yourself and ask permission to perform the examination.
- Ask the patient to stand (veins are collapsed when the patient is supine) immediately so that the veins can start to fill whilst you are preparing to examine.
- Ask the patient if there is any pain anywhere.
- Expose both lower limbs, whilst maintaining dignity by keeping the external genitalia covered.
- Remember:
  - as with examination of peripheral occlusive arterial disease (see 3.5.8), there are three main objectives (the **3S**s) for each the inspection and palpation components of the examination
  - compare left and right legs.

Inspection

Whilst kneeling in front of the patient, look for the **3S**s.

1. **S**ite and **s**ize of varicosities, including the presence of a saphena varix:
   - establish that any visible veins are varicosities (dilated and tortuous) as opposed to physiological (dilated only, as in athletes)
   - determine whether there are varicosities in the distribution of the long saphenous vein (LSV)
   - ask the patient to turn around and inspect for varicosities in the distribution of the short saphenous system (SSV)
   - try to decide whether the varicosities are long or short saphenous in origin, commenting that the distinction may be difficult below the knee
   - examine the groins for the presence of a saphena varix. This will be located at the saphenofemoral junction (SFJ) (see below)
   - are there spider or reticular veins?
2. **S**kin for changes and scars:
   - look for scars indicating previous surgery, especially hidden in the groin creases or previous fracture fixation
   - determine whether there are signs of chronic venous insufficiency, using the acronym **LEGS**:
     - **L**ipodermatosclerosis
     - **E**czema
     - **G**aps in the skin (i.e. ulceration) — active and healed (the latter causing a white patch called atrophie blanche)
     - **S**welling (pedal oedema).
   - inspect specifically around the medial malleolus (the 'gaiter' area) for evidence of these changes if there is evidence of ulceration, describe its characteristics fully (see 3.5.7).
3. **S**welling of the ankle:
   - look for asymmetry between the lower limbs and establish the height and severity of the swelling.
4. Is there a mismatch in the size of the limb to suggest a congenital abnormality such as Klippel-Trenaunay-Weber syndrome (characterised by a triad of port-wine

stain, varicose veins, and bony and soft tissue hypertrophy involving an extremity)?

Palpation

Proceed to palpate using the **3S**s.

1. **S**tate of the skin/subcutaneous tissues:
   - palpate the skin for the presence of pitting oedema
   - woody, non-pitting oedema is suggestive of lipodermatosclerosis
   - feel along the course of the long and short saphenous veins, determining whether there is induration of the subcutaneous tissues.
2. **S**ites of fascia defects:
   - feel along the medial aspect of the leg for defects in the fascia on the medial aspect of the leg below the knee suggestive of large, incompetent perforating veins
   - these sites are frequently tender.
3. **S**ite of incompetence:
   - palpate the saphenofemoral junction (SFJ), which is located 3.5 cm (approximately 2 finger breadths) below and lateral to the pubic tubercle
     - feel for the smooth swelling and palpable thrill of a saphena varix. If present, the cough test may be positive (Cruveilhier's sign)
   - the Trendelenburg test is performed with the patient first lying down:
     - elevate the leg to gently empty the veins
     - palpate the SFJ and ask the patient to stand while maintaining direct pressure over the SFJ
     - if the veins do not refill then the SFJ is incompetent. Should the veins fill, then the SFJ may or may not be competent, but there are certainly distal incompetent perforators.
   - The tourniquet test is performed at the level of the upper thigh and then moved distally to identify incompetent perforators in the mid-thigh and above and below knee regions:
     - again empty the leg in the supine position and apply the tourniquet (e.g. a single use examination glove)
     - then ask the patient to stand and inspect for filling and collapse above and below the position of the tourniquet
     - collapsed veins below the tourniquet indicate that the incompetent vein is at/above the level of the tourniquet
     - rapid filling of veins below the tourniquet indicates that the incompetent vein is below the level of the tourniquet
     - use a hand-held Doppler (if provided) to identify SFJ/popliteal fossa reflux by squeezing the muscle of the thigh or calf, listening proximally as blood flows up the leg (normal) and then for a second 'swoosh' in incompetent veins as blood refluxes down the leg.

Completion

1. Tell the examiner you would:
   - perform a tap test (Chevrier's tap sign)
   - auscultate the vein for bruits (indicating the presence of arteriovenous fistulae)
   - examine the abdomen for masses (including a digital rectal examination) to ascertain whether the varicose veins are primary or secondary.

The discussion

1. Do you think this patient has chronic venous insufficiency? Why?
   - Yes, the hallmark signs in addition to varicose venis are present, specifically:
     - **l**ipodermatosclerosis
     - **e**czema
     - **g**aps in the skin (i.e. ulceration) — active and healed (the latter causing a white patch called atrophie blanche)
     - **s**welling (pedal oedema).
2. How would you want to investigate this patient?
   - Hand-held Doppler (see palpation above).
   - Duplex scanning (B-mode USS with Doppler ultrasound) to look for:
     - abnormal venous anatomy (e.g. absent saphenopopliteal junction/presence of vein of Giacomini)
     - the presence of venous reflux
     - evidence of DVT
     - incompetence in the deep and superficial venous system
     - competence of perforators.
   - Venography if duplex scanning findings are equivocal or technically difficult (morbid obesity).
   - Functional calf volume measurements to ascertain anatomical and functional information (e.g. plethysmography) if evidence of superficial *and* deep venous incompetence.
3. What are the possible causes for this patient's chronic venous insufficiency?
   - In the CEAP classification (American Venous Forum 1994), which refers to **c**linical — **e**tiology — **a**natomy — **p**athophysiology, the etiology is classified as **c**ongenital (E_C), **p**rimary (E_P) or **s**econdary (E_S), anatomy as **s**uperficial (A_S), **d**eep (A_D) or **p**erforator (A_P) and pathophysiological condition reflux (P_R) or obstruction (P_O).
   - Superficial venous reflux:
     - long saphenous
     - short saphenous.
   - Deep venous reflux and obstruction:
     - primary (idiopathic)
     - secondary to DVT or injury.
   - Perforating vein reflux.
   - Abnormal calf pump:
     - neurological
     - musculoskeletal.
   - Combinations of the above.
4. What treatment options are there for this patient?
   - General measures:
     - elevation of affected limbs
     - treatment of comorbidities (e.g. CCF)
     - weight management.
   - Graduated compression therapy:
     - multi-layer, elastic compression is superior to single-layer, non-elastic compression in the healing of ulcers
     - class II (25–35 mmHg pressure at the ankle) compression stockings prevent ulcer recurrence.

- Surgical intervention:
  - superficial venous surgery — high ligation of the SFJ with stripping of the LSV and multiple stab avulsions (see 4.4.16, high ligation of the long saphenous vein)
  - perforator vein surgery — subfascial endoscopic perforator vein surgery (SEPS).

3.5.11 Median nerve palsy

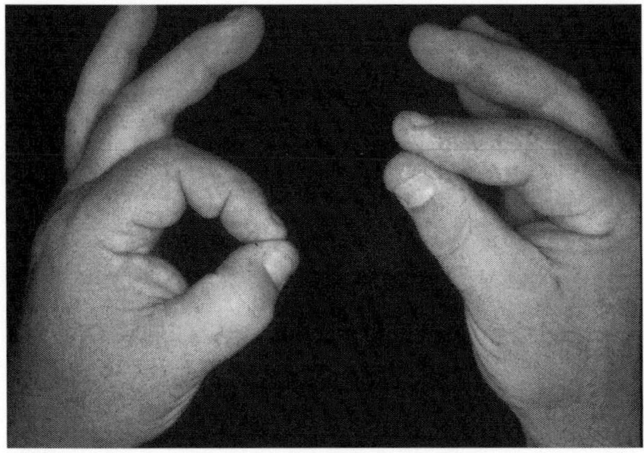

Figure 3.5.11
Right median nerve palsy (Source: *Peripheral Nerve Surgery, Practical Applications In The Upper Extremity*. Slutsky D J, Hentz V R. 2006, Churchill Livingstone: an imprint of Elsevier, Fig 21-12, p 337.)

Instruction

'This patient has been complaining of weakness in her right hand and numbness affecting her thumb and middle finger. Her symptoms are worse at night. Please examine her hands and tell me the diagnosis.'

Approach

- Wash your hands or use the hand sanitiser.
- Introduce yourself and ask permission to perform the examination.
- Ask the patient if there is any pain anywhere.
- Expose to elbows and ask the patient to place her hands palm upwards on a pillow (if available).

Look

1. Asymmetry, deformity.
2. Wasting of the thenar muscles (in advanced cases).
3. Scars from previous surgery over the transverse carpal ligament.

Feel

1. Sensory assessment:
   - ask the patient to outline the area of numbness on her hand
   - test light touch over the palmar aspects of the thumb, index and middle fingers of the involved hand — deficiency implies median nerve involvement. Compare this with the other fingers, proceeding to other sensory modalities such as pain only if the examiner wishes you to
   - the autonomous area of sensory innervation of the median nerve is to the distal phalanges of index and middle fingers.

Move

2. Motor assessment.
   - Test the power of muscles innervated by the median nerve (**LOAF**):
     - **l**ateral two lumbricals — difficult to test
     - **o**pponens pollicis — oppose the patient's thumb and the little finger and ask the patient to stop you pulling the fingers apart
     - **a**bductor pollicis brevis — place dorsum of hand on a flat surface and ask the patient to lift her thumb to the ceiling against resistance, feeling the thenar eminence for the power of abductor pollicis brevis
     - **f**lexor pollicis brevis — not an autonomous muscle (innervation varies).
   - The autonomous motor supply of the hand of the median nerve is the abductor pollicis brevis (as above).

Completion

1. Say that you would like to perform the following special tests:
   - Tinel's sign — tapping over the median nerve at the wrist reproduces tingling sensation in the distribution of the nerve
   - Phalen's test — maximal flexion of the wrist for 1 minute exacerbates symptoms which are promptly relieved when flexion is discontinued
   - flexion compression test (also known as Duran's test) — maximal flexion of wrist and direct digital compression of the median nerve at the wrist reproduces symptoms (if symptoms appear within 20 second, sensitivity = 82% and specificity = 99%)
   - assess the effect of the symptoms on the patient's quality of life (e.g. symptoms are usually worse at night and first thing in the morning — sleep quality may be affected).

The discussion

1. Summarise the findings. For example, 'This patient has symptoms and signs consistent with carpal tunnel syndrome. I would further confirm this diagnosis by requesting a nerve conduction study.
2. What are the causes of carpal tunnel sydrome?
   - The most common cause is *idiopathic*. The other causes can be classified as follows:
     - anatomical abnormalities:
       - bone — previous wrist fractures (e.g. Colles fracture, acromegaly)
       - soft tissue — lipomas, ganglia

  - physiological abnormalities:
    - inflammatory conditions — rheumatoid arthritis, gout
    - alterations of fluid balance — pregnancy, menopause, hypothyroidism, obesity, amyloidosis, renal failure
    - neuropathic conditions — diabetes mellitus, alcoholism.
3. How would you treat this lady?
   - Non-surgical — removal of underlying causes, splinting of the wrist in a neutral position (especially at night-time), and local steroid injections just proximal to the carpal tunnel.
   - Surgical — carpal tunnel decompression (division of the flexor retinaculum under tourniquet control) can be performed either as an open or endoscopic procedure.

3.5.12 Ulnar nerve palsy

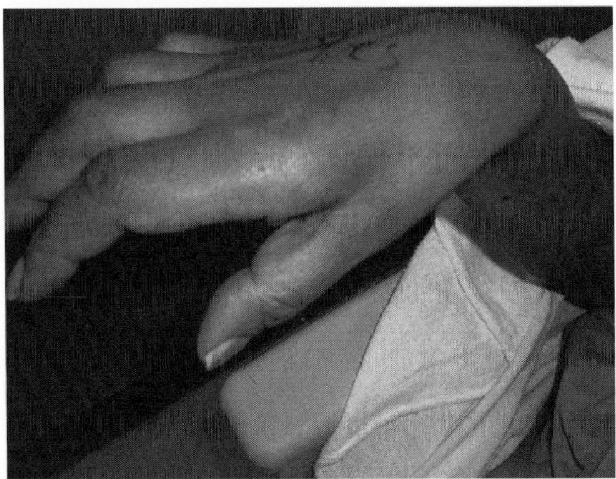

Figure 3.5.12
Right ulnar nerve palsy (Source: *DeLee and Drez's Orthopaedic Sports Medicine*, 3rd edn. DeLee J C et al. 2009, Saunders: an imprint of Elsevier, Fig 19I-3, p 396.)

Instruction

'Please examine this lady's hands and tell me the diagnosis.'

Approach

- Wash your hands or use the hand sanitiser.
- Introduce yourself and ask permission to perform the examination.
- Ask the patient if there is any pain anywhere.
- Expose to elbows and ask the patient to place her hands palm upwards on a pillow (if available).

Look

1. Asymmetry, deformity — there is a unilateral deformity of the right hand, leading to a claw hand appearance. Examine the palm, noting the wasting of the hypothenar eminence (all muscles here are supplied by the ulnar nerve; Fig 3.5.12).

2. Ask the patient to turn her hands over and observe the guttering between the metacarpals as the interossei are wasted (best seen in the first dorsal webspace).
3. Scars from previous surgery, including around the elbows.

Feel

1. Sensory assessment.
   - Ask the patient to outline the area of numbness on her hand.
   - Test light touch over the palmar and dorsal aspects of the of little and medial half of the ring finger. Compare this with the other fingers, proceeding to other sensory modalities such as pain only if the examiner wishes you to.
   - The autonomous area of sensory innervation of the ulnar nerve is to the middle and distal phalanges of the little finger.

Move

1. Motor assessment.
   - Test the **p**almar interossei (which **ad**duct the fingers — **PAd**):
     - ask the patient to hold a piece of paper between two fingers while you attempt to pull it away — you have now tested the autonomous motor supply.
   - Continue to test the **d**orsal interossei (which **ab**duct the fingers — **DAb**):
     - ask the patient to spread the fingers and prevent you from pushing them together.
   - Assess for weakness of flexor digitorum profundus to the ring and little fingers:
     - get the patient to place the hand flat with the palm facing upwards
     - fix the PIPJ by holding it on either side and test active flexion of the distal interphalangeal joint (DIPJ) with the proximal interphalangeal joint (PIPJ) in full extension.

Completion

1. Say that you would like to perform the following special tests.
   - Froment's sign — based on the fact that adductor pollicis is supplied by the ulnar nerve, and if there is an ulnar nerve palsy, the only way to adduct the thumb is by using flexor pollicis longus to compensate (this muscle is supplied by the median nerve).
     - Ask the patient to hold a piece of paper between the thumb and radial aspect of the index finger and as you pull this piece of paper away from the patient, observe the thumb.
     - The distal phalanx will flex if the patient is using flexor pollicis longus to hold the piece of paper.
   - Elbow flexion test:
     - fully flex the elbow for one minute
     - the patient will complain of numbness and tingling in the ring and little fingers
     - this test may be quite uncomfortable for the patient, and therefore you are better off describing it first to the examiner.

The discussion

1. What are the causes of an ulnar nerve lesion?
   - Anatomical — cubital tunnel syndrome at the elbow.
   - Trauma — typically supracondylar fractures and dislocations of the elbow.
   - Degenerative arthritis — with compressing proliferative synovitis and osteophytes or loose bodies.

- Rarer causes — compression from tight fascia or ligaments, tumour masses, aneurysms, vascular thromboses, or anomalous muscles.

2. How do you differentiate clinically between a high and a low ulnar nerve lesion?
   - Low lesions (below elbow):
     - more marked clawing as unopposed action of the long flexors and extensors (e.g. flexor digitorum profundus to ring and little fingers is still functioning).
   - High lesions (above elbow):
     - paralysis of flexor digitorum profundus to ring and little fingers leads to less marked clawing of these fingers as the flexion component of the clawing is less prominent — this is known as the 'ulnar paradox'
     - decreased sensation over ulnar border of the hand
     - otherwise as for low lesion.

3.5.13 Abdominal mass

Read in conjunction with Chapter 3.3.8.

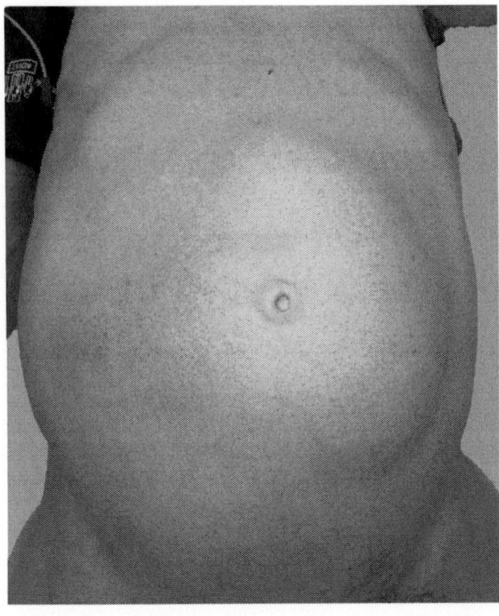

Figure 3.5.13
Massive splenomegaly

Instruction

'Please examine this patient's abdomen.'

Listen carefully to the examiner's instructions. You have been told to examine the patient's *abdomen*, so begin with the abdominal examination itself. By contrast, if you are told to examine the patient's *abdominal system* (as in Chapter 3.3, section 3.3.8) then you commence with the hands and complete an examination of the entire patient.

Approach

- Wash your hands or use the hand sanitiser.
- Introduce yourself and ask permission to perform the examination.
- Lay the patient flat with one pillow beneath the head.
- Expose the patient from nipples to knees, whilst maintaining the patient's dignity.
- Ask the patient if there is any pain anywhere.

Inspection

Note: the appearance of a healthy patient without any abdominal scars should raise the suspicion that the case is 'an abdominal mass'. Conversely, the presence of scars should raise the suspicion that the case is an 'incisional hernia'.

1. Stand back from the patient and observe both the patient and abdomen for signs that may indicate the underlying pathology. Comment on general features such as cachexia, jaundice, pallor.
2. Move closer to the patient and undertake a careful inspection of the patient's abdomen. Often the mass will be obvious by kneeing beside the patient with your eyes level with the abdomen.
3. Comment on any scars or skin lesions. Look for prominent abdominal wall veins (portal hypertension and caput medusae or IVC compression).
4. Masses can be visible especially in thin patients as (a) generalised distension of the abdomen or (b) localised irregularity or protrusion of abdomen.
5. If the mass is visible, describe its features on inspection according to the mnemonic 'Should The Children Ever Find Lumps Readily' (see below, and 'exam technique' in Chapter 3.4).
6. Look for movement of the mass with respiration.
7. Ask the patient to cough and lift off the bed to enhance the observation and examination of any pathology.

Palpation

1. Ask the patient if he/she has any pain and if so to show you where it is located. Commence palpation away from this site.
2. Systematically palpate the abdomen beginning with superficial palpation to detect any tenderness and then deep palpation to identify masses. Take care to avoid causing pain.
3. Attempt to assess normal anatomy. Examine hernia orifices. Palpate for AAA.
4. On identification of a mass, it must be carefully characterised. Abdominal masses can be classified on the basis of:
   - location:
     - anterior abdominal wall
     - intra-peritoneal or
     - retroperitoneal
   - region: the 9 regions of the abdomen are created by two vertical lines (passing between the mid-clavicular and mid-inguinal points) and two horizontal lines (one passing through the transpyloric plane and the other passing between the tubercles of the ileum — the intertubercular line).

Right hypochondrium	Epigastric	Left hypochondrium
Right lumbar	Umbilical	Left lumbar
Right iliac	Suprapubic	Left iliac

5. Define the location/relationship of the mass to the anterior abdominal wall. When you ask the patient to lift their head to tense the abdominal wall,

intra- and retroperitoneal masses are more difficult to feel, whilst masses arising in the abdominal wall become more prominent.

6. If the mass is arising deep to the anterior abdominal wall, go on to establish which region it is in.
7. Complete the description of the features of the mass according to the mnemonic 'Should The Children Ever Find Lumps Readily' (see below, and 'exam technique' in Chapter 3.4):
   - site — does not always reveal the likely organ of origin of pathology in isolation
   - single or multiple
   - shape and size — the splenic notch of an enlarged spleen gives it a characteristic shape
   - contour: is it smooth or irregular? Irregular masses are suspicious for malignancy. Benign masses or fluid filled/cystic masses are more likely to have a smooth surface
   - consistency of the mass (hard or soft and compressible). Hard masses are suspicious for malignancy.
8. In addition, it is crucial to assess the following to help distinguish the aetiology of an abdominal mass. Use the acronym **SPRUE** as an *aide memoire*:
   - **S**ite of enlargement
   - **P**ercussion note (below in percussion)
   - **R**espiratory movement (organs attached to diaphragm i.e. spleen and liver will tend to move downwards with inspiration)
   - **U**nable/able to get above it — can you palpate the upper and lower margins of the mass? You cannot get above an enlarged spleen or liver and conversely you may not be able to get below a mass arising from a pelvic organ
   - **E**dge characteristics — smooth, irregular, tender, notched etc.
9. Is the mass ballotable — retroperitoneal masses (i.e. arising from kidney) may be made more obvious by balloting.
10. Is it pulsatile/expansile. An AAA is expansile. If a AAA is identified, the femoral and popliteal pulses should also be assessed looking for symmetry and for other sites of aneurysmal disease.

Percussion

1. Percussion of the abdomen to further characterise the mass.
2. Dullness in the right and left upper quadrants and extending above the costal margin is characteristic of hepatomegaly or splenomegaly
3. Resonance can imply overlying bowel gas and make a retroperitoneal mass more likely. Alternatively, in the setting of distension, it may represent an obstructed loop of bowel (e.g. volvulus).
4. Percuss from the midline at the umbilicus out to the left flank. If dullness is encountered laterally, help the patient to move to the right lateral position and percuss again at the point dullness was encountered to check for shifting dullness, indicating the presence of ascites.
5. Check for a fluid thrill (ascites).

Auscultation

1. Auscultate for bowel sounds (present or absent, high pitched in small bowel obstruction). Bowel sounds over a hernia implies bowel in hernia contents.
2. Listen for a succussion splash (gastric outlet obstruction).
3. Bruits (AAA/vascular tumour) as appropriate.

Completion

1. Say that you would like to perform:
   - a digital rectal/pelvic examination
   - examination of the external genitalia
   - urinalysis.

The discussion

1. Present your findings and differential diagnosis according to the location and region of the mass and its characteristics.
   - Knowledge of the anatomy of the abdominal viscera is crucial to facilitate this.
   - Use of a surgical sieve will allow you to generate a list of possible differential diagnoses for the viscus. Examples include:
     - trauma
     - infective/inflammatory
     - neoplastic
     - connective tissue diseases
     - arteriovenous
     - nutritional
     - biochemical
     - endocrine/metabolic
     - degenerative/drugs.
   - For example:
     - 'I identified a mass in the right iliac fossa, arising deep to the anterior abdominal wall. Possible intraperitoneal structures that this is arising from include the: terminal ileum, appendix, caecum/right colon and right adnexal structures (in a woman). Very occasionally gross enlargement of upper abdominal structures, typically the liver, can occur into this region. Retroperitoneal structures include: right kidney and ureter and right iliac vessels. Causes for the enlargement of such structures would include: traumatic, infective, neoplastic, etc. In this situation the most likely diagnosis is X.'
2. What is the mass in the right hypochondrium?
   - Cases of hepatosplenomegaly are very commonly encountered in the short cases.
   - Demonstrate to the examiner that the mass you have identified *is* an enlarged liver using the acronym **SPRUE** (SPRUE = gastrointestinal disease = causes of gastrointestinal visceral enlargement).
   - For example, there is a mass arising in the right hypochondrium that is enlarging towards the right iliac fossa, it is dull to percussion, it descends with respiration and I am unable to get above it. The edge is irregular.
   - The same acronym can also be used to confirm the presence of splenomegaly.
3. What are the causes of hepatomegaly?
   - Physiological:
     - Reidel's lobe
     - hyper-expanded chest (displacing the liver inferiorly).
   - Pathological:
     - use the acronym **CHIASMA** as an '*aide memoire*' for the causes of hepatomegaly. The same acronym can be used for causes of splenomegaly (see below):
       - **C**ongestive — cardiac failure, Budd-Chiari syndrome
       - **H**aematological — reticuloses
       - **I**nfection — viral, bacterial, protozoal

    - **A**myloid
    - **S**torage disorders — Wilson's disease, haemochromatosis
    - **M**asses — primary/secondary neoplasia
    - **A**utoimmune/**a**lcohol (fatty liver/cirrhosis).
4. What are the causes of splenomegaly?
   - Again, use the acronym CHIASMA:
     - **C**ongestive — portal hypertension
     - **H**aematological — reticuloses
     - **I**nfection — viral, bacterial, protozoal
     - **A**myloid
     - **S**torage disorders — Gaucher's disease
     - **M**asses — primary/secondary neoplasia
     - **A**utoimmune — Felty's syndrome.
   - Causes of massive splenomegaly (>1000 g and beyond the umbilicus) are much fewer and include:
     - visceral leishmaniasis (kala-azar)
     - chronic myeloid leukaemia
     - myelofibrosis
     - malaria
     - primary lymphoma of the spleen.
5. For the clinical profile, examination, investigations, aetiology and discussion points for intra-abdominal masses please see Chapter 3, Tables 3.3.8 A, B, C and D.

Section 4

The *viva voce* examination

Chapter 4.1

Surgical anatomy

I must confess that a man is guilty of unpardonable arrogance who concludes because an argument has escaped his own investigation that therefore it does not really exist. (David Hume, 1711–76)

The examination format

The examination in anatomy, along with the operative and pathophysiology examinations, has become very structured, standardised and reproducible. The surgical anatomy examination is an applied anatomy exam assessing knowledge of the anatomy of surgical procedures. Commonly, candidates are assessed on knowledge relating to:

- the specific organs/structures encountered during specific operations and important relations with structures susceptible to injury and how to avoid this; for example, the rectosigmoid and the left ureter, thyroid gland and the recurrent laryngeal nerve
- surgical approaches to certain organs; for example, the adrenal gland (anterior or posterior)
- the limits of dissection; for example, in axillary dissection, including which nerves can be injured.

The surgical anatomy viva comprises:

- five computer images in 12.5 minutes
- five wet specimens in 12.5 minutes.

Frequently, computers are set up on benches on one side of the anatomy room and wet specimens can be found on tables opposite. Multiple candidates are examined at the same time. Half the candidates commence with the computer images whilst the other half start with the wet specimens with rotation at 'halftime'. Candidates usually don a gown and gloves and are led to a station where they wait for the bell to ring, which signifies the start of the examination. Candidates remain standing during the entire examination.

Exam technique

> If the examiners *don't* speak, *start* talking. If they *start* talking, be *silent* and *listen* to the statement or question.
>
> Use the structured approach of '*Listen, think, pause, speak*'.

Computer images

The examiners usually introduce themselves and stand on one side of the computer screen and bring up the first image when the exam starts. Frequently, the examiners will set the stage for you with a short statement such as:

- 'This is a trauma patient with a stab wound. Which structures could be injured?'
- 'This is an image of the right recurrent laryngeal nerve during a thyroidectomy'
- 'This is an operative image of the left axilla. Can you tell me about the structures that you see?'

Preferably, you should state what the image shows; for example, 'this shows a mass in the left posterior triangle' or 'this is a barium swallow demonstrating a probable oesophageal cancer in the mid oesophagus'.

If you are correct the examiners will move on to questions, such as 'tell us about the anatomy of the posterior triangle?', or 'tell us about the blood supply of the oesophagus'. If you cannot identify the organ or area of anatomy, just say you don't know. The examiners want the exam to proceed and find out what you do know, not what you don't know. Therefore, they will usually tell you what the organ is or the area of anatomy that you're looking at, to give you the opportunity to answer the question that they have just asked. The examiners move you along and keep to time. A bell rings at 12.5 minutes and you cross the room to the other section of the anatomy exam.

Wet specimens

You are given a wooden pointer and the examiners will usually point at structures and ask 'what is that?'. After the examiners point at a structure (e.g. the diaphragm), you should state what it is and then start talking about it. The first structure that the examiners point at may simply serve as a starting or reference point for further questioning. For example, after pointing at the diaphragm the examiners may ask about the abdominal aorta and its branches, and then the course of an aberrant right hepatic artery (from the SMA) and the course of an aberrant left hepatic artery (from the left gastric artery).

It is crucial to remember that the examination is on *surgical* anatomy. For instance, when shown an axilla, the discussion nearly always relates to the anatomy of an axillary clearance. The examiners want to know that you understand that the axillary vein is the upper limit of a level II dissection. They will also want you to point out the thoracodorsal and long thoracic nerves and subscapular vessels and how you would protect them. For the femoral triangle, the examiners will normally want you to talk about the surgical anatomy of saphenofemoral junction ligation or common femoral artery access. You should describe the boundaries, floor, contents, and the saphenofemoral junction or common femoral artery as directed by the examiners.

> For the anatomy viva it is often useful to describe what you will (i) dissect, (ii) divide and (iii) preserve during an operation on that area.

Preparation and practising

Often it is said that there is no excuse for failing anatomy. This is the core knowledge of surgery and you must know it well from the perspective of someone who has performed, or is going to perform, surgery on the structure or the area being examined. Accordingly, it is imperative that you have a good grasp of the entire contents of an anatomy text, and an in-depth knowledge of the list of common anatomy topics, as listed in Chapter 1.3.

While the use of an anatomy atlas will help you prepare for the viva, you must go and practise on the wet specimens; e.g., prosections available in your closest anatomy laboratory. They are different to what you see in theatre and textbooks. Wet specimens are often grey in colour, without any colouring of the vessels or nerves, and it is easy to get confused if you are not familiar looking at such specimens. Once the examiners point at a structure you must identify it. As previously stated, you must frequently practise viva technique (especially with respect to surgical anatomy) if you are to be successful in the fellowship examination.

Chapter 4.2

Common surgical anatomy viva topics: model answers

In the pages that follow, we have taken the most commonly examined topics during the last 10 years and attempted to provide 'model answers' to help you structure and organise your revision. It is important to point out that the viva usually involves a series of questions from examiners and once each question is answered correctly the candidate is moved along rapidly to another question. We have provided a few 'model answers' in this format. However, we have varied the style of the individual worked answers to try to provide as much diversity as possible with respect to anatomy topics. We have also tried to provide more complete answers than you would be expected to deliver or could conceivably be provided within the time limits of the examination, so that you can refer to them during your revision to acquire key learning points.

4.2.1 Extraperitoneal inguinal region anatomy

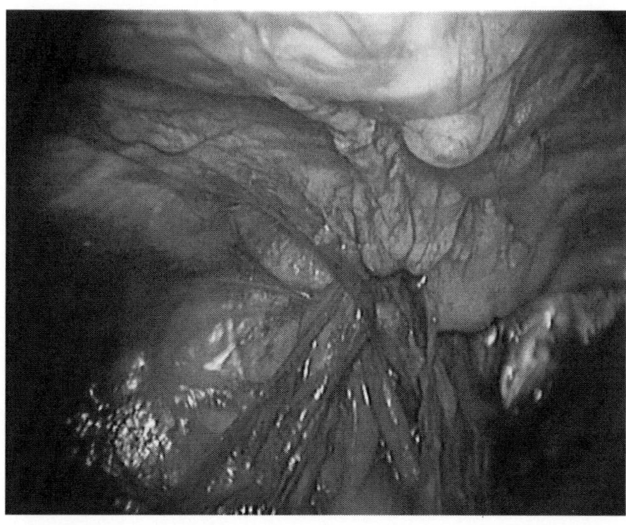

Figure 4.2.1
Left extraperitoneal hernia repair anatomy

Examiner question: can you identify what area you are looking at?

Candidate answer

This is the view encountered in the totally extraperitoneal laparoscopic approach to the inguinal region.

The critical landmarks for orientation are:

- the iliopubic tract (this demarcates the landmark for safe conduct of dissection)
- the pubic symphysis
- the inferior epigastric vessels
- the external iliac vessels
- the gonadal vessels
- the vas deferens.

The critical landmarks for hernia classification are as follows:

- the deep internal ring is located *above* the iliopubic tract *lateral* to the inferior epigastric vessels; an indirect sac will pass into the deep ring lateral to the epigastrics
- the '*direct* space' is located *medial* to the inferior epigastric vessels *above* the iliopubic tract, although this can be difficult to appreciate unless a direct hernia is present
- the *femoral* ring is located just *medial* to the external iliac vessels *below* the iliopubic tract.

Examiner question: what is the iliopubic tract?

Candidate answer

The iliopubic tract is a thickening of the fascia transversalis, extending from the iliopectineal arch to the pubic ramus. It curves around the medial surface of the femoral sheath to attach to the pectineal ligament. It is not the same as the inguinal ligament which is the rolled inferior aspect of the external oblique aponeurosis, which is more superficial and not visualised in the extraperitoneal approach.

Examiner question: can you identify important landmarks here that are relevant to the safe conduct of inguinal hernia repair?

Candidate answer

The iliopubic tract is the key landmark. Structures below the iliopubic tract (external iliac and gonadal vessels and nerves) must not be damaged by placing tacks into them inadvertently. The two most important areas are the triangles of 'doom' and 'pain'.

Triangle of doom: bounded medially by the vas deferens and laterally by the gonadal vessels with the deep ring at its apex. The reflected peritoneal edge forms the posterior border. The external iliac vessels course through this area and tacks placed here risk major haemorrhage.

Triangle of pain: bounded medially by the gonadal vessels and superolaterally by the iliopubic tract. The lateral border is formed by the reflected peritoneal edge. The femoral branch of the genitofemoral nerve or the lateral femoral cutaneous nerve are at risk of injury when tacks are placed in this triangle.

4.2.2 Axillary anatomy

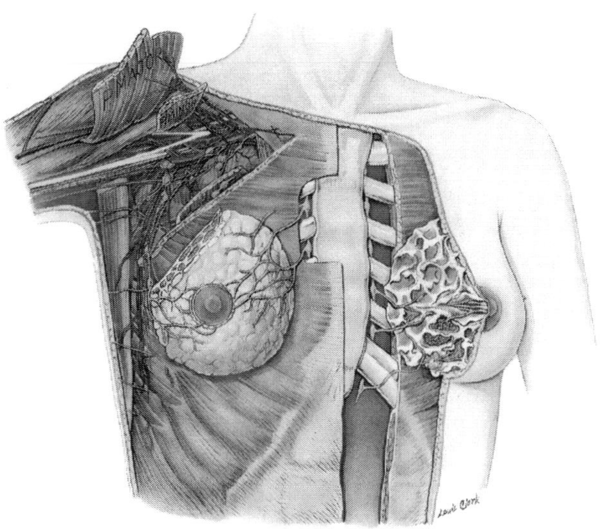

Figure 4.2.2
Right breast and axilla (Source: *The Breast*, 4th edn. Bland K I. 2009, Elsevier, Fig 2-7, p 27.)

Examiner question: what are the borders and contents of the axilla?

Candidate answer

- The axilla is a pyramidal shaped space that lies between the upper arm and side of chest. It is a passage from the root of the neck to the upper limb through which nerves, blood vessels, and lymphatics travel to and from the arm.
- The apex of the axilla is bounded anteriorly by the clavicle, posteriorly by the upper border of the scapula and medially by the outer border of the first rib.
- The base or lower end of the axilla is bounded anteriorly by the axillary fold and lower border of pectoralis (pec.) major muscle, posteriorly by the latissimus (lat.) dorsi and teres major muscles and medially by the chest wall.
- Clinically, the axilla is divided into three levels using pec. minor as a reference:
  1. level I is below
  2. level II is posterior
  3. level III is superior.

WALLS OF THE AXILLA

- Anterior wall: pec. major, pec. minor and subclavius muscles.
- Posterior wall: subscapularis, lat. dorsi and teres major muscles.
- Medial wall: upper 4–5 ribs and intercostal muscles covered by serratus anterior.
- Lateral wall: coracobrachialis and biceps muscles, and the bicipital groove of the humerus.

CONTENTS OF THE AXILLA

- Axillary artery and vein along with their branches and tributaries.
- Cords and branches of the brachial plexus (Intercostobrachial nerve, nerve to lat. dorsi, long thoracic nerve).
- Lymphatics.

Examiner question: tell us about the axillary artery.

Candidate answer

The axillary artery:

- begins at the lateral border of the first rib as a continuation of the subclavian artery and ends at the lower border of teres major — it is divided into three parts by pec. minor:
  1. first part lies proximal to pec. minor and gives off one branch: the superior thoracic artery
  2. second part lies behind the pec. minor and gives off two branches: (i) thoracoacromial trunk (clavicular, humeral, acromial, and pectoral branches) and (ii) lateral thoracic artery
  3. third part lies between the lateral border of pec. minor and medial border of teres major. It gives off three branches: (i) the subscapular artery; (ii) anterior artery; and (iii) posterior circumflex humeral artery.

Examiner question: what are the boundaries of an axillary dissection?

Candidate answer

Once the axilla is entered and the axillary fat exposed, the boundaries of the dissection can be defined as follows.

- Medial boundary: after entering the axilla the medial extent of the dissection is defined by incising the fascia 1 cm below the lateral edge of pec. major. This ensures that the medial pectoral nerve is not injured. This dissection is continued cranially with simultaneous lateral retraction of the axillary fat to help expose the muscle edge. Once the lateral border of pec. major has been exposed it is then retracted anteriomedially to expose pec. minor underneath. The dissection is continued cranially by a combination of sharp and blunt dissection, freeing the axillary fatty nodal tissue from the lateral edge of pec. minor.
- Lateral boundary: this is defined by the lateral border of lat. dorsi. The fascia overlying the lateral edge of the muscle is incised parallel to the muscle 1 cm anterior to its edge. This incision is continued cranially until the tendon of the muscle or axillary vein is seen. The thoracodorsal neurovascular bundle can be identified lying below the fascia overlying the lat. dorsi muscle (approximately 2 cm medial to the lateral edge of the muscle). The neurovascular bundle should be identified and protected during dissection of the lateral boundary of the dissection.
- Superior boundary: this depends on whether the axillary dissection is being performed for breast cancer (level II) or malignant melanoma (level III). Retracting pec. minor anteriomedially with the elbow flexed and the shoulder abducted allows exposure, identification and dissection of the axillary vein. If this is inadequate, pec. minor should be transected. The dissection is continued cranially by a combination of careful sharp and blunt dissection

until the axillary vein is identified behind the medial edge of the pec. minor muscle. Once the vein is encountered all fat and nodal tissue is dissected off the vein and swept laterally. The superior dissection is continued laterally along the axillary vein, peeling down all the lymphatic tissue and ligating all venous tributaries encountered until the lateral extent of dissection is reached. Of note, the thoracodorsal nerve emerges from beneath the axillary vein and courses laterally to meet the thoracodorsal vessels. Ligation of the lateral thoracic vein is necessary to expose the thoracodorsal neurovascular bundle.

- Inferior boundary: This is identified where the angular veins drain into the thoracodorsal vein. Note, when creating the medial and lateral boundaries of your dissection it frees the inferior boundary of the axillary fat.

Examiner question: how can the axillary vein be reliably identified?

Candidate answer

Identification of the axillary vein can be difficult at times and three main techniques can be employed to identify it.

1. Retrograde dissection by identification of the angular veins draining into the thoracodorsal vein. The thoracodorsal vein is then followed cranially until it enters into the axillary vein. Also, if the lat. dorsi muscle tendon is encountered it can be followed cranially to the axillary vein.
2. Palpation of the axillary artery at the apex of the axilla can help locate the axillary vein. The vein lies anterior to the artery and posterior to the junction of the clavicle and first rib.
3. Retraction/transaction of the pec. minor muscle will allow identification of the vein which is located posterior to the medial edge to the muscle.

Examiner question: what are the important nerves encountered during axillary dissection and how can they be reliably identified?

Candidate answer

The three relevant nerves that travel through the axilla and which are encountered during an axillary dissection are (i) the long thoracic, (ii) thoracodorsal and (iii) intercostobrachial nerves.

(i) The long thoracic nerve passes vertically downward to enter the axilla. In the proximal axilla, the long thoracic nerve runs superficial to the serratus anterior fascia and is embedded within the fatty tissue. It then travels medially and at the level of the fourth and fifth intercostal spaces, it pierces the superficial fascia to lie on the serratus anterior muscle deep to the fascia. It courses behind the mid-axillary line and posterior to the lateral thoracic perforating vessels. The search for the long thoracic nerve begins high in the axilla where it is found embedded within the axillary tissue lying approximately 1 cm away from the chest wall. The thin layer of adventitial tissue enveloping the lymphatic tissue is incised laterally and parallel to the long thoracic nerve, thus freeing the nerve, which can then be pushed medially toward the chest wall. Injury to this nerve will result in winging of the scapula.

(ii) The thoracodorsal nerve originates from the posterior cord of the brachial plexus and passes below the axillary vein to enter the axilla. It then passes laterally to meet the subscapular vessels, and forms a triangular space over the subscapularis muscle. The base of the triangle is formed by the axillary vein, the medial border by the thoracodorsal nerve, and the lateral border by the subscapular vessels. The thoracodorsal nerve is superficial to the subscapular artery as it descends along the anteromedial aspect of the lat. dorsi muscle, which it supplies. The lateral thoracic vein, a large venous tributary of the axillary vein, is an important landmark for identification of the thoracodorsal nerve. The thoracodorsal bundle containing the nerve and the vessels are located approximately 1 cm deep and medial to this vein. The lateral thoracic vein must be ligated and transected to expose the thoracodorsal neurovascular bundle which can then be followed and protected as the dissection continues inferiorly. Injury to this nerve will result in weak adduction of the shoulder.

(iii) The intercostobrachial nerve: During dissection of the lateral and medial boundaries of the axilla, the lower branch of the intercostobrachial nerve will be encountered running across the axilla, high up within it. It runs from the chest wall to the upper arm. Care should be taken to preserve it unless it is involved in the malignant process. Injury to this nerve will result in numbness or paraesthesia on the posteriolateral aspect of the upper arm.

4.2.3 Thyroidectomy anatomy

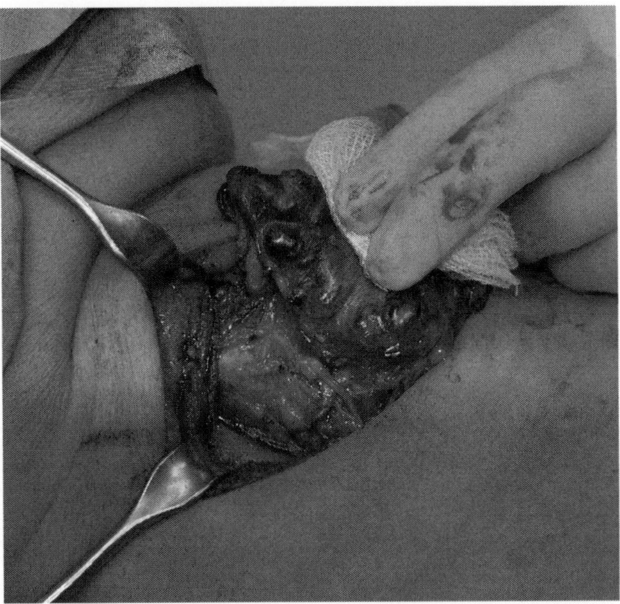

Figure 4.2.3
View from right side of a thyroidectomy

Examiner question: can you identify what area you are looking at?

Candidate answer

This is the view encountered in thyroidectomy. This is the cephalic (to the left of the image) and this is the caudal part (to the right of the image) of the patient.

Note: although every effort is made to ensure that the images are obvious, it may not always be clear to the candidate what they are looking at. It is acceptable to ask the examiner to orientate you if this is the case. The image is only a primer for subsequent questions and you are unlikely to suffer any penalty if your subsequent answers demonstrate a good understanding of the topic.

Examiner question: what is the course of the recurrent laryngeal nerve in this region?

Candidate answer

- The left recurrent laryngeal nerve (RLN) originates from the vagus nerve in the superior mediastinum and loops under the aorta limited by the ligamentum arteriosum. It passes into the root of the neck moving from the left towards midline to enter the tracheo-oesophageal groove.
- The right RLN originates from the vagus nerve in the neck and courses around the right subclavian artery. It ascends in the tracheo-oesophageal groove pursuing a more vertical course than on the left. Both branches pass behind the lateral lobe of the thyroid gland in close association with the branches of the inferior thyroid artery in the region of the Tubercle of Zuckerkandl.
- The RLN enters the larynx under the inferior constrictor of the pharynx to supply all the intrinsic muscles of the larynx with the exception of the cricothyroid (supplied by the external branch of the superior laryngeal nerve). It supplies sensation to the infraglottic larynx.

Examiner question: are these relationships between the RLN and the thyroid constant?

Candidate answer

No, in fact there is considerable anatomical variation. However, the RLN *usually* passes close to and behind the Tubercle of Zuckerkandl.

Examiner interrupts: what is the Tubercle of Zuckerkandl?

Note: If the examiner interrupts you at a point like this, he/she is probably trying to give you an opportunity to excel, rather than trying to fail you!

Candidate answer

- This is a lateral or posterior projection from the lateral lobe of the thyroid. It originates from the ventral portion of the ultimobranchial body.
- In more than 90% of cases, the RLN runs posterior to the tubercle, either in the tracheo-oesophageal groove (~60%), posterior (~24%) or lateral to the trachea (~5%). Only in a small number of cases (~5%) does it pass completely anterior to the thyroid (usually re-operative surgery).
- The relationship to the inferior thyroid artery (ITA) is also variable: in 85% of cases it is posterior and intertwined between branches of the ITA and in 15% it is anterior (more common on the right).
- There are instances of non-recurrent RLN. This affects about 1:200 of the population. It is more common on the right and associated with a retro-oesophageal subclavian artery. In about one-third of people, the RLN branches outside the larynx. If this is the case, the posterior branch is sensory and the (more vulnerable) anterior branch is motor.

Examiner question: is the RLN the only nerve commonly encountered around the thyroid gland?

Candidate answer

When the superior pole of the gland is dissected, the external branch of the superior laryngeal nerve (ESLN) is encountered. This supplies the cricothyroid muscle (which tense the vocal cord). The nerve originates from the vagus and is closely associated with the superior thyroid artery. The relation is categorised into three types (Cernea Classification):

1. Type I: the nerve crosses the superior thyroid vessels >1 cm above the upper pole of the thyroid
2. Type IIa: it crosses the superior thyroid vessels <1 cm above the upper pole of the thyroid
3. Type IIb: it crosses at or below the level of the upper pole of the thyroid.

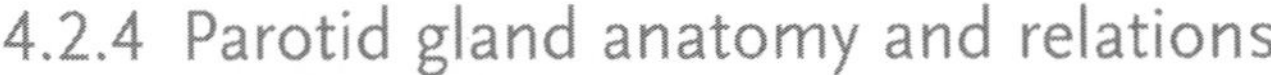

4.2.4 Parotid gland anatomy and relations

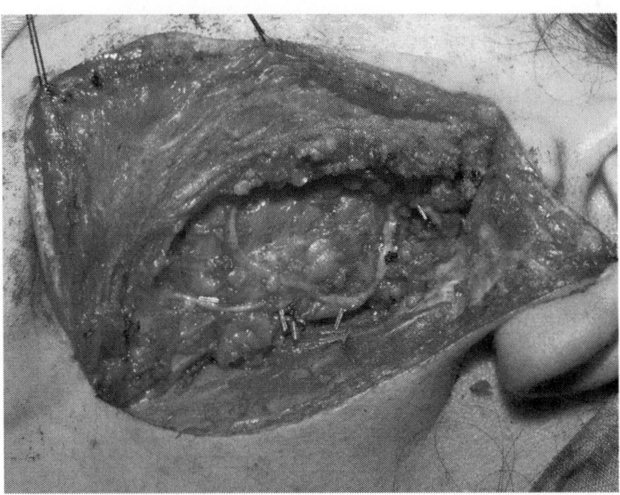

Figure 4.2.4
View following superficial parotidectomy on the left

Examiner question: which structures can you identify here?

Candidate answer

This is an image after a patient has undergone a superficial parotidectomy. The sternocleidomastoid (SCM) muscle can be seen along the inferior border of the image. The anterior branch of the greater auricular nerve can be seen lying on that muscle. The superficial part of the parotid muscle has been removed to reveal the branches of the facial nerve. The posterior belly of the digastric (PBD) muscle can just be seen attached to the inner aspect of the mastoid process. I can see the nerve branching into upper and lower main divisions.

Examiner question: what are the relationships of the parotid gland?

Candidate answer

- The gland lies between the mastoid process posteriorly (with the SCM and PBD attached to its superficial and deep surfaces, respectively) and the ramus of the mandible (with the masseter and medial pterygoid attached to its superficial and deep surfaces, respectively).
- The gland spills over all these muscles to a variable extent. Deep to the posterior part of the gland is the styloid process and its attached muscles and ligaments.
- Surgeons often consider the gland to have a superficial and a deep part separated by the plane of the facial nerve.
- Deep to the facial nerve is the retromandibular vein, which is in turn superficial to the external carotid artery.
- The gland is contained within the investing layer of the deep cervical fascia (known as the parotid sheath). A condensation of this fascia is attached from the styloid process to the mandible and is known as the stylomandibular ligament. This partitions the parotid gland from the posterior aspect of the submandibular gland.

Examiner question: what relationships help you identify the facial nerve during surgery?

Candidate answer

- The facial nerve's main trunk emerges from the stylomastoid foramen and winds lateral to the styloid process just above the tendon of the stylohyoid muscle. The relationship of the stylomastoid foramen and the tympano-mastoid fissure can be used as an operative landmark.
- The main trunk of the facial nerve is less than 1 cm deep to the tympano-mastoid suture line at the level of the digastric muscle. The facial nerve enters the parotid gland then usually bifurcates into an upper division (giving rise to the temporal and zygomatic branches) and a lower division (forming buccal, mandibular and cervical branches). The temporal branch usually lies in front of the superficial temporal artery. The buccal branch runs parallel to the parotid duct. The branches emerge from behind the anterior border of the gland. No branches emerge from the superficial aspect of the gland.

Examiner question: which structures lay deep to the facial nerve in the parotid gland?

Candidate answer

- Major vascular structures course through and lie deep to the gland.
- The superficial temporal and maxillary veins join within the gland to form the retromandibular vein. This divides into anterior and posterior divisions. The former division passes forward and unites with the anterior facial vein to form the common facial vein. The posterior division is joined by the posterior auricular vein to become the external jugular vein.
- Deep to the retromandibular vein is the external carotid artery.

Examiner question: can you describe the nerves that control parotid secretion in response to a meal?

Candidate answer

Fibres arise from the inferior salivatory nucleus of the glossopharyngeal nerve in the medulla. These preganglionic fibres are carried by the glossopharyngeal nerve and its tympanic branch. The latter gives rise to the tympanic plexus on the promontory of the cochlear in the middle ear. These fibres pass via the lesser petrosal nerve to synapse in the otic ganglion. Postganglionic secretomotor fibres reach the parotid via the auriculotemporal nerve (a branch of the mandibular division of the trigeminal nerve).

4.2.5 Submandibular gland and relations

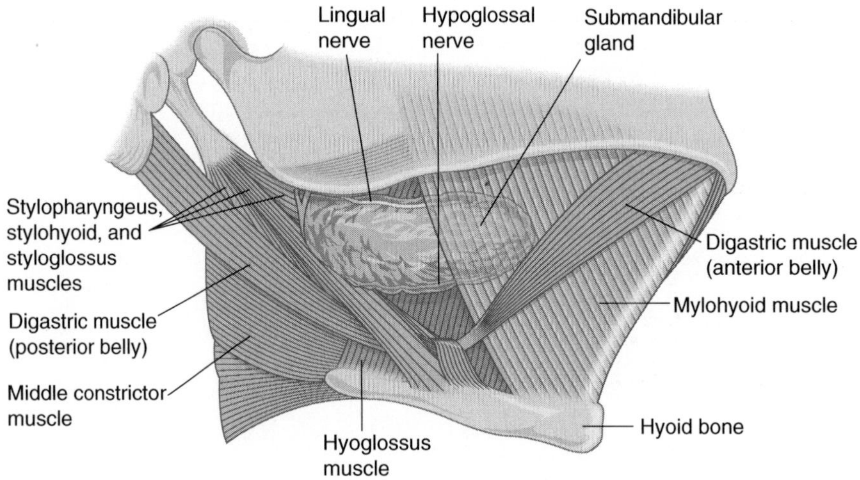

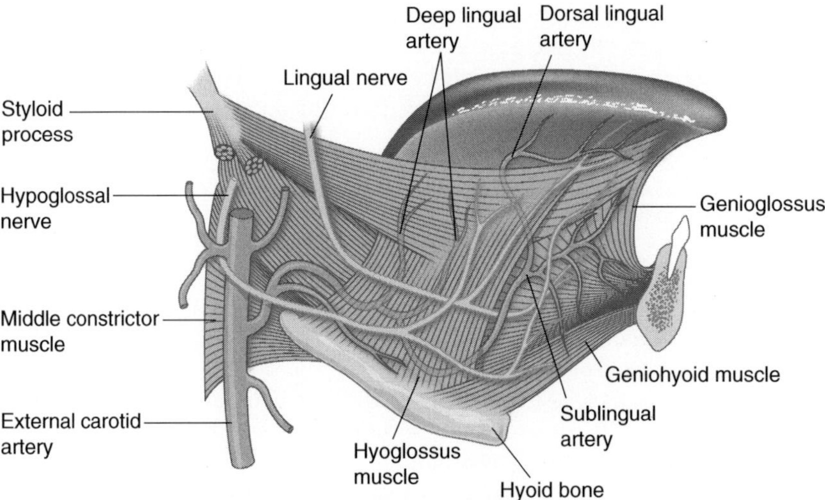

Figure 4.2.5

Submandibular gland anatomy (Source: *Cummings Otolaryngology: Head & Neck Surgery*, 5th edn. Flint P W et al. 2010, Mosby: an imprint of Elsevier, Fig 96-4, p 1296.)

Examiner question: what does this image show?

Candidate answer

This is an image of the right submandibular gland.

- The submandibular glands are paired and constitute the second largest salivary gland. Each gland is divided into a larger superficial portion and a deep portion by the mylohyoid muscle. Emerging from its deep part is the submandibular duct known as Wharton's duct, which opens at the base of the frenulum of the tongue.
- The submandibular gland is located in the digastric triangle, bordered anteriorly by the anterior belly of the digastrics, posteriorly by the posterior belly of the digastrics and laterally by the lower border of mandible and medial pterygoid muscle. The floor of the digastric triangle is made up of the hyoglossus and mylohyoid muscles. The roof is made up of skin, platysma muscle and the investing layer of cervical fascia.
- The blood supply is from branches of the facial and lingual arteries and the venous drainage mirrors this.
- The secretomotor supply is from the VII cranial nerve via submandibular ganglion and chorda tympani.

Examiner question: what are the important anatomical relations of the gland that must be considered during a submandibular gland excision?

Candidate answer

The important anatomical relations that must be considered include those detailed below.

1. Superficial: the mandibular and cervical branches of the facial nerve.
   - The mandibular and cervical branches of the VII nerve emerge from the parotid gland near the angle of the mandible.
   - The mandibular branch runs downwards and forwards deep to platysma and then curves upwards to cross the mandible close to the facial artery.
   - The mandibular nerve is protected during surgery by making the incision 4 cm below the mandible.
2. On the gland: the facial artery and vein.
   - The facial artery arises from the external carotid artery and passes upwards and can be identified at the posterior aspect of the submandibular gland. It passes forwards above the gland and emerges beneath the lower border of the mandible and curls upwards along the face.
   - The facial vein descends along the face from anterior to posterior and crosses the mandible about 2 cm in front of the angle. It then runs along the external surface of the submandibular gland and receives the submental vein, forming the common facial vein which then continues on to drain into the internal jugular vein.
   - The facial vein and artery are usually encountered after identification and preservation of the mandibular nerve. They are usually ligated at this point and again at the posterior aspect of the gland.
3. Deep: the lingual and hypoglossal nerves and the submandibular ganglion.
   - The lingual nerve lies deep to the mylohyoid muscle, and above the deep part of the gland. It runs forward between the mylohyoid and hyoglossus

muscles. It passes around the submandibular duct by initially passing from medial to lateral above the duct, then curving underneath the duct from lateral to medial, emerging at the medial side of the duct. During ligation of the submandibular duct care must be taken to identify the lingual nerve so that it is not damaged at this point. More proximally, the lingual nerve is identified by retracting the submandibular gland laterally and the mylohyoid muscle anteriorly. The lingual nerve is freed from the submandibular gland by dividing between the nerve and the submandibular ganglion.

- The hypoglossal nerve lies deep and below the submandibular gland. It also runs between the mylohyoid and hyoglossus muscles. The nerve is identified after the posterior border of the gland is mobilised and retracted upwards. The mylohyoid muscle is also retracted anteriorly to expose the hypoglossal nerve as it emerges from the posterior belly of digastric.

4.2.6 Blood supply of the stomach

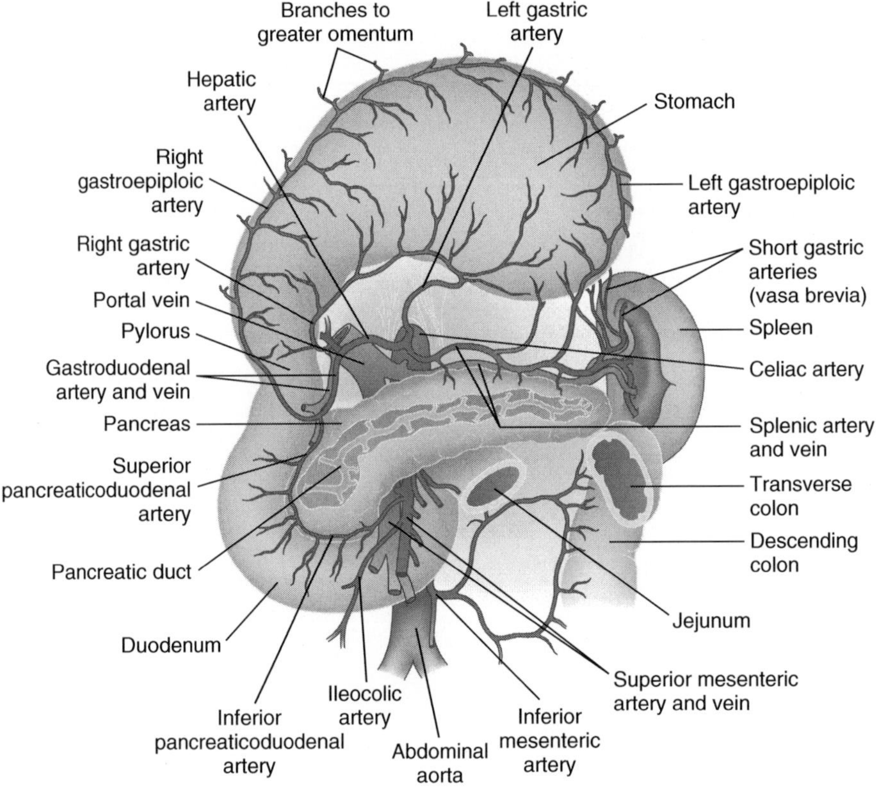

Figure 4.2.6

Stomach anatomy (Source: *Sabiston Textbook of Surgery*, 19th edn. Townsend C M. 2012, Saunders: an imprint of Elsevier, Fig 49-2, p 1183. From *Shackelford's Surgery of the Alimentary Tract*, 6th edn. Yeo C et al. 2007, WB Saunders: an imprint of Elsevier.)

Examiner question: describe the blood supply of the stomach.

Candidate answer

The stomach consists of the greater and lesser curvatures, the cardia, the fundus, the body, and the pyloric antrum and canal. The arterial supply is from three major branches of the coeliac trunk, namely the common hepatic, splenic and left gastric arteries.

- The fundus and upper left part of the greater curvature is supplied by the short gastric arteries, which are branches of the splenic artery, and run in the gastrosplenic ligament.
- The lesser curvature is supplied by the left gastric artery and right gastric artery (a branch of the hepatic or gastroduodenal arteries), which run between the two layers of the lesser omentum.
- The greater curvature is supplied by the left gastro-omental (or gastroepiploic) artery (a branch of the splenic artery) and the right gastro-omental artery (a branch of the gastroduodenal artery) which run between the two layers of greater omentum 1 cm from the gastric wall.
- Both sets of arteries anastomose with each other on their respective gastric curves and then again with the supply of the other curve via a rich anastomosing network at three levels in the gastric wall: the mucosal, submucosal and intramuscularly. The network is well developed everywhere except along the lesser curvature where anastomosing channels are of a finer calibre and are more likely to be end arteries.

Examiner question: how do you use this knowledge when performing an oesophagectomy?

Candidate answer

Knowledge of the stomach's blood supply is important when fashioning a neo-oesophagus following oesophagectomy.

- The short gastric, left gastro-omental and left gastric arteries are divided to mobilise the upper portion of the stomach so it can be pulled up to form an oesophageal substitute and to allow clearance of the lesser curve lymph nodes, which is important oncologically for distal oesophageal cancers. The short gastric vessels are ligated away from the greater curvature to avoid damage to the intramural network. The left gastric artery is ligated at its origin for oncological reasons, since there is no evidence that its branches need to be preserved to maintain viability of the stomach.
- The right gastro-omental and right gastric arteries are preserved to maintain viability of stomach.

4.2.7 Cholecystectomy anatomy

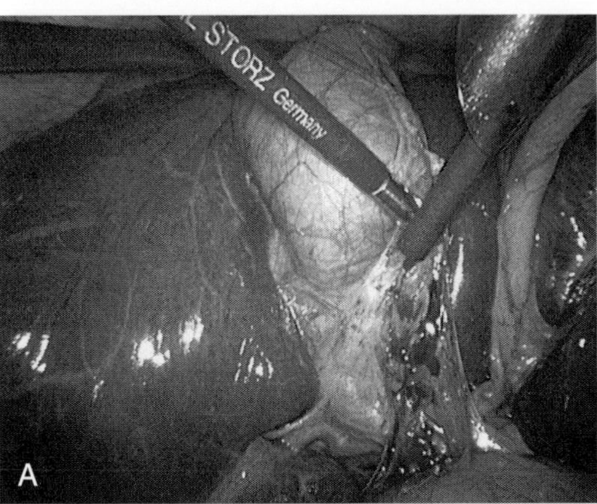

Figure 4.2.7A
Laparoscopic cholecystectomy

Examiner question: describe the important surgical anatomical landmarks that you see.

Candidate answer

- The image above shows a view at the start of a gallbladder (GB) dissection. There is a fissure visible between the right lobe (segment V) and the caudate process through which the right hepatic pedicle passes. The space between the infundibulum of the gallbladder and this sulcus is superior to the plane of the common bile duct and relatively safe for commencing dissection.
- The gallbladder rests on the cystic plate and the main strictures of the *porta hepatis* enter the liver at the hilar plate. The region of the hilar plate can be identified by noting the quadrate lobe, which is bounded by the falciform ligament on the left side and the gallbladder on the right. At the base of the quadrate lobe (segment IVb) the hilar plate is seen.

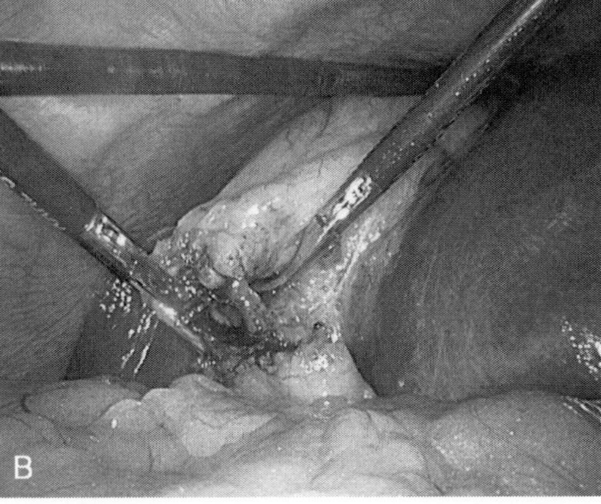

Figure 4.2.7B
Cystic artery

Examiner question: what is the artery you can see here (in figure 4.2.7B)? Can you describe the origin of the artery?

Candidate answer

This is the cystic artery.

- The cystic artery (CA) usually arises from the right hepatic artery (RHA) in Calot's triangle and ascends on the left side of gall bladder in 70% of cases.
- In 20% of cases the CA arises from the common hepatic artery (CHA), its bifurcation or the left hepatic artery.
- In 10% the CA arises from an accessory RHA.
- Occasionally (< 2.5%), it arises from the gastro-duodenal artery (GDA)

Examiner question: what is the significance of these variations in cholecystectomy?

Candidate answer

- The RHA passes close to the GB (10% of patients) with short arterial 'twigs' entering the GB, rather than a single cystic artery. The RHA can then thus be damaged when mistaken for the CA or when the 'twigs' are divided.
- An accessory RHA arises low from the SMA running through Calot's triangle posterior and parallel to the cystic duct (8% of patients). This can be mistaken for a posterior branch of the cystic artery.

4.2.8 Intra-operative cholangiogram

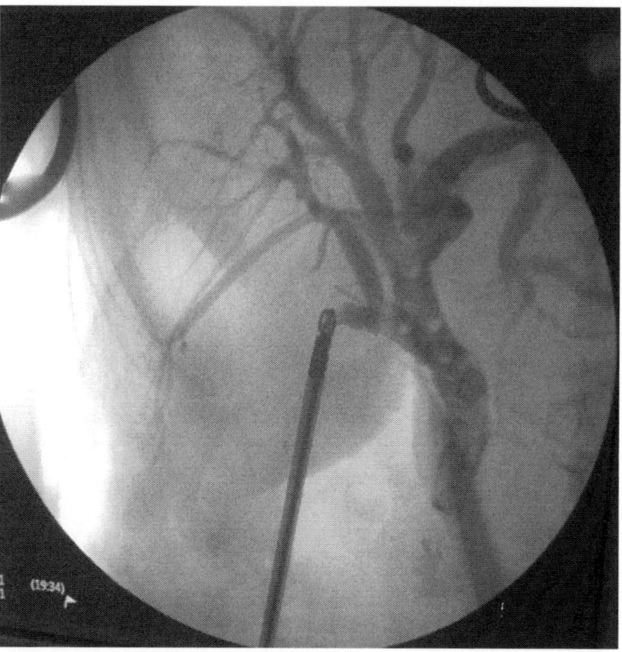

Figure 4.2.8
Cholangiogram of cystic duct inserting into the right posterior sectoral duct, and duct stones

Examiner question: describe what you see in this cholangiogram.

Candidate answer

The cystic duct inserts into the right posterior sectoral duct (RPSD), as a consequence of the RPSD joining very low.

Examiner question: what are the common variations in biliary anatomy that are important in cholecystectomy?

Candidate answer

There are variations of the cystic duct and of aberrant hepatic ducts.

- The three major variants in cystic duct anatomy are angular (75%), parallel (20%) and spiral (5%).
- An aberrant hepatic duct is defined as a duct draining a normal portion of the liver that joins the biliary tree outside the liver.
- In about 2% of cases, the cystic duct joins the right hepatic duct or right posterior sectoral duct and is particularly at risk during cholecystectomy.
- If the cystic duct was dissected beyond the union with the aberrant hepatic duct or sectoral duct, this portion of the liver would not be opacified by the cholangiogram. However, it would be possible to misinterpret a cholangiogram as satisfactorily showing a normal intrahepatic biliary tree. The only clue would be the relative paucity of ducts on the right inferior part of the liver shadow. This type of injury, unrecognised would lead to excision of the distal end of the RPSD without realising it, leading to obstruction or leakage.

4.2.9 Liver anatomy

Examiner question: can you please describe the important surgical anatomy of the liver?

TOP TIP

It is best to pick up the liver and have a methodical approach, as there is a lot to say!

One approach is: surfaces → lobes → ligaments → segments → fissures → porta hepatis.

The time spent in each part depends on the interest shown by the examiners.

Candidate answer

SURFACES

- The liver has a diaphragmatic and a visceral surface.
- The diaphragmatic surface is covered with peritoneum except for the bare area (containing IVC and hepatic veins).
- The visceral surface is related to the stomach, duodenum and hepatic flexure.

LOBES

- Liver lobar anatomy can be described morphologically and functionally.
- Traditionally, based on external appearance, four lobes are distinguishable: right, left, quadrate, and caudate. On the diaphragmatic surface, the falciform ligament divides the liver into the right and left lobes. On the visceral surface the ligamentum venosum and ligamentum teres fissures provide the demarcation. The quadrate lobe is demarcated on the visceral surface by the gallbladder fossa, porta hepatis and ligamentum teres. The caudate lobe is demarcated by the inferior vena cava groove, porta hepatis and venous ligament fissure.
- Alternatively, the liver anatomy can be described functionally. The initial classification was based on biliary ducts and hepatic artery branching using Cantlie's line to divide the liver into left and right and five segments: medial, lateral, posterior, anterior and caudate. Cantlie's line passes along the left side of gallbladder fossa and the left side of the inferior vena cava. The left liver is divided into medial and lateral segments by a plane defined by the falciform ligament on the diaphragmatic surface and round ligament on the visceral surface. The right liver consists of anterior and posterior segments, divided by the right fissure. Each segment is further divided into superior and inferior subsegments by a transverse line. Latterly, this has given way to Couinaud's classification (see below).
- The quadrate lobe is bounded by gallbladder and its bed on the right and the fissure for the ligamentum teres on the left.
- The caudate lobe bounded by IVC on the right and ligamentum venosum (continuation of umbilical fissure) on the left.

LIGAMENTS

- The falciform ligament (vestigial of ventral mesogastrium) attaches the front of the liver to the anterior abdominal wall, descending to attach to the umbilicus.
- The ligamentum teres (obliterated umbilical vein) lies within the free edge of the falciform ligament. The ligamentum teres acts as a guide to the ductal system of segment III, as it separates segment III from the segment IV of right lobe (quadrate lobe).
- The ligamentum venosum is a cord formed by the obliteration of the ductus venosus.
- The coronary and triangular ligaments attach the posterior surface of the liver to the diaphragm. The coronary ligament lays to the right, consisting of a superior and inferior leaf; where they meet forms the right triangular ligament.

FISSURES

- Main fissure: divides right and left side of the liver. It separates segment IV from V and VIII. The middle hepatic vein and gallbladder fossa is in this plane.
- The left fissure separates the left lateral sector from the medial sector. The left hepatic vein is in this plane.

- The right fissure is between the right anterior and posterior sector and corresponds to the right hepatic vein.
- The umbilical fissure is where the falciform ligament reaches the anterior border of the liver. It separates segment III from IV.
- The fissure venosum is a continuation of the umbilical fissure on the posterior surface of the liver. The lesser omentum passes into this fissure. It was the ductus venous in fetal life, which connected the left branch of portal vein to left hepatic vein.
- The dorsal fissure separates segment IV from I.

SEGMENTS

- Segmental anatomy of the liver (eight segments as described by Couinaud) is based on the intrahepatic distribution of the portal trinity, the principle component of which is the portal vein and its division.
- In both the traditional and the Couinaud classifications, the plane defined by the middle hepatic vein subdivides the liver into the true right and left lobes. A standard right or left (hemi) hepatectomy requires division along the plane of the middle hepatic vein.
- Segments numbered in anti clockwise fashion around the portal vein. The left lobe consists of segments II, III and IV and the right lobe segments V, VI, VII and VIII.
- In Couinaud nomenclature, the plane defined by the right branch of the portal vein divides the anterior and posterior divisions of the right liver superiorly and inferiorly, thus dividing the right lobe into four segments (V-VIII). The medial segment of the left lobe can also be divided into two segments by the plane of the portal vein (IVa and IVb) [Bismuth].
- The caudate lobe (segment I) is autonomous in that it receives arterial blood from both right and left hepatic arteries and its venous blood drains directly into the IVC.

PORTA HEPATIS

- This is the fissure in the liver between the quadrate lobe in front and the caudate process and lobe behind. It receives the hepatic pedicle and two ligaments (teres and venosum). The hepatic pedicle consists of the portal vein posteriorly, hepatic artery antero-medially and common bile duct antero-laterally. These are surrounded by Glissonian sheath, which forms the anterior border of foramen of Winslow (used in the Pringle manoeuvre).

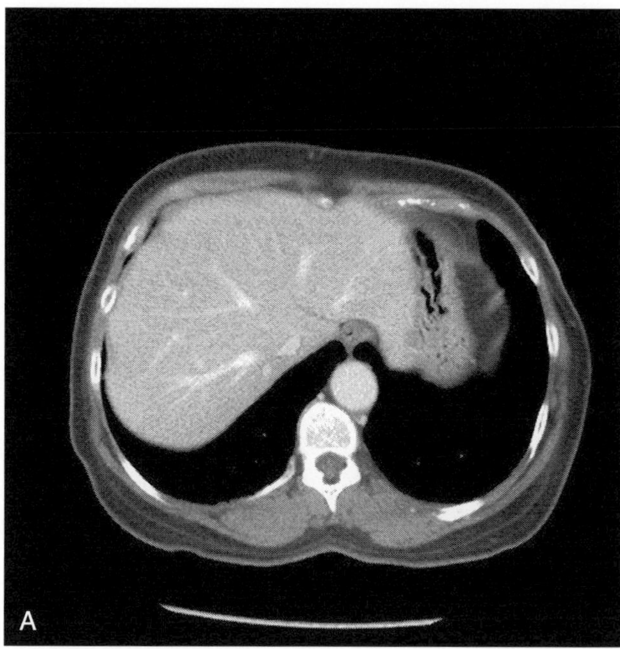

Figure 4.2.9A
CT scan of liver

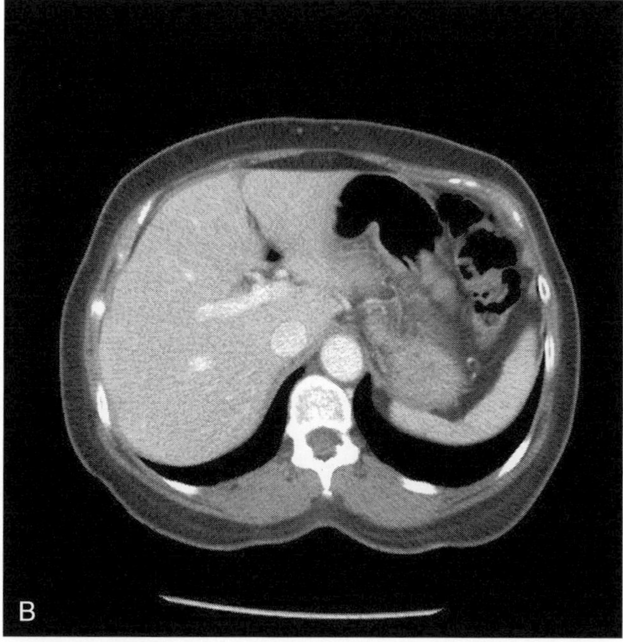

Figure 4.2.9B
CT scan of liver

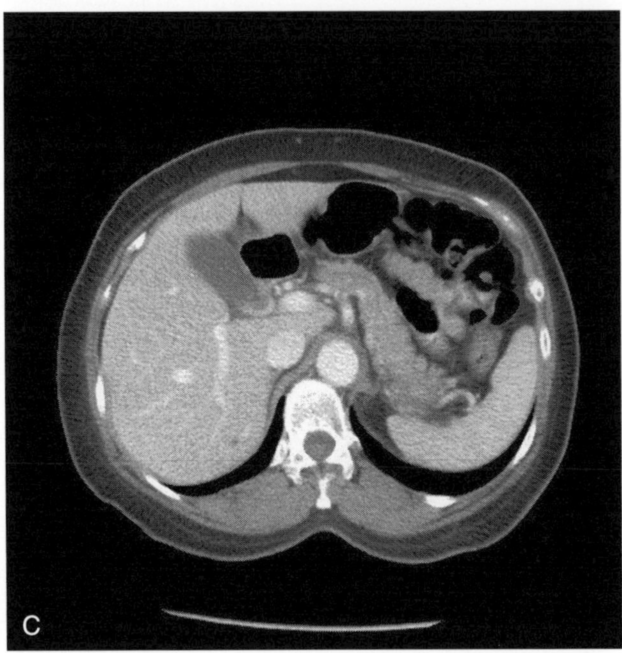

Figure 4.2.9C
CT scan of liver

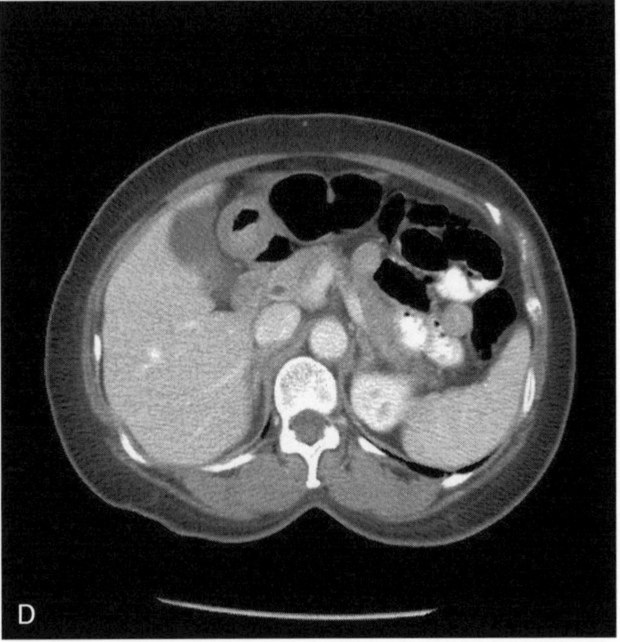

Figure 4.2.9D
CT scan of liver

Examiner question: can you define the segments of the liver on this CT scan?

Candidate answer

The key anatomic landmarks are set out below.

- The plane of division of the portal vein within the liver = horizontal plane.
- The course of each of the right, middle and left hepatic veins = vertical planes.
- Superior to the plane of the portal vein:
  - segment II lies medial to the left hepatic vein
  - segment IVa lies between the left and middle hepatic veins
  - segment VIII lies between the middle and right hepatic veins
  - segment VII lies posterior or postero-lateral to the right hepatic vein.
- Inferior to the plane of the portal vein:
  - segment III lies medial to the left hepatic vein
  - segment IVb lies between the left and middle hepatic veins
  - segment V lies between the middle and right hepatic veins
  - segment VI lies posterior or postero-lateral to the right hepatic vein.
- Segment I (the caudate lobe) lies superior and medial to the GB, and posterior to segment 4a.

Examiner question: what is the surgical relevance of the segmental anatomy of the liver?

Candidate answer

- For the liver to remain viable, resections must proceed along the vessels that define the peripheries of these segments. In general, this means resection lines run parallel to the hepatic veins while preserving the portal veins, bile ducts, and hepatic arteries that provide vascular inflow and biliary drainage through the centre of the segment.
- It is possible to remove any single segment of the liver without jeopardising the blood or biliary drainage of the rest.
- Right (hemi) hepatectomy involves resection of segments V to VIII whereas left (hemi) hepatectomy involves resection of segments ii to iv. According to the Brisbane terminology, Healey's functional classification of *sections* defines right anterior, right posterior, left medial or left lateral *section*ectomy. Couinaud's *segmental* classification allows more precise definition of individual (or combination) *segment*ectomy.

4.2.10 The pancreas and its relations

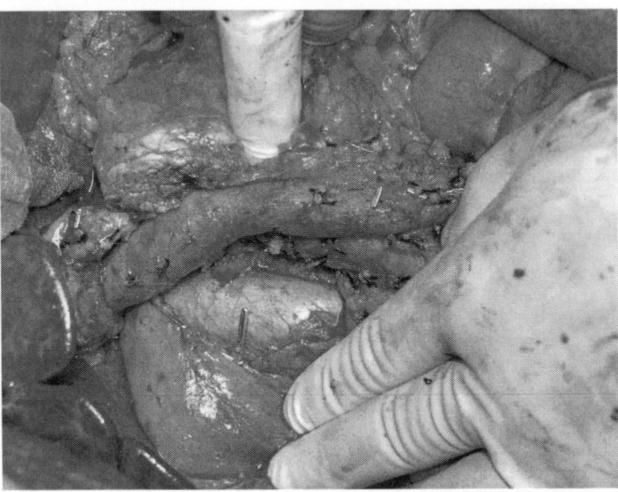

Figure 4.2.10
View immediately after pancreaticoduodenectomy

Examiner question: can you identify the key structures in this image?

Candidate answer

This image appears to be taken during a pancreaticoduodenectomy (Whipple's procedure). The pancreas is under the surgeon's finger and I can also see the superior mesenteric vein and portal vein and the IVC.

Examiner question: can you discuss the important relations of the pancreas with respect to pancreaticoduodenectomy?

Candidate answer

- The pancreas is entirely retroperitoneal and thus operative procedures require mobilisation from this position. The plane lateral to the duodenum is avascular and employed for this purpose (Kocher's manoeuvre). The inferior border of the pancreas is also relatively avascular, although the inferior mesenteric vein may be encountered to the right of the spine.
- The pancreas has a head, neck, body and tail. It is encased within major blood vessels. The vena cava and aorta occupy its posterior surface in the midline.
- The head fits into the C shape concavity of the duodenum and the neck is the narrower part of the pancreas that lies over the portal vein. The head lies over the IVC and renal veins and the neck lies over the confluence of the SMV and splenic vein as they form the portal vein.
- The uncinate process (an extension of the head of the pancreas) passes behind the superior mesenteric vessels and in front of the IVC.
- Posteriorly, the body of the pancreas is related to the origin of the SMA and the aorta.
- The body of the pancreas is related anteriorly to the lesser omentum and stomach. The transverse mesocolon divides into two leaves, the superior leaf

covering the anterior surface and the inferior leaf passing inferior to the pancreas. The middle colic artery (a branch of SMA) emerges from beneath the pancreas to travel between the leaves of the mesocolon.

- The splenic vein occupies the posterior surface of the body and tail of the pancreas.
- The splenic artery runs in a tortuous fashion along the superior border of the pancreas towards its tail. It gives off the dorsal pancreatic artery, a varying number of smaller pancreatic branches and a larger branch (great pancreatic artery).
- The tail of the pancreas is relatively mobile and has variable relationships with the splenic hilum. The two layers of splenorenal ligament contain the tail as well as the splenic artery, origin of the splenic vein and lymphatics. The tail of the pancreas lies within 1 cm of the spleen hilum in approx 70% of patients and is in direct contact with the spleen in 30%.
- The distal portion of CBD may lie behind the pancreas in a groove or more commonly embedded in the pancreatic substance.
- There are usually two ducts draining the pancreas:
    - the major duct of Wirsung, which opens as major papilla (about 7 cm distal to pylorus in the second part of duodenum)
    - the accessory duct of Santorini which opens as a minor papilla (2 cm proximal to the opening of main duct)
- There is significant variation in the relationship between the main and accessory duct.
- The major duct and common bile duct run parallel in the head of the pancreas before joining to form the ampulla of Vater.

Examiner question: what is the blood supply to the pancreas?

Candidate answer

- The arterial supply of the pancreas is mainly from the splenic artery via one of its largest branches known as the arteria pancreatica magna. However, the head is supplied by the superior and inferior pancreaticoduodenal arteries (from the gastroduodenal and superior mesenteric arteries, respectively).
- Venous return is by numerous small veins into the splenic vein, which is formed within the splenorenal ligament and receives the left gastroepiploic vein. The head is also drained by the superior and inferior pancreaticoduodenal veins into the portal and superior mesenteric veins, respectively.

Examiner question: tell us about the portal vein.

Candidate answer

- The portal vein is an important landmark in pancreaticoduodenectomy. It is formed by the confluence of the splenic vein and SMV at the neck of the pancreas.
- The IMV drains at right angles into the splenic vein or sometimes directly into the SMV.
- The portal vein receives the majority of venous drainage of the gastrointestinal system and supplies 70% of the blood flow to the liver. It receives the left and right gastric veins and the superior pancreaticoduodenal veins.

- Most of the tributaries of the portal vein enter on its sides or posteriorly. Accordingly, there are usually minimal/no branches anteriorly, so that a space can be created bluntly between the portal vein/SMV and neck of the pancreas during pancreaticoduodenectomy.
- The portal vein then ascends to join the porta hepatis in the free margin of epiploic foramen lying behind the CBD and hepatic artery. At the porta hepatis it divides into a shorter but wider right branch and longer but narrower left branch.

Examiner question: what is pancreas divisum?

Candidate answer

- The pancreas develops from two buds — the ventral and dorsal mesogastrium during the 4th–7th week of fetal life, which eventually fuse.
- Pancreatic divisum occurs if the two buds don't fuse. The small ventral duct (of Wirsung) drains via the major papilla and the large dorsal duct (of santorini) drains via the minor papilla. The high ductal pressure may result in recurrent pancreatitis.
- An annular pancreas occurs if the ventral bud, which tends to bi-lobed, migrates in different directions to fuse with the dorsal bud around the second part of the duodenum. It can present in utero or during infancy, although approximately 50% present later in life with recurrent pancreatitis or duodenal obstruction.

4.2.11 Superficial venous system of the lower limb

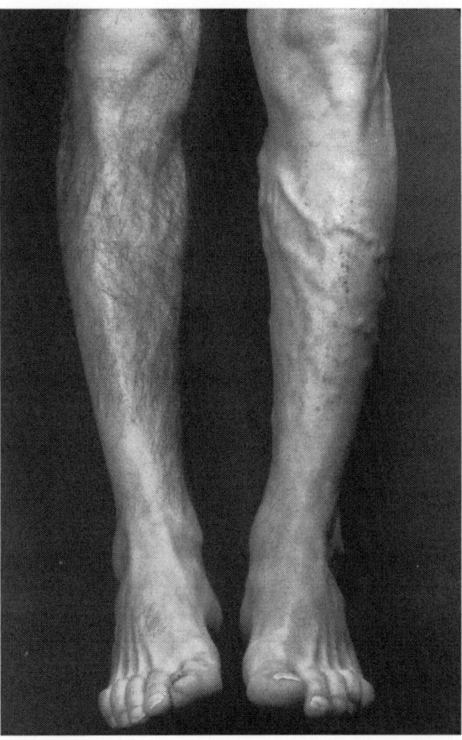

Figure 4.2.11
Varicose veins lower legs

Examiner question: please describe the important surgical anatomy when performing varicose vein surgery.

Candidate answer

Varicose vein surgery involves the ligation of the saphenofemoral junction (SFJ) and stripping of the long saphenous vein. Other important superficial veins include the short saphenous vein and perforators. When performing this surgery one must be aware of the cutaneous nerves associated with the veins, namely the saphenous and sural nerves.

THE LONG SAPHENOUS VEIN (LSV)

- The longest vein in the body begins as an upward continuation of the medial marginal vein of the foot. It courses upwards in front of medial malleolus and then a hands-breadth behind the medial border of patella. It ends by passing through the cribriform fascia which is 3.5 cm below and lateral to the pubic tubercle. It has up to 20 valves, mainly in the 'below knee' segment. Its tributaries include:
  - the anterolateral and posteromedial branches
  - the superficial circumflex, superficial epigastric, and superficial and deep external pudendal veins.
- During surgery it is important to differentiate between the LSV and the femoral vein. The LSV has a greater number of tributaries and a greater amount of adventitial tissue surrounding it. However, the only safe way is to dissect the femoral vein 1–2 cm above and below the SFJ.

THE SHORT SAPHENOUS VEIN (SSV)

- Is an upward continuation of lateral veins of the foot. It passes behind the lateral malleolus into the posterior aspect of the lower leg and penetrates the deep fascia of the calf and has an intrafascial segment before emerging to terminate in the popliteal vein.
- Unlike the SFJ, the saphenopopliteal junction (SPJ) is highly variable; in fact in 25% of the population it does not terminate in the popliteal vein directly. Therefore, pre-operative ultrasound directed marking of the junction is critically important.
- The Da Vinci vein (also known as vein of Giacomini) is the posterior vein that joins the LSV to the SSV.

PERFORATORS

- These are veins that connect the superficial and deep venous systems. There are three large ones on the medial aspect of the calf (Cockett's perforators), occurring at approximately 3, 6 and 9 cm above the medial malleolus. These perforators usually terminate in the posterior tibial veins and may connect directly to LSV. There are various other perforators described (e.g. Hunterian perforator above the knee).

CUTANEOUS NERVES

- The saphenous nerve is the largest cutaneous branch of the femoral nerve (L3, L4). It arises in the femoral triangle and then descends lateral to the femoral vessels in the adductor canal. It then crosses medially and descends on the medial side of the knee where it pierces the fascia lata in between the tendons of sartorius and gracilis. It is then closely related to LSV (anteriorly) below the knee. Hence the LSV is stripped only to the knee to minimise inadvertent injury to this nerve. It innervates the skin on the anteromedial aspect of the knee and the medial and dorsal side of the lower leg and foot.

- The sural nerve (S1, S2) supplies the lateral part of the foot and lower third of the leg. It has contributions from both tibial and common peroneal nerves via communicating branches. It arises in the popliteal fossa and pierces the deep fascia to have a variable relationship with the SSV.
- In SPJ ligation, it is important to appreciate the anatomy of the common peroneal nerve (L4, 5 and S1, 2). It penetrates the intermuscular septum and is closely related to the periosteum of proximal fibula (in fact it can be palpated at the head of the fibula). It divides into superficial and deep peroneal nerves. Its lateral sural cutaneous nerve branch joins the medial sural cutaneous nerve (from the tibial nerve) to become the sural nerve.

4.2.12 The parathyroid glands

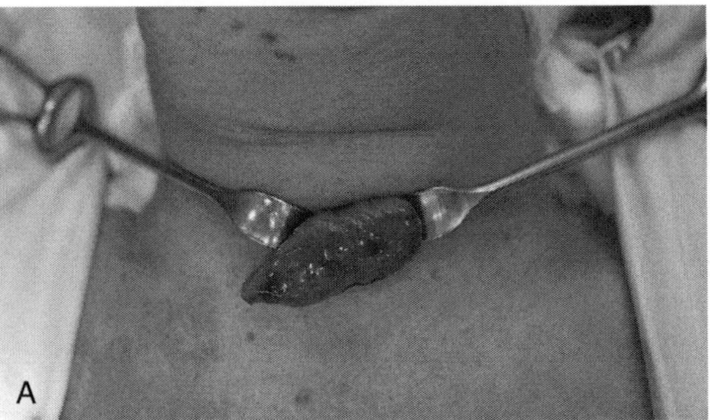

Figure 4.2.12A
Large inferior parathyroid gland

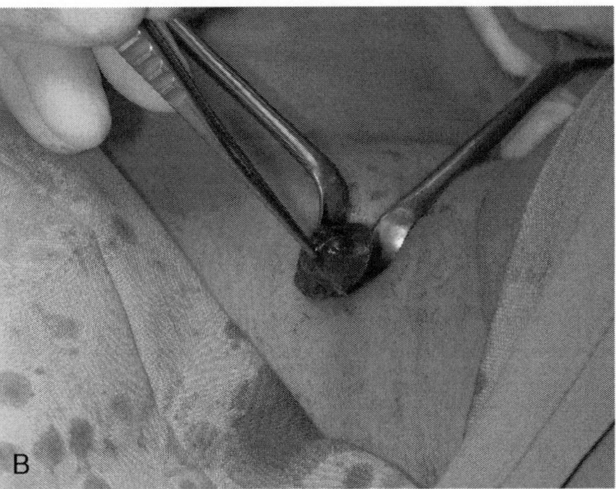

Figure 4.2.12B
Parathyroid gland delivery in MIPS

Examiner question: what do you see here?

Candidate answer

- Parathyroid glands being removed during minimally invasive surgery. There are generally four in total; two on the left and two on the right.
- They are generally small in size and lie within their own capsule. The classical colour description is a 'London tan' colour with the weight of the glands ranging between 25–35 mg.
- Histologically, the parathyroids are composed of chief cells and oxyntic cells. The chief cells are responsible for producing parathyroid hormone which is responsible for calcium regulation.

Examiner question: can you describe the embryology and position of the parathyroid glands?

Candidate answer

- Parathyroid tissue arises from the interaction of neural crest cells and third and fourth branchial pouch endoderm.
- The superior parathyroid glands (P IV) arise from the fourth pharyngeal pouch.
- The inferior parathyroid glands (P III) arise from the third pharyngeal pouch.
- The significance of this is twofold:
  1. both parathyroid glands derive their blood supply from the inferior thyroid artery (ITA) with third order branching
  2. the inferior parathyroid glands have a longer distance to descend during organogenesis and hence the superior parathyroid tissue has a more constant location, while the inferior parathyroid glands are more variable.
- The superior parathyroid glands are usually located adjacent to the inferior cornu of the thyroid cartilage adjacent to the recurrent nerve and cranial branch of the inferior thyroid artery
- When enlarged they migrate posteriorly and downwards:
  - posterior to junction of RLN and inferior thyroid artery
  - retropharyngeal
  - retrolaryngeal
  - retro-oesophageal
  - posterior mediastinum (very rare).
- The location of the inferior parathyroid glands is more variable. The search usually begins at the posterior aspect of the thyroid lobe from the inferior thyroid artery to the lower pole of the lobe. Here it is usually in front of the recurrent nerve.
- When it is tumoural, the exploration must continue around the inferior pole of the lobe, inspecting the lateral, anterior and inferior aspects in turn. They may be located in the:
  - thyrothymic ligament
  - thymus
  - superior mediastinum — if the inferior glands fail to separate from the thymus
  - rarely they are located within the thyroid gland itself.

Examiner question: what is the relevance of this with regard to performing a minimally invasive parathyroidectomy (MIP)?

Candidate answer

- It requires appropriate positioning and dual localisation of the parathyroid gland(s) with sestamibi and ultrasound.
- Adequate localisation of the gland enables a small 2.5 cm collar incision on the side of the gland, followed by division of platysma with flaps raised and division of the investing layer of deep cervical fascia. The sternohyoid and sternothyroid muscles are retracted medially.
- With the knowledge of location of parathyroids I will:
  - identify (serpiginous, vasa nervorum, white) and preserve the recurrent laryngeal nerve (RLN)
  - identify the inferior thyroid leash
  - generally, the parathyroids sit around this bifurcation (of ITA and RLN)
  - superior glands tend to sit superior and posterior to this bifurcation and then in a line with fourth branchial pouch derivatives
  - inferior glands tend to sit below and anterior to this bifurcation in a line with third branchial pouch derivatives
  - on assessment for the inferior parathyroid, check inferior and anterior to ITA and RLN and then anterior gland of thyroid, then thyrothymic ligament, and finally thymus
  - if there is doubt about location, recheck pre-operative sestembi and ultrasound and then explore the other thyroid lateral lobe through an anterior approach
  - if still not present may need to perform hemithyroidectomy on the side of the parathyroid adenoma.

4.2.13 Median nerve

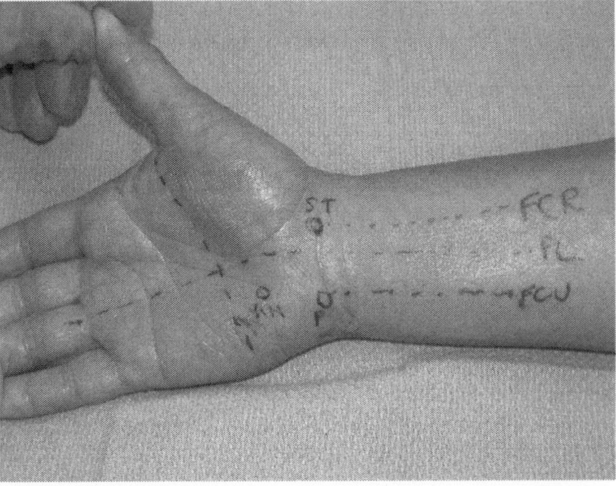

Figure 4.2.13

Surgical landmarks in forearm and hand for median nerve, carpal tunnel release (Source: *Textbook of Arthroscopy*. Miller M D et al. 2004, Saunders: an imprint of Elsevier, Fig 40-3A, p 396.)

Examiner question: you are performing a carpal tunnel decompression. Please take us through the important anatomical structures relevant to this procedure.

Candidate answer

- To perform this procedure safely, one must be aware of the important neuro-vascular structures that maybe endangered, namely:
  - the median nerve
  - the palmar cutaneous branch of median nerve (sensation to the thenar eminence)
  - the recurrent branch of median nerve (motor supply to thenar muscles)
  - the superficial palmar arch (blood supply to hand)
  - the ulnar nerve as it passes through flexor retinaculum (if the incision it placed too far towards the ulnar side).
- The important landmark of carpal tunnel is the flexor retinaculum, a fibrous band attached radially to the tubercle of scaphoid and ridge of the trapezium and to the pisiform and hook of the hamate on the ulnar side.
- The muscles of hypothenar and thenar muscles arise from the flexor retinaculum. The tendon of palmaris longus is fused with the retinaculum in the midline.
- The ulnar nerve and artery lie on the retinaculum, in the small canal of Guyon.
- The contents of carpal tunnel are:
  - the median nerve
  - long flexors of fingers and thumb — flexor digitorum superficialis and profundus and flexor pollicis longus
  - flexor carpi radialis.

THE MEDIAN NERVE (C5–T1)

- It leaves the axilla in front of brachial artery, lies medial to the brachial artery deep to bicipital aponeurosis at the elbow and descends between the two heads of pronator teres and beneath the fibrous arch of flexor digitorium superficialis.
- It emerges between the flexor carpi radialis and palmaris longus before entering the carpal tunnel.
- It gives off muscular branches to the forearm muscles, as well as cutaneous branches.
- It also supplies the radial two **l**umbricals and the thenar muscles (**o**pponens pollicis brevis, **a**bductor pollicis brevis and **f**lexor pollicis brevis) — remembered by the acronym **LOAF**.
- The palmar cutaneous branch is given off *proximal* to the flexor retinaculum and pierces the deep fascia.
- In the carpal tunnel, the median nerve divides into lateral and medial branches. The lateral branch gives off the muscular recurrent branch (T1) which supplies the thenar muscles. Usually this branch is extraligamentus (i.e. it emerges at the distal border of the retinaculum and curves around) and it is uncommonly transligamentus. The lateral branch then breaks up into three palmar digital branches. The medial branch divides into two palmar digital nerves.

4.2.14 Ulnar nerve

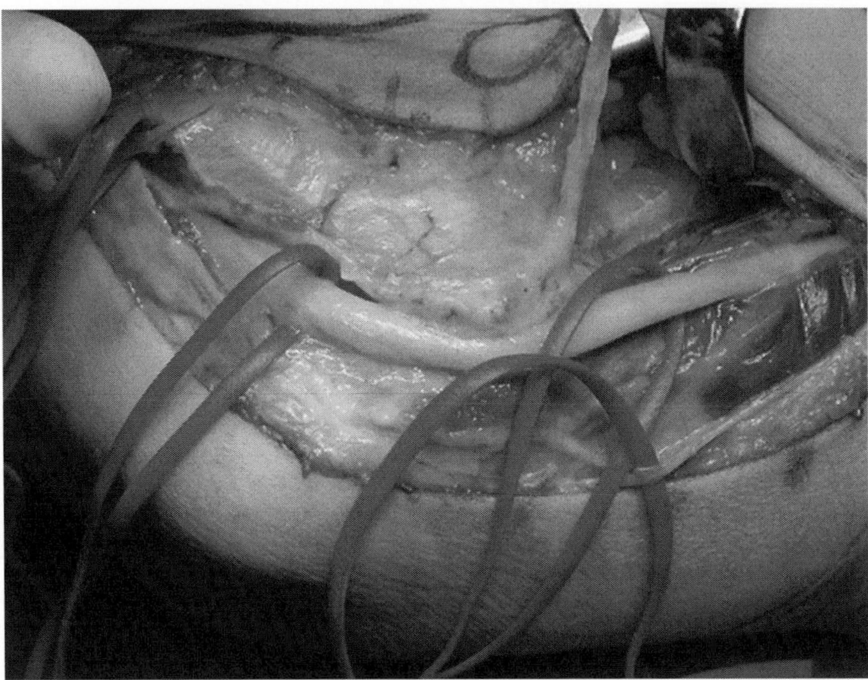

Figure 4.2.14
The ulnar nerve after in situ release. The roof of the tunnel has been removed (Source: *DeLee and Drez's Orthopaedic Sports Medicine*, 3rd edn. DeLee J C et al. 2009, Saunders: an imprint of Elsevier, Fig 19I-2, p 396.)

Examiner question: the structure in this image was damaged following a supracondylar fracture, are you able to identify it?

Candidate answer

- The image shows the ulnar nerve (C7–T1).
- It runs down between the axillary artery and vein behind the medial cutaneous nerve of the forearm. It continues downwards and backwards posterior to the brachial vessels to pierce the medial intermuscular septum. It then descends along the triceps by lying on the shaft of the humerus between the medial epicondyle and the olecranon, where it is susceptible to injury in supracondylar fractures and elbow dislocations.
- The surface marking of the nerve is along a line from the groove behind coracobrachialis to the point where the medial epicondyle of the humerus is palpable.

Examiner question: what is the course of the nerve in the forearm?

Candidate answer

It enters the forearm from the extensor compartment by passing between the humeral and ulnar heads of flexor carpi ulnaris. In the forearm it descends on flexor digitorum profundus (FDP) under cover of the flexor carpi ulnaris (FCU); here it is joined by the ulnar artery. The two emerge from beneath the tendon of flexor carpi ulnaris, passing distally over the flexor retinaculum alongside the pisiform bone, where it divides into superficial and deep branches.

Examiner question: what does the nerve supply?

Candidate answer

The nerve supplies:

- the flexor muscles of the ulnar side of the forearm (flexor carpi ulnaris [FCU] and the ulnar half of flexor digitorum profundus [FDP])
- the skin of the ulnar one and a half digits
- the intrinsic muscles of the hand concerned with fine movements:
  - adductor pollicis
  - flexor pollicis brevis
  - *all* dorsal and palmar interossei
  - third and fourth lumbricals
  - abductor/opponens/flexor digiti minimi.
- It has no branches in the upper arm, but gives a branch to the elbow joint and a motor branch to supply FCU and the ulnar half of FDP.
- The superficial branch supplies palmaris brevis and is carried as digital nerves to supply the skin of the ulnar one and a half digits.
- The deep branch passes deep into the palm between the two heads of flexor and abductor digiti minimi and through the origin of opponens digiti minimi to give off motor branches to the three hypothenar muscles, two lumbricals, all interossei and both heads of adductor pollicis.

Examiner question: how do you clinically differentiate between a high and a low ulnar nerve lesion?

Candidate answer

Low lesions (below elbow):

- more marked clawing as flexor digitorum profundus to ring and little fingers still functions.

High lesions (above elbow):

- paralysis of flexor digitorum profundus to ring and little fingers leads to less marked clawing of these fingers as the flexion component of the clawing is less prominent — this is known as the 'ulnar paradox'
- decreased sensation over ulnar border of the hand
- otherwise as for low lesion.

4.2.15 Femoral triangle

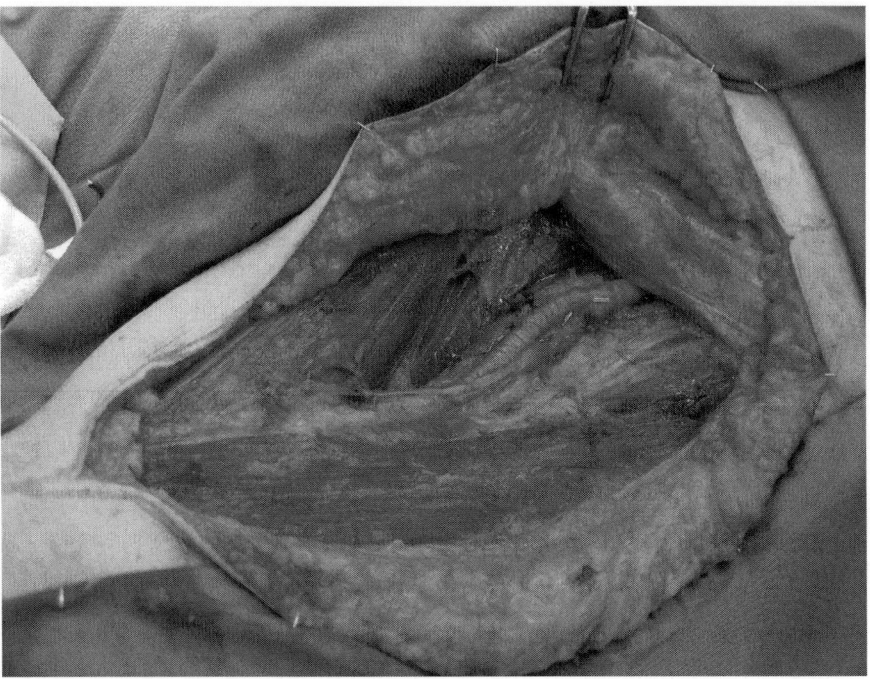

Figure 4.2.15
Left femoral triangle following radical lymph node dissection

Examiner question: what do you see in this image?

Candidate answer

The femoral triangle with the inguinal and femoral region on the left after a lymph node dissection.

Examiner question: tell me about the anatomy of the femoral triangle?

Candidate answer

BOUNDARIES

- The lateral boundary is formed by the medial border of sartorius.
- The medial boundary is formed by the medial border of adductor longus.
- The base is formed by the inguinal ligament.

FLOOR

- The floor is formed from medial to lateral by adductor longus, adductor brevis, pectineus and iliopsoas muscles.

CONTENTS

- From medial to lateral at the inguinal ligament are the femoral canal, common femoral vein, common femoral artery and the femoral nerve.
- The superficial draining lymph nodes lie subinguinally and along the long saphenous vein (LSV) and drain the leg, buttock, lower abdominal wall and the perineal area. They then drain to deep inguinal lymph nodes and into the pelvis to the external iliac nodes.
- Deep inguinal nodes lie within the femoral canal (Cloquet's node) and between the femoral vessels. These nodes drain to the pelvis along the obturator and internal iliac vessels.
- The common femoral artery (CFA) branches into the superficial femoral artery (SFA) and profunda femoris artery (PFA) within the triangle. The PFA travels deep to adductor longus.
- Smaller branches of the CFA just inferior to inguinal ligament are the superficial epigastric artery, superficial circumflex iliac artery, and superficial and deep external pudendal arteries.
- The long saphenous vein drains into the femoral vein at the saphenofemoral junction where it pierces through the cribriform fascia at the fossa ovalis. Other veins draining into the saphenofemoral junction include the superficial epigastric vein, superficial circumflex iliac vein and the superficial external pudendal vein. The superficial external pudendal artery may be encountered during dissection of saphenofemoral junction running between tributaries to the LSV.
- The femoral nerve lies lateral to the femoral artery and divides into anterior and posterior divisions within the triangle. Its terminal motor branches supply quadriceps, sartorius, pectineus and the gracilis muscles. It lies in a deeper plane to the artery and vein, is covered by fascia and is not usually seen during a groin dissection. Cutaneous branches of the femoral nerve are the intermediate and medial femoral cutaneous nerves. It continues on as the saphenous nerve.
- Also, the lateral femoral cutaneous nerve lies laterally within the triangle.
- The superficial femoral artery and vein along with the saphenous nerve exit the femoral triangle at its apex and enter the subsartorial canal or adductor hiatus.

Examiner question: what is removed during a subinguinal lymph node dissection?

Candidate answer

- A subinguinal lymph node dissection is the removal of all superficial and deep lymph nodes within the femoral triangle along with the LSV. The margins of the dissection extend past the borders of the triangle superiorly to include the lymphatic tissue overlying the external oblique aponeurosis in the lower abdominal wall and laterally to include the fascia overlying the sartorius muscle.

4.2.16 Popliteal fossa

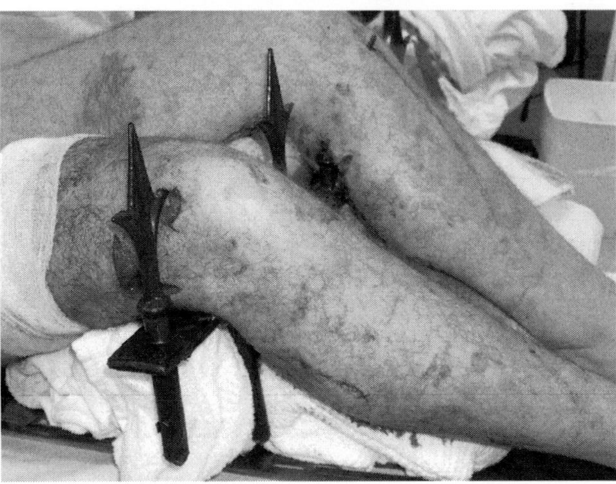

Figure 4.2.16
Popliteal artery injury

Examiner question: what do you see in this image? It happened after this man fell off a balcony.

Candidate answer

It appears to be an image of a person who has been impaled on top of a gate or fence at the level of the popliteal fossa.

Examiner question: assuming there is concern regarding an arterial injury, how would you access the popliteal vessels?

Candidate answer

- I would make a curved incision along the anterior border of sartorius, extended across the knee joint and along the posteromedial edge of the tibia.
- The long saphenous vein (LSV) passes a hands-breadth behind the medial border of patella.
- The saphenous nerve exits the adductor canal between the sartorius and gracilis, gives off an infrapatellar branch then passes down the medial aspect of the lower leg with the LSV.
- I would then make an incision through the deep fascia.

Examiner question: once you have incised the deep fascia, which muscles do you encounter?

Candidate answer

- Sartorius (arises from the ASIS, crosses the thigh obliquely and inserts into the upper part of medial surface of tibia).

- Gracilis (most superficial muscle on medial side of thigh arising from the inferior pubic ramus and ischial ramus and inserts into the tibia just behind sartorius).
- Semimembranosus and semitendinosus (hamstring muscles, arise from the ischial tuberosity; semimembranosus inserts into the back of the medial tibial condyle, semitendinosus inserts into the upper part of the medial surface of tibia).
- Medial head of gastrocnemius (arises from the back of the medial femoral condyle and shaft of the femur and joins with the lateral head to form the Achilles tendon).
- Once these muscles are retracted, the adductor magnus comes into view. This is formed by fusion of adductor and hamstring parts and inserts into the medial supracondylar line and linea aspera of the femur.

Examiner question: what is the opening in the tendon of adductor magnus? Name the structures passing through the adductor canal.

Candidate answer

- The opening is the adductor hiatus and it represents the lower opening of the adductor canal.
- The canal contains the femoral artery and vein and the saphenous nerve. The nerve to vastus medialis is present in the upper part.

Examiner question: what are the branches of the popliteal artery?

Candidate answer

Five genicular arteries:

- superior and inferior medial
- superior and inferior lateral
- middle.

Examiner question: can you name the other nerves in the popliteal fossa?

Candidate answer

- The tibial nerve (runs vertically down through the middle of the popliteal fossa to pass between the heads of gastrocnemius). The branches of the tibial nerve are:
  - the sural nerve (runs between the two heads of gastrocnemius)
  - three genicular nerves
  - motor branches to muscles in the popliteal fossa.
- Common fibular (peroneal) nerve (passes medial to the biceps femoris tendon and enters peroneus longus to lie on the neck of fibula). The branches of the common fibular nerve are:
  - the sural communicating nerve (pierces roof of fossa to join sural nerve)
  - lateral cutaneous nerve of the calf (pierces roof of fossa over lateral head of gastrocnemius)
  - genicular nerves.

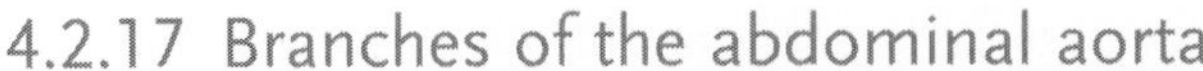

4.2.17 Branches of the abdominal aorta

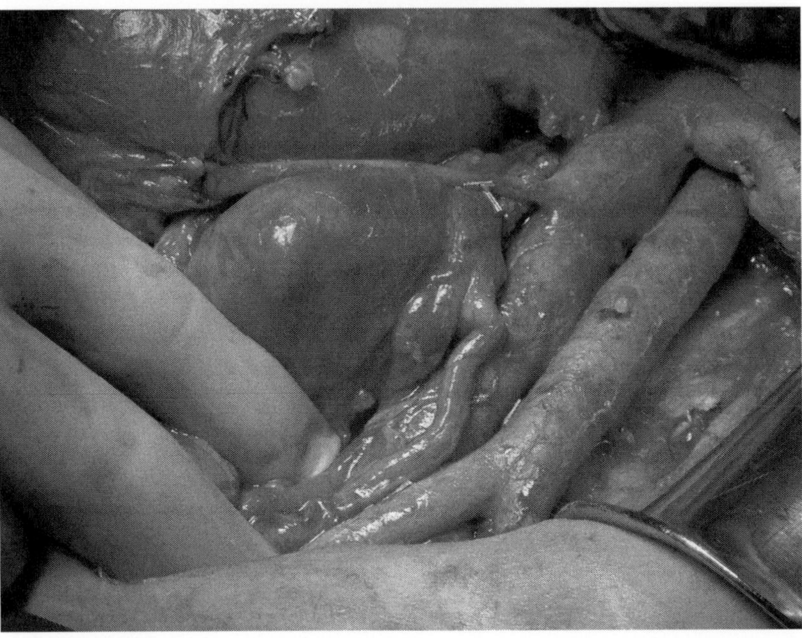

Figure 4.2.17
Aorta and branches after retroperitoneal lymph node dissection

Examiner question: what is this structure and where does it begin and end in the abdomen?

Candidate answer

- It is the abdominal aorta and it begins by passing behind the median arcuate ligament and between the crura of the diaphragm in front of the body of T12. It passes downwards on the bodies of the lumbar vertebrae, inclining slightly to the left with the left sympathetic trunk at its left margin.
- It terminates by dividing into the two common iliac arteries on the body of L4.

Examiner question: what branches does it give off in the abdomen?

Candidate answer

- From the posterior surface at its bifurcation it gives off the small median sacral artery.
- It also gives off:
  - three single ventral branches to the gut
  - three paired branches to other viscera
  - three paired branches to the anterior abdominal wall.

SINGLE VENTRAL BRANCHES TO THE GUT

- The coeliac trunk:
  - the artery of the foregut
  - arises just below the arcuate ligament at the level of T12 and branches at the upper border of the pancreas
  - branches to form the left gastric, splenic and common hepatic arteries.
- The superior mesenteric artery:
  - the artery of the midgut
  - arises 1 cm below the coeliac trunk at the level of L1
  - it branches to give off (i) the inferior pancreaticoduodenal, (ii) jejunal and ileal branches, (iii) the ileocolic, (iv) the right colic and (v) the middle colic arteries.
- The inferior mesenteric artery:
  - the artery of the hindgut
  - arises at the inferior border of the third part of the duodenum at L3
  - it gives off the (ascending) left colic artery and the sigmoid arteries before continuing as the superior rectal artery.

PAIRED BRANCHES TO OTHER VISCERA

- Suprarenal arteries:
  - arise between the inferior phrenic and renal branches
  - run laterally across the crura of the diaphragm to divide into small branches upon reaching the gland.
- Renal arteries:
  - arise at right angles from the aorta at the level of L2
  - the left renal artery crosses the left crus behind and above the left renal vein, covered by the tail of pancreas and spleen
  - the right renal artery passes behind the IVC and right renal vein.
- Gonodal arteries:
  - arise below the renal arteries (L2) but above the IMA (L3)
  - they slope steeply downwards over the psoas and cross the ureters.

PAIRED BRANCHES TO THE ANTERIOR ABDOMINAL WALL

- Subcostal arteries:
  - strictly arise from the thoracic aorta but they enter the abdomen beneath the lateral arcuate ligament
  - pass into the neurovascular plane of the anterior abdominal wall (between internal oblique and tranversus).
- Inferior phrenic arteries:
  - arise from the aorta at the aortic opening
  - slope upwards over the crus of the diaphragm, which they supply. They also give off suprarenal branches.
- Lumbar arteries:
  - four in number, arising at the level of the bodies of L1–L4
  - they pass beneath the lumbar sympathetic trunks and psoas (and IVC on the right) to enter the neurovascular plane.

4.2.18 Diaphragm

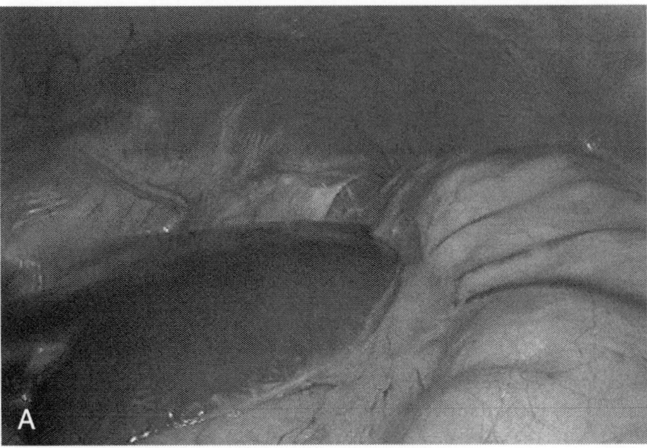

Figure 4.2.18A
Diaphragm anterior to liver

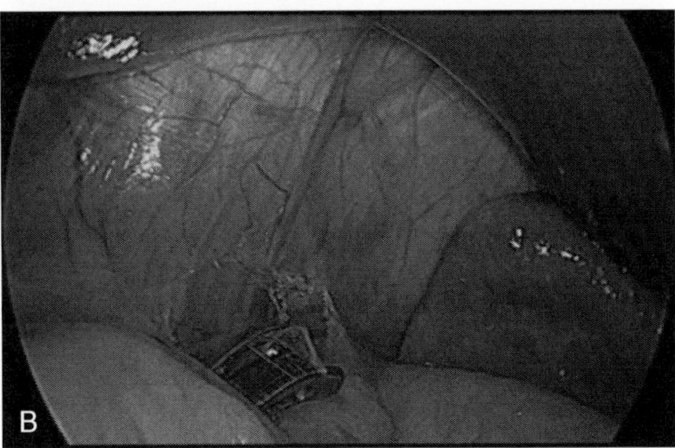

Figures 4.2.18B
Diaphragm between liver and stomach during laparoscopic gastric banding

Examiner question: the first image was taken during a routine laparoscopy and the second image during a laparoscopic gastric band procedure. What do they show?

Candidate answer

I can see the diaphragm and upper abdominal organs in both images.

Examiner question: tell me about the diaphragm?

Candidate answer

EMBRYOLOGY

The adult diaphragm is derived from four embryological structures:

1. septum transversum (anterior)
2. dorsal mesentery of foregut (central and posterior)

3. pleuropericardial membranes (lateral)
4. body wall myotomes (lateral).

FUNCTION

- The diaphragm functions to assist inspiration; it increases intra-abdominal pressure with straining.
- Developmental anomalies of the diaphragm can result in hypoplasia of the lungs.

ATTACHMENTS

- Anteriorly: xiphoid process, slips of muscle from ribs and costal cartilages 7–12.
- Posteriorly: right and left crura, medial and lateral arcuate ligaments.
- Laterally: ribs.
- Median arcuate ligament: formed by fibres of the left and right crus.
- Medial arcuate ligament: thickening of psoas fascia, attached from body of L1 to the transverse process of L1.
- Lateral arcuate ligament: thickening of quadratus lumborum fascia attached to the 12th rib laterally.
- Muscle fibres pass upwards and inwards to insert into the central tendon. The central tendon has no bony attachment and is fused with the fibrous pericardium.

OPENINGS AND STRUCTURES PASSING THROUGH THEM

- T8: lateral aspect of the central tendon (approx 1 cm right of midline):
  - IVC
  - Right phrenic nerve.

  (Note: the left phrenic nerve passes through the left dome of diaphragm.)
- T10: oesophageal hiatus (just left of the midline):
  - oesophagus (reinforced inferiorly by fibres from the right crus which form a sling)
  - left and right vagus nerves
  - oesophageal branch of left gastric artery
  - oesophageal lymphatics.
- Superior epigastric arteries pass through parasternal spaces.
- T12: aortic hiatus behind the median arcuate ligament:
  - aorta with the thoracic duct and azygous vein.
- Greater, lesser, least splanchnic nerves pass behind or through the arcuate ligaments.
- Sympathetic chain — behind medial arcuate ligament.

BLOOD SUPPLY

- Inferior phrenic arteries (left and right) — first branches of the abdominal aorta and lie on the inferior aspect (main blood supply).
- Pericardiophrenic artery and musculophrenic artery — branches of the internal thoracic artery.
- Superior phrenic artery branch of thoracic aorta.
- Lower five intercostal arteries and subcostal artery (laterally).

NERVE SUPPLY

- Left and right phrenic nerves (C3, C4, C5):
  - sensory and motor
  - the only motor nerve to the diaphragm.
- Branches of intercostal nerves give some sensory fibres to the lateral diaphragm.
- Pain from the diaphragm is referred to the tip of the shoulder.

Examiner question: what structures are related to the diaphragm?

Candidate answer

Superiorly:

- left and right lung bases
- pericardium of the heart fused with central tendon.

Inferiorly:

- liver — bare area adherent to under surface of the diaphragm, right and left lobes
- falciform ligament
- coeliac artery and coeliac plexus
- spleen
- oesophagus
- cardia/fundus of stomach
- right and left subdiaphragmatic spaces — peritoneal spaces on either side of the bare area divided by the falciform ligament — potential spaces for infected intra-abdominal fluid
- right and left kidneys.

4.2.19 Retroperitoneal anatomy

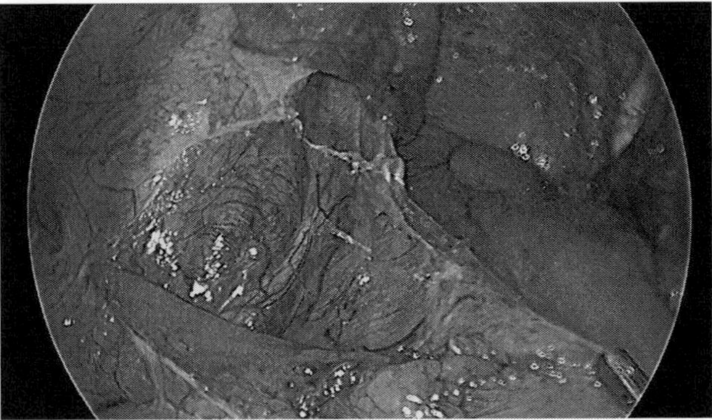

Figure 4.2.19
Left ureter at laparoscopic rectal mobilisation

Examiner question: what is the important structure in this image that is at risk of division in pelvic surgery?

Candidate answer

The left ureter.

Examiner question: could you tell me about the ureter and its course?

Candidate answer

- The ureter is a smooth muscle tubular structure that propels urine from the kidneys to the urinary bladder. In the adult, they measure 25–30 cm in length and 4 mm in diameter.
- They arise from the renal pelvis and descend towards the bladder on the anterior surface of the psoas major muscle. The ureters cross the pelvic brim and then run posteroinferiorly on the lateral walls of the pelvis, and curve anteromedially to enter the posterior aspect of the bladder at the vesico-ureteric junction.
- The ureter is divided into an abdominal part and pelvic part. The abdominal part lies behind the peritoneum, on the medial part of the psoas major muscle and is crossed by the gonadal vessels.
- At its origin, the right ureter is covered by the duodenum (descending part), lies to the right of the IVC and is crossed by the right colic and ileocolic vessels. The left ureter is crossed by the left colic vessels and passes posteriorly to the sigmoid colon and its mesentery.
- It enters the pelvis by crossing the division of the common iliac vessels. The pelvic part runs downward on the lateral wall of the pelvic cavity, along the anterior border of the sciatic notch. It lies anterior to the hypogastric artery and medial to the obturator nerve. It inclines medially and enters the bladder at the lateral angles of the trigone.
- In females, the ureters pass under the uterine arteries ('water under the bridge').
- In males, the ureters pass under the vas deferens.

Examiner question: could you tell me about the relations, blood supply and nervous innervations of the ureter?

Candidate answer

- The anterior relations of:
  - right ureter include: the duodenum, right gonadal artery, right colic artery, ileal mesentery, SMA
  - left ureter include: the left gonadal artery, left colic artery, sigmoid mesentery.
- The posterior relations include:
  - psoas muscle, genitofemoral nerve, sacroiliac joint, bifurcation of common iliac artery.
- The blood supply of the ureter is from:
  - branches of the renal, gonadal, common iliac, vaginal, hypogastric and inferior vesicle arteries.
- The nervous innervation:
  - inferior mesenteric, spermatic and pelvic plexuses (autonomic).

4.2.20 Transpyloric plane

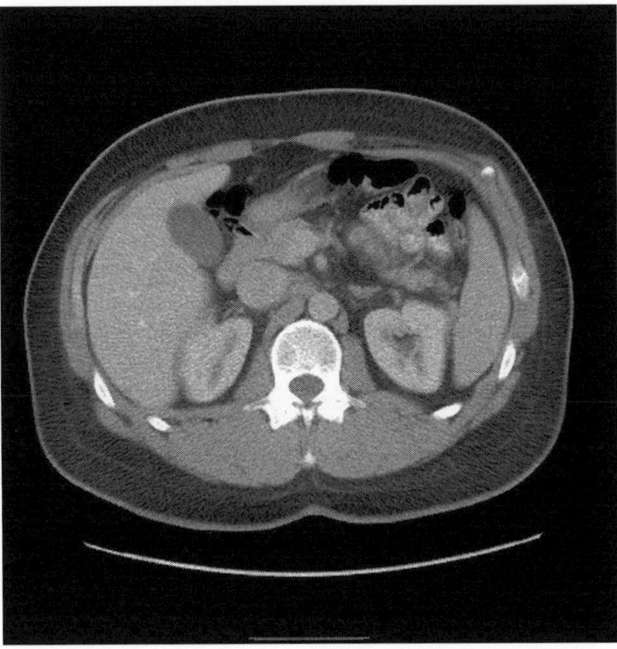

Figure 4.2.20
CT scan of transpyloric plane (L1)

Examiner question: what does this image show?

Candidate answer

Noting the kidneys and fundus of the gallbladder, I would say that it is a CT scan at the level of L1 or the transpyloric plane.

Examiner question: what can you tell me about the transpyloric plane and the structures that are normally found on that plane?

Candidate answer

- The transpyloric plane of Addison is located halfway between the jugular notch and the pubic symphysis and is named as it passes through the pylorus of the stomach.
- Alternatively, its surface anatomy can be defined as the intersection of the linea semilunaris with the costal margin at the level of the ninth costal cartilage.
- Structures that are normally found in the transpyloric plane include:
  - first lumbar vertebra L1
  - the pylorus of the stomach which will lie at this level approximately 5 cm to the right of the midline
  - first part of the duodenum
  - duodenojejunal flexure

- the fundus of the gallbladder
- the neck and body of the pancreas
- the spleen
- the origin of the superior mesenteric artery from the abdominal aorta
- confluence of the superior mesenteric vein with the splenic vein to form the portal vein
- root of the transverse colon mesentery (which divides the abdomen into supra- and infra-colic compartments)
- left and right colic flexures
- hilum of the left kidney
- upper pole of the kidney on the right
- tips of the ninth costal cartilages
- the termination of the spinal cord.

4.2.21 Transtubercular plane

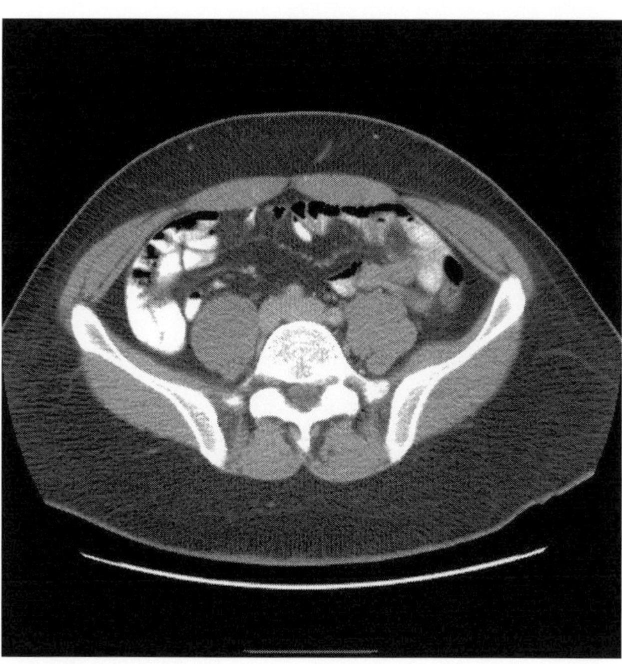

Figure 4.2.21
CT scan of transtubercular plane (L5)

Examiner question: what does this image show?

Candidate answer

This is an axial CT scan taken at the level of the iliac tubercles, denoting the transtubercular plane.

Examiner question: what vertebral level does that make it then?

Candidate answer

L5

Examiner question: what else can you tell me about this plane and the important structures that lie on it?

Candidate answer

- The transtubercular plane is a plane uniting the two tubercles of the iliac crests. The iliac tubercles lie slightly posterior to the anterior superior iliac spines along the iliac crest.
- It marks the start of the inferior vena cava at the confluence of the common iliac veins, a surface marking for which is 2.5 cm to the right of midline.

4.2.22 Internal iliac artery branches

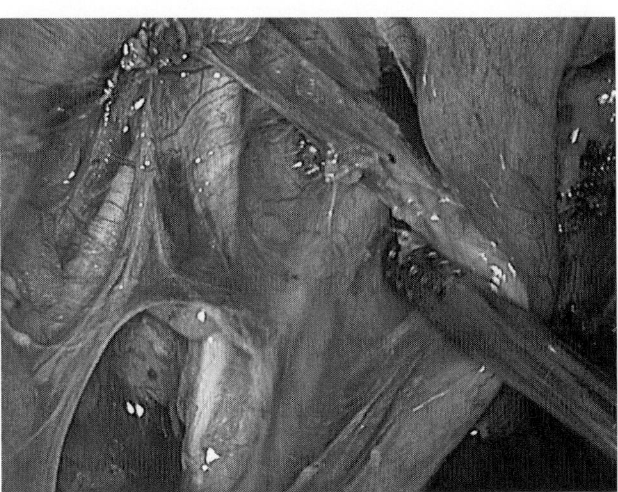

Figure 4.2.22

Laparoscopic image of two branches of the anterior trunk of the left internal iliac artery (the uterine artery and the umbilical artery), seen medial to the left obturator nerve. The nerve lies on the obturator internus muscle. The ureter is retracted by the instrument (Source: *Clinical Reproductive Medicine and Surgery*. Falcone T, Hurd W W. 2007. Mosby: an imprint of Elsevier, Fig 7-6, p 120.)

Examiner question: what does this image show?

Candidate answer

It is a laparoscopic image of the pelvic side wall showing two branches of the anterior trunk of the left internal iliac artery.

Examiner question: where does the internal iliac artery begin and what are its divisions?

Candidate answer

- The internal iliac arteries commence at the bifurcation of the common iliac arteries at the pelvic brim opposite the sacroiliac joint.
- The internal iliac artery supplies the pelvic walls and viscera via its branches, which lie within the parietal pelvic fascia and only their branches that pass out of the pelvis need to pierce this fascia.
- Shortly after its origin, the internal iliac artery bifurcates into a short posterior and a longer anterior division.

Examiner question: what are the branches of these divisions of the internal iliac artery?

Candidate answer

The posterior division divides into three parietal branches:

- iliolumbar — passes out of the pelvis behind the lumbosacral trunk to supply the lumbar muscles and iliac fossa
- lateral sacral — runs in front of the roots of the sacral plexus, supplying it and the piriformis
- superior gluteal — leaves the pelvis through the greater sciatic foramen to enter the buttock.

The anterior division divides into nine branches:

- three associated with the bladder
  - superior and inferior vesicle
  - obliterated umbilical
- three other visceral branches
  - middle rectal
  - uterine
  - vaginal
- three parietal branches
  - obturator
  - internal pudendal
  - inferior gluteal.

Chapter 4.3

Operative surgery

The enemy of good is better. Presumed original source of this quote in French is 'Le mieux est l'ennemi du bien', from Voltaire's *Dictionnaire Philosophique* (1764), which literally means 'The best is the enemy of good'.

The examination format

The operative surgery viva consists of two sections:

- one section involves a 10-minute discussion based around a scenario and
- five computer images are shown and discussed over 20 minutes.

These images serve as a 'primer' for the discussion, which may include examination of:

- general operative principles, such as valid informed consent
- pre-operative decision making and work up
- operative technique and strategy
- management of intra-operative and post-operative complications.

A bell rings to signal the start of the exam and you will enter the room where you will meet the examiners, who will show you images on a computer screen. The 10-minute scenario begins as a computer presentation that contains brief information relating to the case and a selection of clinical/radiological/operative images pertinent to the case. For example, the presentation may contain details of a 64-year-old man with RIF tenderness, abdominal distension and an AXR revealing large bowel obstruction. Subsequently, you may be shown a gastrografin enema performed in the same patient. The examiners will ask you 'what would you do?' as you progress.

After 10 minutes, another bell rings and you move to the next section of the surgical anatomy viva where you will be shown five images in a 20-minute period. Usually, the questions are quite specific and the examiners may lead you to the procedure they want you to discuss; for example, lateral internal sphincterotomy after being shown an image of a fissure-in-ano.

Exam technique

Remember: 'Listen, think, pause, speak'.

During the viva you are being examined on the operative management of surgical conditions. You may elect to 'perform' (discuss) just about any appropriate procedure. The focus of the examination is to assess what *you* can/are going to do. Whilst it may be okay to consult a colleague, the examiners want to know the safest and most appropriate intervention in *your* hands. For example, if the examiners present you with a scenario where you have to explore a common bile duct due to stones (maybe because ERCP is not available) and you can't or have not performed a laparoscopic exploration, than you need to describe what is possible and safe in your hands and that you would perform *open* exploration and removal of the stone(s).

The 10-minute scenario will usually evolve with more clinical and radiographic information being revealed as the scenario progresses. Importantly, you should have a structured approach and present your thoughts in a coherent and methodical manner. The model answers presented in Chapter 4.4 will help you achieve this. You should aim to score points at every step along the way during this process. In the example of large bowel obstruction used above, after telling you the clinical summary and showing you the AXR demonstrating large bowel obstruction, the examiners will likely ask '*what would you do?*'. You should take the opportunity of scoring points by stating that you would:

- fully resuscitate the patient using CCrISP principles
- organise baseline investigations (urine/bloods etc.)
- commence initial treatment by decompressing the bowel and achieving fluid and electrolyte replacement with the insertion of a nasogastric tube, iv fluid resuscitation and insertion of a urethral catheter
- initiate additional investigations to establish a definitive diagnosis — in this case a CT scan of the abdomen and pelvis with oral, rectal and IV contrast.

The examiners might say that you cannot have a CT scan and instead show you a Gastrografin enema. You should start to describe the image in as much detail as possible using a structured approach, including the name and the date/nature of the study (if present) and describe what you see and what the diagnosis is. If you do not start talking, they will probably tell you that it is a Gastrografin enema showing a large bowel obstruction, so that you can progress to discuss the surgical options. At this point, they will ask '*what would you do?*'. Now you can discuss operative options, demonstrating your appreciation of the importance of:

- patient factors
- disease factors
- findings at laparotomy (e.g. presence/absence of perforation/caecal ischaemia).

You finish by stating how much bowel needs to be resected and considerations related to stoma formation/possible anastomosis.

In the next section of this viva you will be shown five images. You need to say what the image shows and this will usually initiate a discussion about how you would manage that condition. As mentioned, the examiners will usually want to keep you to a 'tight script' and will almost certainly have specific procedures in mind that they want you to discuss. After you are shown an image and asked '*What do you think?*', you should start talking and state the diagnosis. If you cannot identify the image, the examiners will often tell you what it shows. You may be asked conservative options, but mostly they want to discuss surgical operations (e.g. lateral internal sphincterotomy for fissure-in-ano). They may say something like '*You are going to do a lateral sphincterotomy, please describe it*'.

Be certain to describe what you would do in *your* hospital/practice, not what someone else may do or what you have read. Wherever possible you should be decisive and start with '*I would*', '*I think*' or possibly '*In my experience*' rather than '*These are the options*'.

Remember, if you are digging a hole for yourself the examiners may ask '*Why do you say that?*', '*Why are you doing that?*', '*Is that what you really think?*' or '*Would you like to rephrase your answer?*'. Just take it for granted that they are trying to help you and modify your answer.

Example of a standard introductory phrase when describing operative surgical procedure

Having fully and adequately prepared the patient for theatre and after taking informed consent, I would prepare and drape, under appropriate anaesthesia and position the patient in the ... position. I would ...

You should aim to begin each response with such a phrase, unless instructed to omit by the examiners.

You should continue with the detail of the procedure, during which the examiners may ask '*Can you draw this on a piece of paper?*'.

A structured approach to your answers will help avoid pitfalls (e.g. forgetting to mention contrast studies prior to closing a temporary defunctioning ileostomy). Due to the potential stop-and-start nature of the examination, you may not get through the following schema. Alternatively, you may be asked to just describe the operation. However, we suggest you keep it in mind as a guide to aid your preparation, practise and recitation of answers in the operative surgery viva; particularly if you get stuck!

a) Indications
b) Contraindications
c) Pre-operative preparation
d) Anaesthesia
e) Position of patient
f) Special equipment (laparoscopic surgery)
g) Incision
h) Exploration
i) Options arising during surgery (what if?) — predict and pre-empt these
j) Drainage etc.
k) Closure
l) Dressing(s)
m) Post-operative instructions

You should have also thought about, prepared and rehearsed responses to address:

- general operative principles/checks
- predictable intra-operative disasters such as major haemorrhage
- post-operative complications.

General operative principles/checks

To ensure that you don't miss things before 'knife to skin', run through the ABCDE checklist to determine if indicated pre-op/at induction:

A: antibiotics/analgesia
B: bowel preparation
C: consent/catheter
D: DVT prophylaxis/drains (NGT)
E: ensure timeout complete.

In the model answers in Chapter 4.4, we will not labour the importance of this checklist in the interests of brevity. Suffice to say that you must consider the list for every procedure that you discuss in the viva.

Predictable intraoperative disasters such as major haemorrhage

Again, you should employ a standardised approach which in the case of major haemorrhage might be based around the *5Ps* incorporating *lights, camera, action*

- **p**repare:
  - lights: improve lighting
  - camera: improve the view/exposure
  - action: improve/seek additional assistance
- **p**ressure/**p**ack
- **p**roducts (blood)
- **p**lan definitive intervention (haemostatic sutures/further mobilisation to gain access/proximal and distal control of named vessels if injured to allow repair)
- **p**atience (*not pray*!)

Post-operative complications

A system for stratification should be employed. This might include:

- immediate, early and late
- superficial (wound), deep (operative site), systemic.

Preparation and practising

As previously stated in Chapter 1.2, frequent practise is imperative. Look at the list of common operative surgery topics in Chapter 1.3, and add to it with reports from previous exam candidates of what they were examined on. While you are in the operating theatre you should pay close attention to *every step* of the operation that you are doing/assisting. It is useful to write a summary of the steps afterwards for reference when you are revising. Read up on the anatomy before any elective surgery list and identify as many structures as you can during the operation. Think about potential pitfalls and how to avoid them and think of alternative operative strategies.

Chapter 4.4

Common operative surgery viva topics: model answers

In this chapter, we have attempted to provide 'model answers' to the commonest topics that are examined in the operative surgery viva to help you structure and organise your revision. Again, we have varied the style of the individual worked answers to try to provide as much diversity as possible with respect to operative surgery topics. We have also tried to provide more complete answers than you would be expected to/could conceivably provide within the time limits of the examination, so that you can refer to them during your revision to acquire key learning points. To avoid repetition, we have omitted to start each description with a 'standard introductory phrase' (see Chapter 4.3), but you should remember to include it in the examination.

4.4.1 Inguinal hernia repair

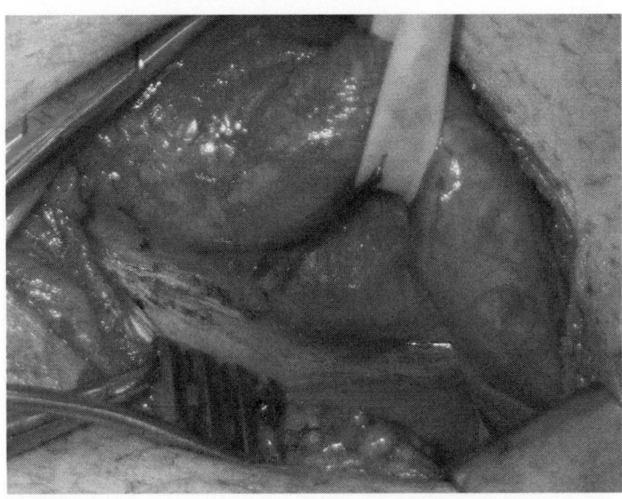

Figure 4.4.1
Open right inguinal hernia repair, canal dissected, sling around spermatic cord

Examiner question: could you tell me what is going on in this image?

Candidate answer

It looks like an open repair of a right inguinal hernia where the inguinal canal has been dissected and a rubber sling has been placed around the spermatic cord structures.

Examiner question: would you please describe an open repair of an inguinal hernia for me?

Candidate answer

- The procedure can be done under general, regional or local anaesthesia. One dose of prophylactic antibiotics is administered at induction.
- The patient is placed supine and prepped and draped
- I make a transverse incision 2 cm above the medial half of inguinal ligament and parallel to it (or skin crease incision).
- The skin, subcutaneous fat, Scarpa's fascia and external oblique aponeurosis are opened in layers.

Procedure

The procedural steps involve:

1. dissection of the hernia sac from surrounding structures
2. reduction of hernia contents
3. repair of the hernia defect.

I would proceed as outlined below.

- Open the external oblique aponeurosis at superficial ring, extending lateral to the deep ring and create a plane beneath it.
- Identify the ilioinguinal nerve → protect or divide.
- Dissect a space in the inguinal canal to accommodate a mesh, as necessary.
- Separate the spermatic cord ± sac from pubic tubercle and encircle the cord with a hernia ring or Penrose drain.
- Dissect the spermatic cord from the hernia sac.
- If it's a direct hernia sac (arising medial to the epigastric vessels) — reduce and plicate the posterior wall.
- If it's indirect hernia sac (arising lateral to the epigastric vessels) — commencing close to the deep ring (rather than the pubic tubercle), peel off the outer (cremasteric) layers of cord using blunt or sharp dissection until the white edge of peritoneal sac is identified. Dissect the sac down to its neck at deep ring.
- Open the sac → inspect and reduce contents → transfix neck of sac with synthetic absorbable suture → excise redundant sac → return stump to peritoneal cavity.
- If sliding hernia → simply plicate without injuring contents or reduce the sac.
- If inguino-scrotal hernia → transect the sac, leaving the distal part open in the scrotum.

- I then perform a *Lichtenstein repair*: tension-free technique involving placement of mesh to reinforce the posterior wall of the inguinal canal, involving:
  - cutting a prosthetic mesh to shape
  - anchoring the mesh medial to the pubic tubercle with synthetic non-absorbable suture to prevent recurrence
  - securing the lower edge of the mesh to the inguinal ligament with a continuous suture (taking care not to injury the femoral vessels or include the cut edge of the external oblique aponeurosis)
  - splitting the mesh to 'fish-tail' around the cord at deep ring and securing it to reduce the size of ring
  - securing the upper border of mesh to the internal oblique muscle with interrupted sutures.
- I then ensure complete haemostasis and close in layers: external oblique aponeurosis (taking care to avoid inclusion of the ilioinguinal nerve), Scarpa's fascia, skin.
- Infiltration with local anaesthesia if performed under GA.

Examiner question: what other methods do you know for hernia repair?

Candidate answer

- *Bassini repair*: approximates the conjoint tendon to the inguinal ligament from the pubic tubercle to the deep ring.
- *Shouldice repair*: modification of Bassini repair, and divides and 'double-breasts' the transversalis fascia using non-absorbable sutures.
- *Stoppa method*: uses an extra-peritoneal approach and employs the use of mesh to fill excess space in the vicinity of the deep inguinal ring.
- *Laparoscopic repair:* (pre-peritoneal [TEP] or transperitoneal [TAPP]), main indications: bilateral or recurrent hernias.

Examiner question: can you list the specific complications associated with the repair of an inguinal hernia?

Candidate answer

- Recurrence
- Chronic inguinal pain
- Infection: wound, mesh
- Seroma
- Haemorrhage
- Ischaemic orchitis
- Femoral vessel injury

4.4.2 Complicated femoral hernia repair

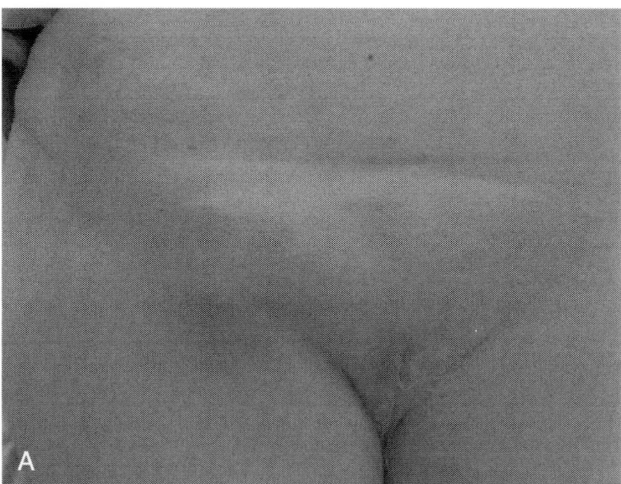

Figure 4.4.2A
Obstructed right femoral hernia

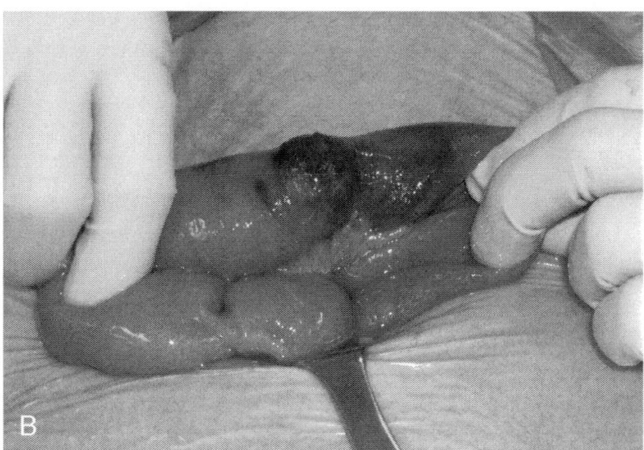

Figure 4.4.2B
Small bowel damage from Richter's hernia

Examiner question: a 78-year-old woman presented to the emergency department with a history of a lump in the groin. She had vague abdominal pain and has vomited once. Her abdomen was mildly distended but not peritonitic. The lump was tender and irreducible. She was taken to theatre and Figure 4.4.2B reveals the contents of her hernia sac. How would you have prepared her for surgery?

Candidate answer

Note: this is an operative viva. The examiner has flagged that this scenario is going to end in an operation. He wants a brief discussion of pre-operative preparation focusing on fluid resuscitation.

- Before theatre, I would resuscitate her using CCrISP principles including administering 1 L of Hartmann's solution over 1 hour and monitoring response.
- I would take an adequate history, including understanding her medical comorbidities and medications (particularly anticoagulants such as warfarin or clopidogrel).
- I would pay careful attention to fluid status during physical examination (BP, pulse, skin turgor, dry tongue, JVP).
- I would order and check electrolytes, urea, creatinine and a full blood count.
- I would insert a urethral catheter to monitor urine output.

Examiner interrupts: given the history and the image, what is the diagnosis?

Candidate answer

It is a complicated groin hernia, which could have been inguinal or femoral. The second image (Fig 4.4.2B) suggests that it was a Richter's hernia with small bowel compromise, making a femoral hernia more likely. Further investigations would not really change my management, so I would take her to the operating room for groin exploration after resuscitation.

Examiner: okay. You are now in the operating room, what procedure would you do?

Candidate answer

Given that she has potential for visceral compromise on the basis of the history, I would employ a high approach (McEvedy) to the right groin. Under general anaesthetic, I would place the patient supine with arms tucked by the side.

Examiner interrupts: that's fine, just describe the operation from the skin incision.

Candidate answer

The procedural steps involve:

1. access to the area
2. delivery/release of hernia sac with inspection of contents
3. reduction of hernia contents with additional intervention to address visceral compromise as indicated
4. repair of the hernia defect.

- Transverse skin crease incision 3 cm above pubic tubercle on the ipsilateral side from close to the midline extending approximately about 8 cm laterally.
- Ligate superficial epigastric veins with 2/0 vicryl ties and divide.
- Open the external oblique aponeurosis in line of fibres extending close to the midline (linea alba) to expose the rectus muscle.
- Get the assistant to retract the rectus medially using a large Langenbach retractor.
- This allows entry into the pre-peritoneal space. Gently move inferiorly towards the pubic tubercle to expose the entire myopectineal orifice. This may require a deeper inferior retractor (such as a Deaver) and a second assistant in a large or muscular patient.

- If the sac is heading above the iliopubic tract, it is an inguinal hernia. I would identify the inferior epigastric vessels and follow them inferiorly using gentle blunt dissection. These vessels provide a guide to the position of the deep ring (laterally) and superficial ring (medially).
- If the sac is heading below the iliopubic tract, it is a femoral hernia.
- A hernial sac will appear as a funnel-shaped structure entering the crural canal.
- If the hernia sac is small it is easily reduced with the dissection or with pressure on the groin.

Examiner interrupts: if the hernia and its contents reduce spontaneously before you have inspected them, what would you do?

Candidate answer

- Given this woman's symptoms, it is mandatory that the contents of the hernia (i.e. viscera) are fully inspected.
- If the sac or its contents slip back into the peritoneal cavity, especially if the sac is empty once opened, I would open the peritoneum in the region immediately below the incision. The large fenestration in the peritoneum can be extended laterally, offering enough space to eviscerate the entire small bowel, allowing its inspection.

Examiner: okay, let's return to the procedure, assuming that you have just identified the hernia sac heading down the femoral canal containing small bowel. What would you do next?

Candidate answer

- I would like to inspect the condition of the hernial contents.
- At this point, it is necessary to open the peritoneum as described above and follow the small bowel loop down to the femoral canal.
- As it is possible that the small bowel has been strangulated with potential for occult perforation into the sac, I would gain control of the small bowel loop disappearing into the hernia before reducing it to avoid potential peritoneal spillage and contamination.
- I would achieve this using nylon tapes in preference to non-crushing bowel clamps. I would make a small window at the mesenteric border of each of the limbs of small bowel and pass the tape through the window to occlude the lumen atraumatically.
- If the small bowel is compromised on reduction, repair/resection can be accomplished through this incision, if necessary (see Chapter 4.4.8 for more detail).
- I would then close the peritoneum using 2/0 vicryl.
- For a femoral hernia, I would close the femoral canal with 2–3 ethibond sutures. I would suture the iliopubic tract to the pectineal ligament, taking care to protect the femoral vein which is lateral.
- For an inguinal hernia, I would place a prolene mesh in the pre-peritoneal plane to cover the myopectineal orifice.
- I would then close the anterior rectus sheath with 0 PDS with subcuticular 3-0 monocryl to skin.

Examiner: when the hernia is chronic and has become complicated, it can be difficult to reduce. What strategies are available to you in this situation?

Candidate answer

Being careful to control the reduction so that contents can subsequently be inspected, I would attempt each of the following in succession.

- Having gently dilated the neck of the hernia with a finger alongside the sac, I would push gently over the hernia externally (from the groin) whilst applying gentle traction from within the (pre-) peritoneal surface.
- Next, I would formally dissect the sac to free the surrounding tissue with blunt and sharp dissection in both the *pre-peritoneal and subcutaneous planes*, whilst leaving the neck of the sac adherent to the crural canal. Occasionally, it is necessary to open the sac layer by layer (in the subcutaneous plane) if it is particularly thickened and oedematous.
- If these measures prove unsuccessful, I would formally divide the lacunar ligament medially, having first made sure that there is *not* an aberrant obturator artery present.

4.4.3 Axillary dissection

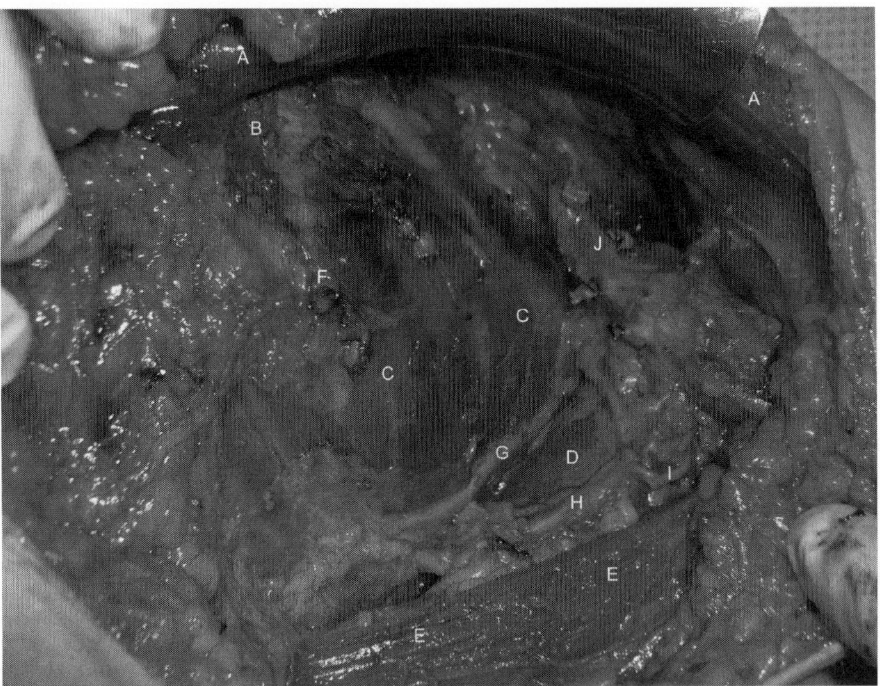

Figure 4.4.3

Left axilla after radical lymph node dissection. Intercostobrachial nerve has been excised. A: pectoralis major muscle, B: divided origin pectoralis minor muscle, C: serratus anterior muscle, D: subscapularis muscle, E: latissimus dorsi muscle, F: divided origin intercostobrachial nerve, G: long thoracic nerve, H: thoracodorsal nerve, I: subscapular artery, J: axillary vein and divided tributaries

Examiner question: this image is of the left axilla during an axillary dissection. Please describe how you would perform an axillary dissection?

Candidate answer

Pre-operative indications for axillary dissection generally include:

- pre-operative involvement of axillary nodes
- a large primary breast tumour
- positive sentinel lymph node biopsy.

Preparation:

- GA
- supine with arm abducted to 80°
- prep and free arm drape.

The procedural steps involve:

1. entry to the axilla
2. define the boundaries of the dissection (see Chapter 4.2.2)
3. identify and preserve important structures
4. excise axillary nodal tissue.

- Transverse axillary incision at inferior aspect of hair line running between pectoralis (pec.) major and Latissimus (lat.) dorsi.
- Raise 'axillary flaps' using cat's paws for retraction.
- Personally, I employ the inferior approach to axillary dissection.
- Identify the pectoralis major and latissimus dorsi muscles, as they define important boundaries of the dissection. The axilla is covered by fascia, which needs to be incised to access the axillary contents. I use a Babcock on axillary tissue to deliver it inferiorly and get my assistant to retract the muscles that form the boundaries to the axilla.
- The medial extent of the dissection is defined by incising the clavipectoral fascia 1 cm below the lateral edge of pec. major. This ensures that the medial pectoral nerve is not injured. This dissection is continued cranially with simultaneous lateral retraction of the axillary fat to help expose the muscle edge.
- Care is taken to identify and preserve the long thoracic nerve, which lies on serratus anterior.
- Once the lateral border of pec. major has been exposed it is then retracted anteriomedially to expose pec. minor underneath. The dissection is continued cranially by a combination of sharp and blunt dissection freeing the axillary fatty nodal tissue from the lateral edge of pec. minor.
- The lateral dissection is along the lateral border of lat. dorsi. The fascia overlying the lateral edge of the muscle is incised parallel to the muscle 1 cm anterior to its edge. This incision is continued cranially until the tendon of the muscle or axillary vein is seen. The thoracodorsal neurovascular bundle can be identified lying below the fascia overlying the lat. dorsi muscle (approximately 2 cm medial to the lateral edge of the muscle). The neurovascular bundle should be identified and protected during dissection of the lateral boundary of the dissection.
- The axillary envelope between the long thoracic and thoracodorsal nerves (which have been identified and preserved) constitutes a level I dissection.

- At this point I aim to define the superior border of my dissection which is the lower border of the axillary vein.
- Cues that I am close to the axillary vein are:
  - superior to medial pectoral pedicle
  - superior to the intercostobrachial nerve
  - palpation of the pulsation of axillary artery which can be a sign dissection is too high.
- Right angle forceps to gently part the tissue to expose the bluish hue of the axillary vein are useful.
- Often there will be tributaries draining into the vein. There is often an unnamed superficial vein which runs anterior to the thoracodorsal leash. However prior to dividing this branch, I will identify the thoracodorsal branch and the deeper plane it runs in.
- All unnamed branches are divided using two ligaclips proximally and one distally with Metzenbaum scissors.
- Between the thoracodorsal and long thoracic nerves, the dissection continues to a plane along the fascia of subscapularis (floor of dissection).
- Generally I divide the intercostobrachial nerves which run parallel to the vein when moving from superior to inferior.
- Attention now turns to level II dissection, which involves dissection behind pec. minor.
- I dissect tissue off the inferior surface of pec. minor and then I carefully dissect inferior to axillary vein, whilst keeping it in my field of vision at all times.
- I ligaclip any tributaries during my dissection, and often sacrifice the medial pectoral leash during this level of dissection.
- After gaining haemostasis, I use a 14 French belovac drain to the axilla and close in two layers.

4.4.4 Ileostomy closure

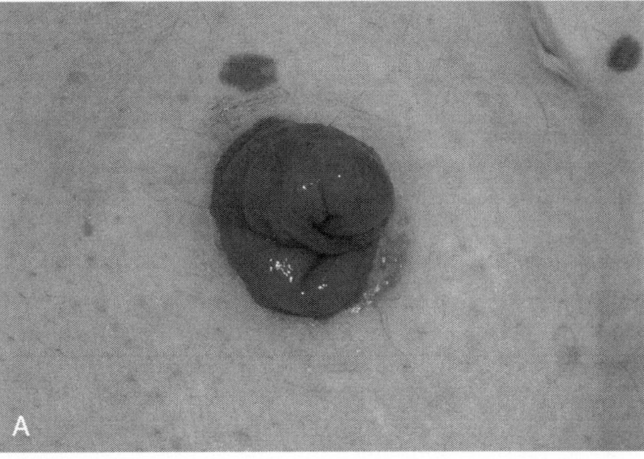

Figure 4.4.4A
Loop ileostomy

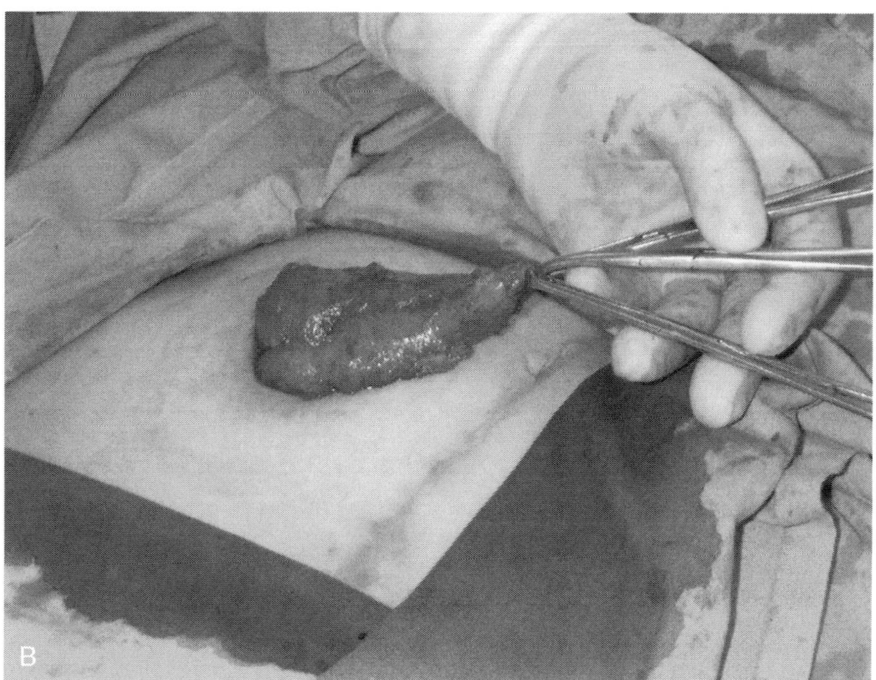

Figure 4.4.4B
Loop ileostomy mobilised for closure

Examiner question: how would you close this stoma?

Candidate answer

This is a loop ileostomy with a 'spouted' proximal limb.

Pre-operative preparation would include:

- in situations where this is a diverting stoma, i would ensure the integrity of the anastomosis by checking endoscopically and/or radiologically (e.g. with gastrografin enema) prior to reversal
- if I am concerned about the continence mechanism then manometric assessment of the sphincter muscles may be helpful.

Preparation:

- prophylactic antibiotics intravenously at induction
- GA
- supine
- remove stoma bag and decontaminate skin/spout
- prep and drape.

The procedural steps involve:

1. circumferential incision to dissect free from subcutaneous tissues
2. mobilisation of limbs
3. anastomosis/closure of enterotomy
4. closure of fascial defect with decontamination of superficial tissues.

- Optional infiltration with local anaesthetic with adrenaline for hydrodissection/haemostasis.
- Circumferential or elliptical incision peristomally staying 1–2 mm away from the muco-cutaneous junction of the ileostomy.
- Dissect down onto small bowel and continue meticulously to separate from the extrafascial subcutaneous tissues using sharp/diathermy dissection without causing serosa injury to the ileum.
- At the level of the fascia, safely enter the peritoneal cavity in one position and continue to free the ileostomy from the fascia circumferentially.
- Ensure good mobilisation is achieved with delivery of a reasonable length of ileum proximally and distally, especially if resection/stapled anastomosis is to be performed.
- Once adequately mobilised and if possible, the spout should be reverted and the 1–2 mm of skin remaining attached to the ileum at the muco-cutaneous junction should be excised, leaving fresh, clean ends for primary anastomosis.
- Anastomosis is ideally performed using 3-0 PDS placed serosubmucosally in an interrupted fashion, whilst adhering to the principles of no tension, adequate blood supply and precise technique.
- In cases where the stoma ends are of dubious quality/viability then a formal small bowel resection and primary anastomosis is performed. The anastomosis can be hand sewn (as above) or a functional end-to-end stapled anastomosis can be fashioned using two fires of a 75 mm linear stapler, one to create a common limb and the second to close the enterotomy created by stapler insertion.
- The fascial defect is then closed using interrupted figure of eight 1 PDS sutures. The skin defect is apposed using a subcuticular absorbable suture in a circumferential purse-string, which can be drawn together to leave a small circular defect which is then left open for free drainage, granulation and epithelialisation (this technique has lowest risk of wound infection 0–4%).

Examiner question: what would you do if you are unable to adequately mobilise the stoma?

Candidate answer

In such settings, where there are extensive adhesions, a formal laparotomy will need to be performed if I am unable to safely mobilise under direct vision.

Examiner question: what would you do if there is an associated parastomal hernia?

Candidate answer

Manage as with any hernia principle. That is I would reduce the contents, excise the sac and close the fascia (primarily with non-absorbable sutures).

4.4.5 Right hemicolectomy/caecal volvulus

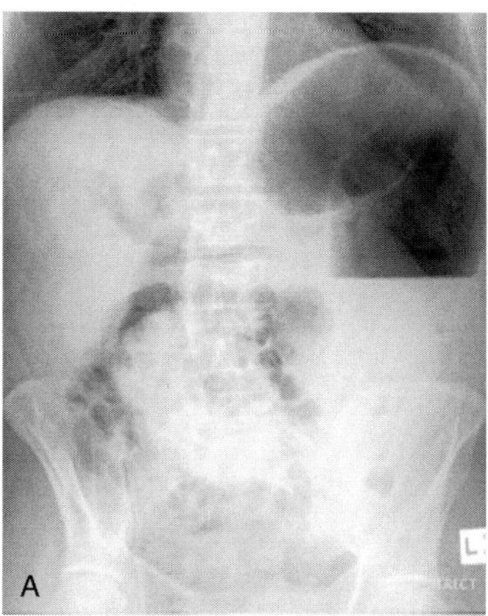

Figure 4.4.5A
AXR of caecal volvulus

Examiner question: this is the x-ray from a 50-year-old patient, otherwise fit and well. The patient presents with severe abdominal pain and vomiting, with no previous surgical history. What do you see here?

Candidate answer

It is a plain abdominal x-ray showing a large dilated closed loop of bowel in the left upper quadrant. I cannot see any gas in the right iliac fossa, so it is probably a caecal volvulus. There is also gas in the biliary system (pneumobilia) evident on the x-ray.

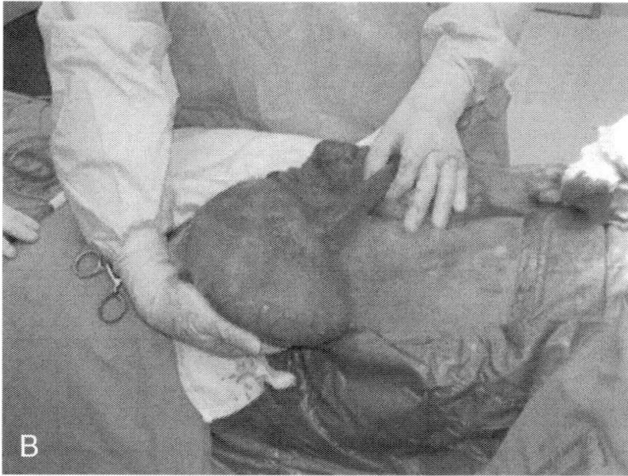

Figure 4.4.5B
Caecal volvulus at operation

Examiner: that is correct. Figure 4.4.5B shows what was found at surgery. Can you describe how you would do an open right hemicolectomy in this case?

Candidate answer

Preparation:

- GA
- prophylactic antibiotics
- thromboprophylaxis
- IDC/NGT if not already inserted
- supine position (occasionally modified Lloyd-Davies if access to the pelvis is anticipated)
- prep and drape.

The procedural steps involve:

1. entry/laparotomy
2. mobilisation of the right colon and terminal ileum (off the duodenum)
3. ligation and division of blood vessels
4. resection
5. anastomosis
6. closure.

- Midline incision (centred above the umbilicus) down to the linea alba with entry to the peritoneal cavity at the cicatrix by dividing the peritoneum between two artery clips.
- Perform a full laparotomy looking for evidence of free fluid, faecal contamination or ischaemic bowel.
- Possible deflation of the caecum using a 16–18 G needle on a 5 ml syringe with the plunger replaced with suction tubing through a taenia coli.
- The caecum and ascending colon will usually be drawn medially in the case of a caecal volvulus.
- The right colon can be mobilised using an inferior, medial (to lateral) or lateral approach. My preference is the lateral approach.
- The key to right hemicolectomy is to mobilise the right colon off the second part of the duodenum.
- The peritoneum lateral to the colon is incised along the white line of Toldt from the caecum to the hepatic flexure.
- Immediately, I seek to identify, dissect, free and preserve the retroperitoneal structures from the right mesocolon. The second part of the duodenum is the key structure as the right ureter/gonadals are only infrequently sought/seen.
- The dissection is continued cephalad and medially until the duodenum is completely free of the mesocolon, dropping back to its native position in the retroperitoneum.

- I know to be careful to not avulse the fragile mesocolic veins at the hepatic flexure with excessive traction on the specimen, particularly when the mesocolon is short. The hepatocolic ligament, containing vessels, often needs to be formally ligated.
- Attention then turns to the transverse colon and mobilisation continues proximally back towards the hepatic flexure until it is completely mobilised.
- Finally, any terminal ileal bands/adhesions are divided so that the whole of the right colon can be lifted from the abdomen.
- With adequate mobilisation of the duodenum away from the mesocolon, identification of the ileocolic artery at its origin from the SMA is usually obvious. Accordingly, it is possible to create mesenteric windows in the peritoneum on either side of the ileocolic pedicle. Large artery forceps are then applied to the pedicle, which is divided and ligated with 0 vicryl.
- The proximal and distal resection margins are then identified on the terminal ileum and colon, respectively. Small windows are made at the mesenteric border of the bowel at such points and the peritoneum scored between the 2 (via the ligated ileocolic pedicle) in a V-shape.
- With my assistant elevating the specimen, I can transilluminate the mesentery to identify the ileal, right colic and other mesenteric vessels prior to their ligation and division. Specifically, the right colics and the marginal artery (or on occasions the right branch of the middle colics) are divided.
- The extent of the resection will usually include approximately 10 cm of terminal ileum and the colon to the mid-third of the transverse colon. Abdominal packs are used to cover the abdomen and a 75 mm linear stapler can be used to divide the ileum and the transverse colon and the specimen removed. The ends to be anastomosed are held using Babcock's forceps and the corners of each are cut so that a 75 mm linear stapler can be inserted and fired on two more occasions to create a functional end-to-end stapled anastomosis. It is important to ensure that the orientation of the bowel is correct so that there is no twist in the mesentery. The internal lumen of the anastomosis is examined to ensure there is no staple line bleeding. A 'crotch' suture is applied using 3-0 PDS for additional support. The staple line is examined for bleeding and oversewn using 3-0 PDS.
- Alternatively, the anastomosis can be hand-sewn using interrupted serosubmucosal sutures.
- Haemostasis should be confirmed, especially in the right paracolic/retroperitoneal space.
- Washout with normal saline can be performed if required.
- Closure of the abdominal fascia is performed using two looped 1 PDS sutures.
- Skin closure using subcuticular 3/0 monocryl.

4.4.6 Hartmann's procedure

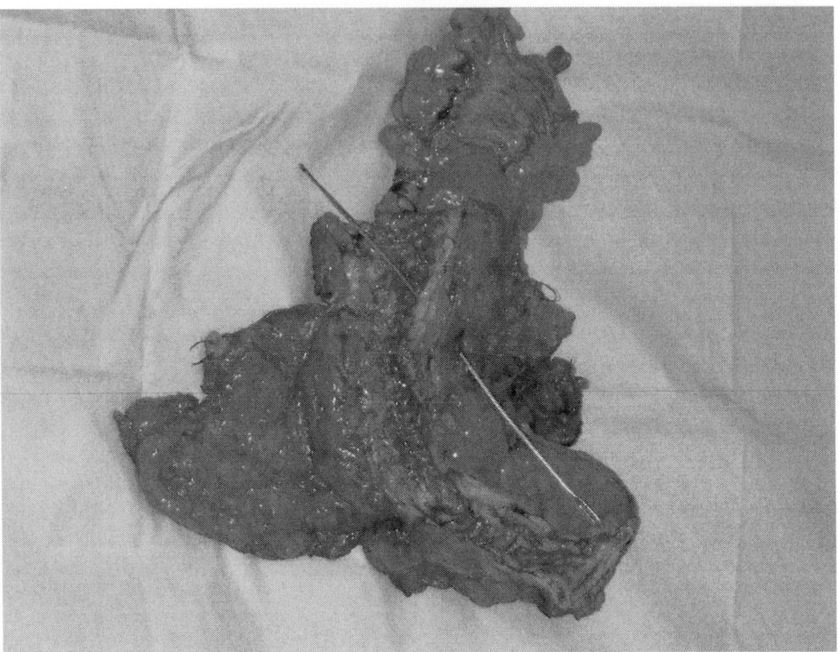

Figure 4.4.6
Hartmann's resection for perforated sigmoid diverticular disease

Examiner question: this specimen is from a 60-year-old patient who presented with an acute abdomen with a history of left-sided lower abdominal pain and evidence of generalised peritonitis. What do you see here?

Candidate answer

Macroscopically, the specimen looks like colon. Additionally, there is evidence of a communication through the layers of the bowel wall, suggestive of a perforation. Given the history, it is probable that this is a perforation of the sigmoid colon.

Examiner: that is correct. The patient underwent a Hartmann's procedure for faecal peritonitis secondary to perforated diverticular disease of the sigmoid colon. Can you describe how you would perform a Hartmann's procedure?

Candidate answer

Preparation:

- GA
- prophylactic antibiotics
- thromboprophylaxis
- IDC/NGT if not already inserted

- modified Lloyd-Davies to allow access to the pelvis with Trendelenburg tilt
- prep and drape.

The procedural steps involve:

1. entry/laparotomy
2. mobilisation of the left colon (and possibly upper rectum)
3. ligation and division of blood vessels
4. resection of diseased segment to control contamination and treat sepsis
5. decontamination of peritoneal cavity
6. closure with formation of end colostomy.

- Lower midline incision down to the linea alba with entry to the peritoneal cavity at the cicatrix by dividing the peritoneum between two artery clips.
- Upon entry into the peritoneal cavity, the degree of contamination is assessed and a thorough exploration of the abdominal contents performed. The site(s) of contamination should be controlled with purse-string sutures/direct closure if possible.
- The small bowel is packed to the right side of the abdomen to improve access and exposure to the left colon and pelvis.
- A large, moistened pack is placed over the left colon and mobilisation is performed using electrocautery and begins by dividing the congenital sigmoid adhesions. The left colon is retracted anteromedially out of the wound to expose the lateral peritoneal attachments. The full-thickness of the peritoneum is incised from sigmoid colon in a cephalad direction. Care is taken to incise the peritoneum alone without entering the fascia of the mesocolon.
- The sigmoid colon is then retracted medially so as to put the V-shaped mesocolon on stretch. The peritoneum at the apex of the mesocolon is incised. The extrafascial plane between the left mesocolon and Gerota's fascia is developed and the gonadal vessels and left ureter are identified. The left ureter can be reliably identified as it crosses the common iliac vessels, its identity can be confirmed by gently compressing it with DeBakey forceps to demonstrate vermiculation.
- Once identified, the gonadals and left ureter are displaced posteriorly and mobilisation continues under the left colon mesentery towards the midline.
- Ideally, it is best to avoid mobilisation of the upper rectum as this makes subsequent reversal more challenging. However, in some instances, it will be necessary to permit distal transection.
- Upon adequate mobilisation, the limits of the resection are marked at the mesenteric border of the sigmoid colon and the peritoneum between the two sites is scored in preparation for vessel ligation. The mesentery is then transilluminated and the vessels individually isolated, ligated and divided using 0 or 2/0 vicryl, as appropriate.
- The diseased sigmoid colon is then resected using a 75 mm linear stapler. At this stage it is important to ensure that there is adequate mobility on the descending colon proximally to allow the colostomy to be fashioned without tension. Formal mobilisation of the splenic flexure is seldom necessary. The distal margin of resection is usually at the rectosigmoid junction. The rectal

stump is oversewn with 3-0 PDS and marked with prolene to facilitate its identification during the reversal procedure. A thorough lavage of peritoneal cavity is then performed using copious volumes of warmed, saline and drains are inserted.

- A trephine is then made in the LIF in preparation for colostomy formation. The skin and fascia are firmly grasped and the skin at the proposed stoma site is grasped with an Allis forceps and a circular incision made with cutting electrocautery. A disc of skin about 3 cm in diameter is then excised. I usually preserve the subcutaneous fat. Using retractors, dissection is continued until the anterior rectus sheath is visualised. The anterior rectus sheath is incised in a cruciate fashion. During this procedure a pack is placed in the abdomen and the abdominal wall elevated using the non-dominant hand to protect the underlying viscera. The rectus muscle is spread transversely and longitudinally to identify the posterior rectus sheath. I protect the inferior epigastric arteries during this step. A similar cruciate incision is made in the posterior sheath. The resulting defect should be large enough to easily accommodate two fingers. Two Babcock clamps are passed through the defect to grasp the colon and are gently drawn through the defect, avoiding any twists or constriction of the mesentery.
- Mass closure of the abdomen is then performed, the skin closed and a dressing applied before creation of the stoma. The stapled end of the colon is excised using Metzenbaum scissors and haemostasis achieved. Finally, the colostomy is fashioned using undyed taper cut 2/0 vicryl. Interrupted sutures are placed between the seromuscular layer of the colon and the dermis. Stoma bag is then applied.
- Post-operatively, the patient will be managed in a HDU setting and oral intake resumed as soon as possible. I usually continue the antibiotics for 5 days post-operatively and ensure patient receives daily mechanical and chemical DVT prophylaxis.

Note: in selective cases a primary anastomosis may be performed but in exam settings you must act as a safe general surgeon, as marks are given for safety and not heroism!

Examiner question: in an emergency setting where the stoma is not marked pre-operatively, how would you site your stoma intra-operatively?

Candidate answer

- If patient is not marked pre-operatively by a stoma therapist then I would mark the site with indelible pen prior to scrubbing. I would avoid bony areas, creases, previous scars. In the presence of panus, the stoma will be sited above it.
- I usually position the stoma within a triangle formed by the anterior superior iliac spine, umbilicus and the pubic symphysis. Ideally the colostomy should be brought out through the fibres of rectus abdominis.

Examiner question: during the mobilisation of the left colon, which anatomical landmarks would you use to identify the ureter?

Candidate answer

It is usually seen at the apex of V-shaped sigmoid mesocolon where it crosses the left common iliac artery. It is a whitish cord-like structure which is non-pulsatile but which vermiculates. It passes down on the psoas major in the retroperitoneum, crossing the genitofermoral nerve, and it is crossed by gonadal vessels.

Examiner question: what is your approach if you identify a ureteric injury intra-operatively?

Candidate answer

- This is an unfortunate predicament and I would do my best to prevent it from happening. However, should it happen I would endeavour to minimise further harm. Upon suspicion of this injury, I would confirm that it is the ureter, assess the level of injury, any evidence of tissue loss and viability of the cut ends. After assessing the severity of the injury, I would contact a urologist for help.
- The options (with the help of the urologist) may include an uretero-ureterostomy repair over a stent when injury is to the mid or upper ureter above the bifurcation of the iliac vessels. If an injury to a ureter is distal enough to allow the proximal ureter to be mobilised and inserted into the dome of the bladder without tension, a uretero-neocystostomy without psoas hitch would be appropriate.
- If a urologist can't attend, I would be guided by him/her over the phone as to how to salvage the situation until it can be definitively repaired by an expert. Options may include placement of a drain tube, a stent or exteriorisation of the cut end.

Examiner question: in a scenario where you have mobilised the splenic flexure in order to bring out a tension free stoma, you notice blood pooling in the left upper quadrant. Discuss your approach in this setting.

Note: the principles for managing intra-operative bleeding are the same, irrespective of the scenario. Refer to Chapter 4.3 for a suggested approach.

Candidate answer

- In this scenario, I suspect that the bleeding is from the spleen. I would first pack the left upper quadrant, improve lighting (including a headlight), get more assistants, and extend the incision. I would also inform the anaesthetic team, ensure blood is available and place an appropriate retractor to assist with exposure.
- There are two ways of injuring the spleen: (i) by traction (most common) and (ii) direct injury from instruments (e.g. retractors). This can result in a capsular tear (most common) or lacerations. Most bleeding ceases with simple packing and placement of topical haemostatic agents (e.g. surgicele or gelfoam). In some cases the use of Tissell or Floseal may be appropriate.
- If there is any doubt, performing a splenectomy is the safest option to ensure haemorrhage control, although I wouldn't undertake this lightly given the potential consequences.

4.4.7 Haemorrhoidectomy

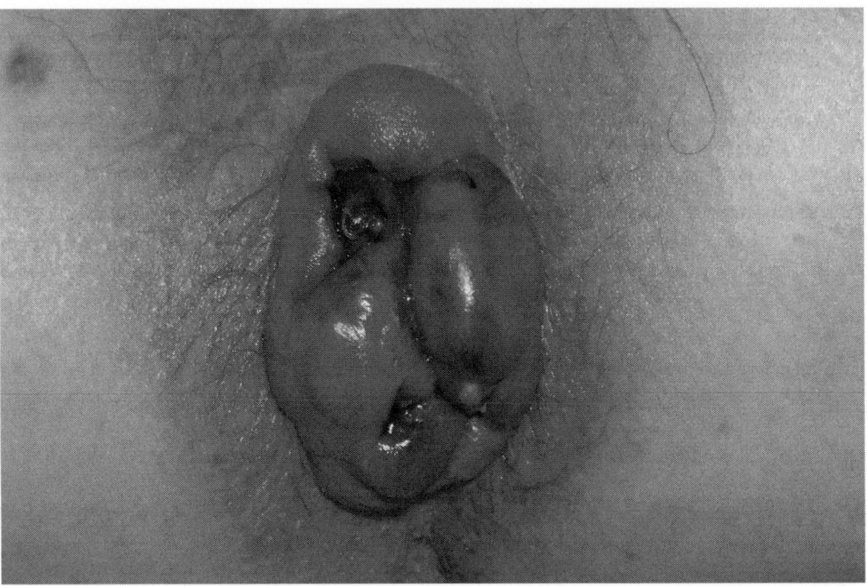

Figure 4.4.7
Prolapsed and thrombosed external and internal haemorrhoids

Examiner question: what do you see here and how would you manage this condition surgically?

Candidate answer

This image illustrates complex strangulated prolapsed haemorrhoids with both external and internal components. After obtaining a full history and examining the patient, I would perform a three-quadrant haemorrhoidectomy in this patient under GA.

Preparation:

- GA
- prophylactic antibiotics
- lithotomy or prone
- prep and drape.

The procedural steps involve:

1. examination under anaesthesia
2. identification and marking of the haemorrhoids, ensuring preservation of adequate mucocutaneous bridges between each
3. dissection of haemorrhoids from the internal anal sphincter
4. ligation and excision of the haemorrhoidal pedicles.

- The objectives of the surgery are to remove the abnormal haemorrhoidal tissue whilst leaving adequate mucocutaneous bridges and preserving continence.

- I routinely perform a haemorrhoidectomy as described by Milligan-Morgan. Anorectal examination is performed using a Hill-Ferguson anal retractor and the three haemorrhoids (right anterior and posterior and left lateral) are identified. I then use coagulating diathermy to 'mark' each of the haemorrhoidal pedicles to ensure that I will preserve an adequate muco-cutaneous bridge between each following excision. I then infiltrating each using Marcain with 0.5% with adrenaline to provide hydrodissection and for post-operative analgesia.
- I usually begin with the right posterior haemorrhoid (to avoid blood entering my field during dissection of subsequent pedicles. I place artery forceps on the associated external component and the internal component as appropriate. Using the previous diathermy marks, I incise the skin and develop the submucosal plane of dissection.
- Immediately, I seek to identify the white, circular fibres of the internal anal sphincter and continue the dissection in a craniad direction separating haemorrhoidal tissue from the underlying sphincter, which is identified and preserved at all times. The dissection is continued until a narrow pedicle remains.
- I suture ligate the pedicle with 0 vicryl. The process is repeated for the other two haemorrhoids, ensuring adequate preservation of mucocutaneous bridges. This will usually result in a haemorrhoidal bed in the configuration of a three-leaf clover.
- I ensure haemostasis and insert a spongostan into the anal canal.
- Post-operatively the patient is provided non-opioid analgesia, metronidazole (to reduce pain) and stool softeners.

Examiner question: what are the potential complications of this surgery?

Candidate answer

These may be early or delayed:

- early:
  - pain (may be severe for several days)
  - urinary retention (10–15%)
  - bleeding (acute 1%, delayed 2%)
  - infection (<1%)
- delayed:
  - anal fissure (1%)
  - anal stenosis (1%)
  - incontinence (<1%)
  - recurrence (1%).

4.4.8 Small bowel resection

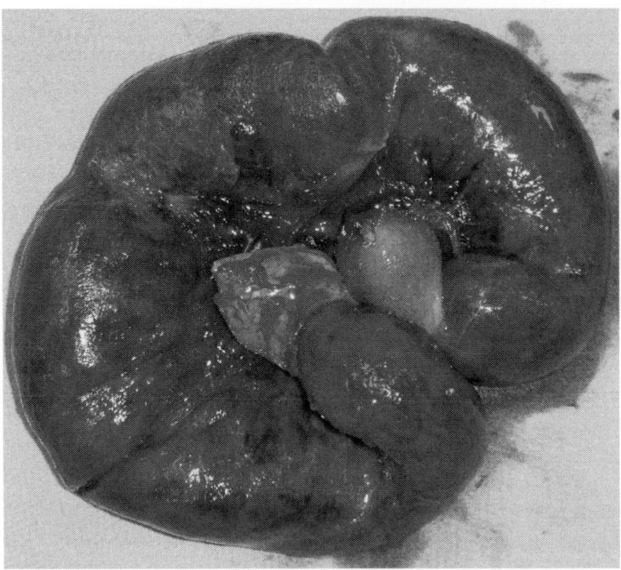

Figure 4.4.8
Small bowel resection specimen

Examiner question: this patient requires a small bowel resection. How would you perform this, assuming that you have already gained access to the peritoneal cavity?

Candidate answer

Assuming that I have already gained entry to the peritoneal cavity, I would proceed as follows:

Preparation:

- ensure prophylactic antibiotics and thromboprophylaxis have been administered
- check to see whether a IDC/NGT have been inserted.

The procedural steps involve:

1. inspection of the entire small bowel from DJ flexure to TI (and abdominal contents)
2. identify limits of resection
3. ligation and division of blood vessels
4. resection of diseased segment
5. anastomosis
6. closure.

- The primary goal of the surgery is to address the obstruction by removing the abnormal segment of small bowel.
- I would begin by examining the entire small bowel from DJ flexure to TI to ensure that there is no other pathology (e.g. this could be multifocal disease such as fibrostenotic Crohn's disease or polyposis).

- I would then isolate the diseased segment by placing packs around the wound edges. I would select the limits of resection of the diseased segment and make mesenteric windows adjacent to the bowel at this point.
- I would then incise only the peritoneum in a V shape between the two sites. I would then transilluminate the bowel to assist with the identification of mesenteric vessels, which I would individually ligate and divide using 2/0 vicryl.
- I would then place soft bowel clamps on either side of the resection site to avoid spillage and contamination when the bowel is transected. The diseased segment is then resected between two crushing (Kocher's) bowel clamps.
- When performing a hand-sewn anastomosis, I ensure that:
  - there is an adequate blood supply (i.e. both limbs of bowel are pink and viable with evidence of bleeding at the cut edge)
  - there is no tension on the bowel ends
  - that there is mucosa to mucosa apposition
  - there is no evidence of disease at the resection margin
  - I employ a precise and meticulous technique.
- I insert two stay sutures, one at the mesenteric and the other at the anti-mesenteric borders and insert interrupted 3-0 PDS sutures in a serosubmucosal fashion, ensuring that I take adequate bites from either end of the small bowel to be anastomosed. I insert the first suture at the midpoint and leave it untied before inserting subsequent sutures equi-distant apart. I suture towards the midpoint, leaving the last few in clips to allow accurate placement of the final sutures prior to tying.
- I then turn the bowel over using the stay sutures and repeat the same along this surface, ensuring that I don't obliterate the lumen. Once this wall is complete, I re-vert the bowel to its normal alignment using the stay sutures.
- **Note:** it does not matter which anastomotic technique you describe (stapled, single/double layer sutured), what matters is that you sound like as if you have done it multiple times before.
- I then close the fascia using loop PDS and close the skin using a continuous subcuticular suture.

Examiner question: are you aware of any ways of testing the integrity of your anastomosis?

Candidate answer

A leak test can be performed by placing a 'mixing' cannula in the last gap before the last suture is tied and attaching this to either (i) a 'giving' set attached to saline or (ii) 50 ml syringe full of air. Non-crushing clamps are placed on both limbs and the anastomotic site is distended with fluid or air, respectively, to check for leaks between sutures.

Examiners: in what situation will you not perform a primary anastomosis?

Candidate answer

I would not perform an anastomosis if there are any factors that may compromise the healing of the anastomosis (in such setting either a planned re-look laparotomy or a stoma is preferred). These include:

- patient factors; for example, in severe septic or cardiogenic shock where high doses of inotropic support is required
- disease factors; for example, SMA embolus requiring vascular intervention. In such setting, a re-look laparotomy is required to assess the extent of the ischaemia.

4.4.9 Thyroglossal cysts

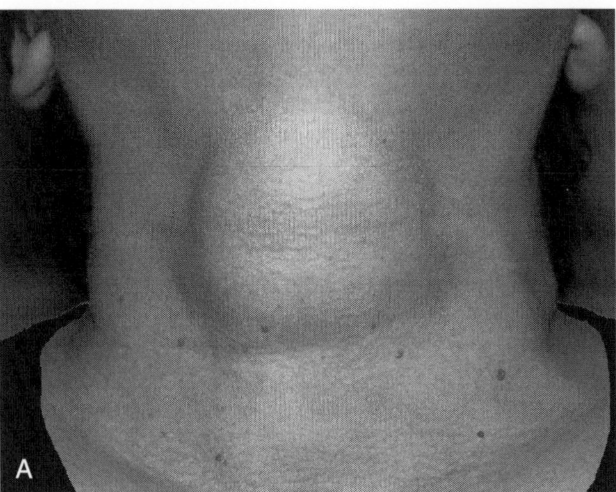

Figure 4.4.9A
Thyroglossal cyst from the front

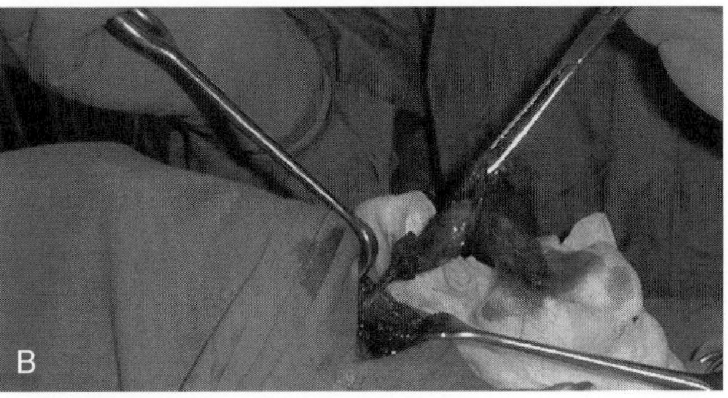

Figure 4.4.9B
Thyroglossal cyst Sistrunk operation

Examiner question: please take a look at these images. The second image is taken from the right side of the neck with the head under the drape on the left. Would you like to tell me what you think is going on here?

Candidate answer

The first image demonstrates an anterior lump in the neck in the midline with a smooth edge and no skin changes and the second image shows a transverse incision in the neck, with the retractors under the skin flaps. A structure is being retracted that appears to be extending towards the cranial end of the wound. I assume that it is an operation for a thyroglossal cyst.

Examiner: that's right, it's an image of a Sistrunk procedure. Can you discuss the relevant embryology please?

Candidate answer

- The thyroid gland develops from the median and paired lateral thyroid anlages.
- Anomalies of development of the median anlage result in thyroglossal duct remnants.
- The median anlage forms most of the adult thyroid. A diverticulum between the muscles of the base of the tongue, marked by the foramen caecum, appears by week 3 of development and becomes displaced and migrates caudally in the midline to the level of the thyroid cartilage to fuse with the lateral anlages.
- It forms the thyroglossal duct (epithelial lined tube) as it descends and it migrates through or anterior to the mesoderm that forms the hyoid bone.
- Normally the duct obliterates and atrophies by weeks 9–10, although normal remnants are the foramen caecum and the pyramidal lobe.
- Failure of the duct to obliterate results in epithelial lined cysts and can also be associated with ectopic thyroid tissue.

Examiner question: can you describe how you would perform an elective resection of an uncomplicated thyroglossal cyst?

Candidate answer

- Treatment requires en bloc excision of the cyst and the duct remnants from the foramen caecum to the pyramidal lobe and includes resection of a central portion of the hyoid bone — a procedure known as the Sistrunk procedure.
- Simple cystectomy without resection of the duct is associated with high rates (up to 80%) of recurrence.

Preparation:

- GA
- patient positioned supine with the neck extended and a shoulder roll positioned between the shoulder blades
- pre-operative intravenous 1 gram cephazolin given.

The procedural steps involve:

1. incision and access
2. identification of the cyst and duct down to the pyramidal lobe
3. hyoid bone identified, muscles separated and central portion resected
4. dissection to the foramen caecum is completed
5. closure.

- A transverse skin crease incision is made inferior to the hyoid bone, usually over the location of the cyst. Skin and platysma flaps are created. The median raphe between the strap muscles of the anterior neck is identified and opened — the cyst is located beneath the median raphe.
- The strap muscles are retracted laterally to allow dissection of the cyst and the thyroglossal duct down to the pyramidal lobe, which if present is resected, up to the level of the hyoid bone.
- Muscles attached to the centre of the hyoid bone are separated and the central portion of the hyoid is resected en bloc (about ¼ of an inch or about 6–7 mm).
- No attempt is made to isolate the duct above the hyoid bone as it is often small and fractures easily. Dissection proceeds at a 45 degree angle created by a horizontal plane through the anterior hyoid and a plane perpendicular to this towards the foramen caecum. A central core of tissue is resected approx ⅛ of an inch (about 3–4 mm) on each side. An index finger inserted into the mouth and placed on the foramen caecum can be used to manipulate the tongue and act as a guide for suprahyoid dissection. This dissection passes though the central portions of the mylohyoid and geniohyoid muscles and the foramen caecum is resected.
- The opening in the mouth is closed with absorbable sutures and the geniohyoid and mylohoid muscles are re-approximated with absorbable sutures with superficial bites to avoid hypoglossal nerve injury. While Sistrunk also originally described approximation of the ends of the hyoid bone, this is thought not to be necessary and I do not do it.
- A small drain can be left in the tract, especially if there was evidence of cyst infection. The median raphe is re-approximated with absorbable sutures. The platysma is closed with absorbable sutures and the skin is closed with an absorbable subcuticular suture.
- If a firm mass is encountered intra-operatively, biopsy can be sent for frozen sectioning as there is a 1% incidence of thyroglossal duct carcinoma.
- If there is ectopic thyroid tissue and the patient has a normal thyroid gland, it can be safely resected. If the patient does not have a normal thyroid gland the patient will require permanent thyroid hormone replacement.

4.4.10 Submandibular gland excision

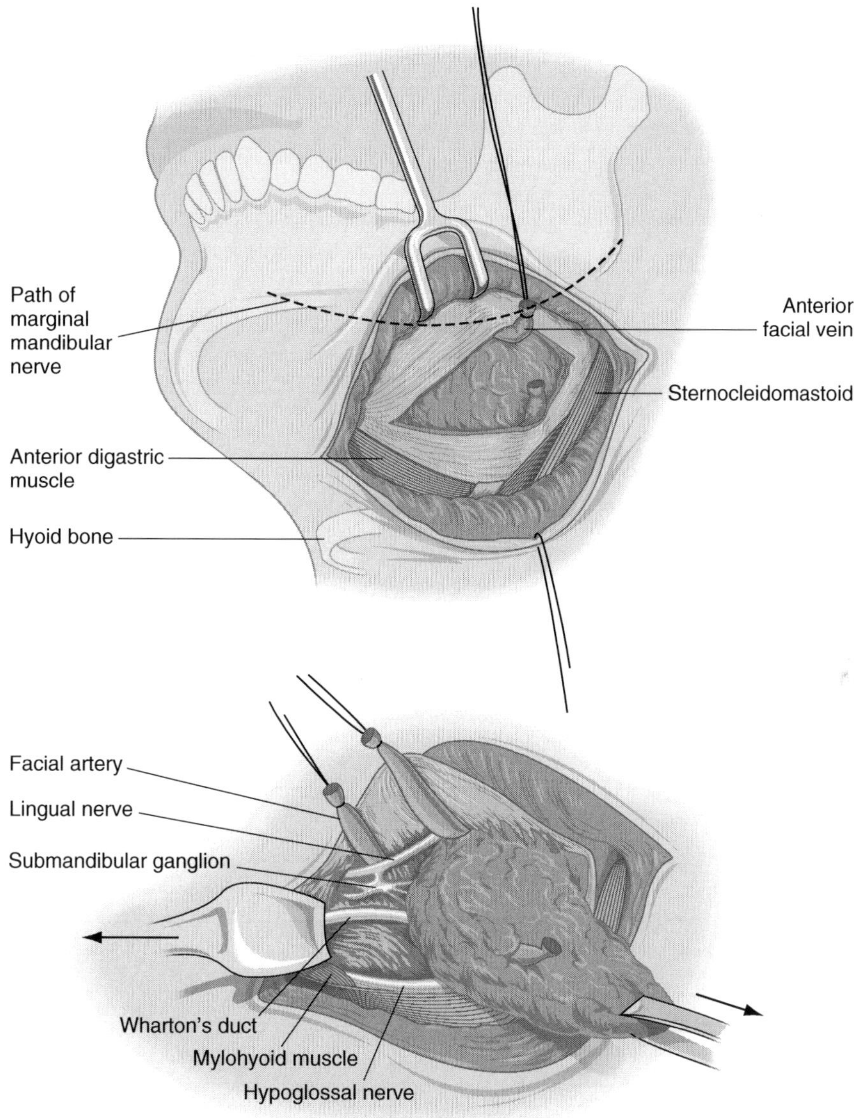

Figure 4.4.10

Excision of the submandibular gland (Source: *Cummings Otolaryngology: Head & Neck Surgery*, 5th edn. Flint P W et al. 2010, Mosby: an imprint of Elsevier, Fig 87-18, p 1174.)

Examiner question: discuss your approach to the removal of the submandibular gland for benign disease. Please highlight the important anatomical structures you encounter and the consequence of injury to these structures.

Candidate answer

- Indications for surgery include submandibular gland stones, sialadenitis.
- To remove the superficial and deep lobes of the submandibular (SMN) gland, the structures that need to be protected are:
  - the marginal mandibular branch of the facial nerve (supplies depressor anguli oris, depressor labii inferioris, risorius and part of orbicularis oris — injury causes facial asymmetry and drooling)
  - the hypoglossal nerve (motor to all intrinsic muscles of the tongue except palatoglossus)
  - the lingual nerve (sensation and taste to anterior two-thirds of the tongue).

Preparation:

- GA
- patient positioned supine with the neck extended and the head turned away on a head ring
- DVT prophylaxis
- pre-operative intravenous 1 gram cephazolin given.

The procedural steps involve:

1. incision and access
2. dissection of the superficial lobe
3. dissection of the deep lobe
4. ligation of the duct and excision of the gland
5. closure.

- A skin crease incision is made from a point 2 cm lateral to the midline extending to angle of mandible. The incision is 4 cm inferior to the lower border of the mandible (to protect the marginal mandibular branch of the facial nerve).
- The incision is deepened through platysma onto the surface of the SMN gland. No flaps are dissected to avoid injury to the marginal mandibular branch of facial nerve.
- The inferior border of the SMN gland is bluntly dissected free and the facial vein is ligated as it is encountered on its superficial surface.
- The posterior aspect of the SMN gland is dissected free. The facial vein and artery are ligated and divided when encountered.
- The superior border of SMN gland is dissected. The facial artery is again ligated on the superior border as it loops around the inferior border of the mandible.
- The superficial lobe is dissected off the mylohyoid muscle. I retract the SMN gland laterally while my assistant retracts the posterior border of mylohyoid medially and I bluntly dissect the deep lobe of the gland free.
- The deep lobe lies between mylohyoid and hyoglossus and is dissected free. The hypoglossal nerve lies on hyoglossus inferiorly and is protected. It is deep to the tendon of the digastric.

- The SMN duct extends from the deep lobe and is closely related to the lingual nerve. The lingual nerve is superior to the duct and is retracted inferiorly with the gland. SMN ganglion fibres attaching the nerve to the duct are divided, freeing the lingual nerve, which is retracted superiorly.
- The SMN duct is ligated with vicryl ties and divided. The gland and duct are excised and checked for stones.
- The wound is washed and a 10 bellovac drain inserted. Closure is performed in layers using vicryl and monocryl.

Examiner question: how does your approach differ in the setting of malignant disease?

Candidate answer

- In the case of malignancy, the aim of the operation is to remove both the submandibular gland and the associated lymphoid tissue in the submandibular triangle.
- Consequently, the initial dissection is carried only through platysma and subplatysmal flaps are created. It is important to stay on platysma while creating the superior flap. The marginal mandibular nerve is then formally identified in the fascia deep to platysma and retracted superiorly.
- Dissection then proceeds to remove all the tissue below the mandible and between the posterior and anterior bellies of digastric. Care is again taken to preserve the lingual and hypoglossal nerves. However, the preservation of the above structures may not be possible depending on the extent of the malignancy being treated.

4.4.11 Tracheostomy

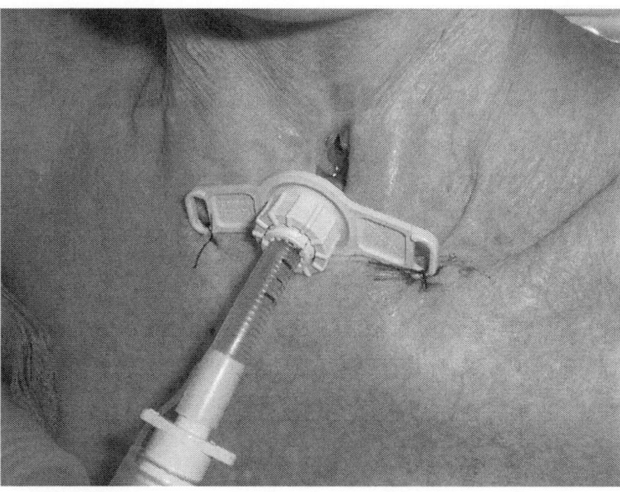

Figure 4.4.11
Tracheostomy with tracheo-oesophageal fistula

Examiner question: can you tell what you see here in this image?

Candidate answer

There is an older patient with a tracheostomy present and sutured to the skin. There appears to be a chronic deep wound and something else going on.

Examiner: the patient has got a tracheoesophageal fistula.

Candidate response

Oh, I see!

Examiner: what are the complications of a tracheostomy apart from a tracheoesophageal fistula?

Candidate answer

- Bleeding — this can occur from thyroid or jugular veins or from a trachea-innominate fistula.
- A dislodged tube — if a Bjork flap has been created this can aid replacement of the tube.
- Creation of a false passage — this can occur if the tube is not placed into the trachea correctly or if there is inadvertent removal and blind replacement.
- Infection — uncommon.
- Obstruction — can occur due to drying of mucus secretions. Therefore, good tracheostomy toilet and humidified air is important. Obstruction can also occur following dislodgement of the tube.
- Subglottic tracheal stenosis — due to pressure effects of the cuff and may require corrective surgery if the tracheostomy is to be removed.
- Vocal cord dysfunction — uncommon.
- Tracheo-innominate fistula — uncommon (~1%). May be preceded by a sentinel bleed, due to erosion of any part of the tube into the brachiocephalic trunk. Rapidly fatal.

Examiner: what are the indications for tracheostomy formation?

Candidate answer

- Patients requiring prolonged ventilation or intubation.
- Supraglottic infection or inflammation in a semi-elective setting.
- Patients requiring protection of their airway (vocal cord paralysis, stroke).
- Patients requiring permanent airway access — oropharyngeal tumours/ resection.
- As an emergency procedure for airway obstruction, although cricothyroidotomy is usually preferred if endotracheal tube (ETT) placement is unsuccessful.
- Increasingly, percutaneous tracheostomy is performed, especially on ICU in patients requiring prolonged ventilation or intubation. Relative contraindications to percutaneous tracheostomy include: obesity, short neck, cervical spine injury, enlarged thyroid.

Examiner: can you describe how you perform a tracheostomy formation?

Candidate answer

Preparation:

- GA
- the patient is usually intubated and ventilated
- patient positioned supine with the neck extended, the head placed on a head ring and a shoulder roll positioned between the shoulder blades
- the skin is prepped and the head draped
- DVT prophylaxis
- pre-operative intravenous 1 gram cephazolin given.

The procedural steps involve:

1. check tracheostomy tubes and their cuffs to ensure that they work and have ventilator extension tubing available
2. incision and access
3. divide thyroid isthmus and expose the 3rd to 6th tracheal rings
4. incise the trachea (inferiorly based Bjork flap)
5. insertion of tracheostomy tube
6. closure.

- My aim is to secure an airway at the 2nd to 4th tracheal rings, whilst avoiding the thyroid ima artery, the anterior jugular veins, thyroid bleeding and the larynx.
- Before I scrub I check the tracheostomy tubes and their cuffs that they work and that I have suction and ventilator extension tubing available. I usually use tracheostomy tube sizes 5–7, one size above and one size below the ETT size.
- Incision in skin crease 2–3 cm (or two fingers) above the sternal notch.
- Raise platysmal flaps superiorly to the cricoid and inferiorly to the sternal notch and retract using Joll's plus Langenbeck retractors.
- Make a longitudinal incision in fascia and separate the strap muscles in the midline and come down onto the thyroid gland.
- Divide the thyroid isthmus — ligate thyroid ima artery, clamp isthmus between artery forceps, divide and oversew edges with 2/0 vicryl.
- Expose the 3rd to 6th tracheal rings and place a 2/0 vicryl stay suture in the trachea.
- Retract cricoid superiorly with a hook.
- I inform the anaesthetist that I going to open the trachea.
- I incise the trachea (inferiorly based Bjork flap) between 3rd and 4th (or 2nd and 3rd) tracheal rings (no diathermy due to risks with 100% oxygen) with a 15 blade and scissors.
- I ensure that the ETT balloon is not ruptured and that the incision does not extend into the posterior trachea and injure the oesophagus behind.
- The opening in the trachea is held open with the stay suture and the tracheostomy tube with the introducer is held ready to be inserted.
- I ask anaesthetist to withdraw the ETT, but *not to remove it*.
- The ETT cuff is deflated and slowly withdrawn. Once the ETT is out of view the tracheostomy tube can be placed. This requires good communication with

the anaesthetist and prior to this a period of ventilation with 100% oxygen maybe appropriate in anticipation of a period of apnoea while the tracheostomy is placed.

- I remove the introducer and inflate the tracheostomy tube cuff and connect to the ventilator.
- Suture Bjork flap to subcutaneous tissue inferiorly.
- Close platysma and then skin with interrupted sutures.
- Secure phalanges of tube to skin with sutures, then with linen tapes around the patient's neck.

4.4.12 Trauma laparotomy

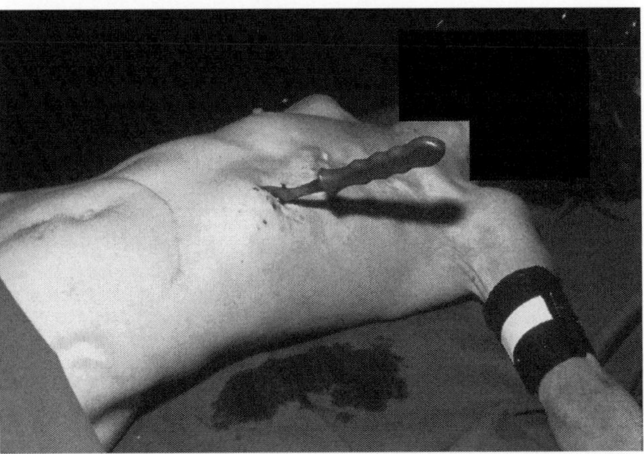

Figure 4.4.12
Penetrating abdominal injury

Examiner question: this patient is haemodynamically unstable in the emergency department and non-responsive to volume resuscitation. How would you manage him?

Candidate answer

- This patient has sustained a low-velocity penetrating injury to the upper abdomen. As this patient is haemodynamically unstable and non-responsive to volume, he requires an immediate laparotomy to achieve definitive haemorrhage control as part of the 'circulation' of the primary survey.
- I would prepare this patient for theatre by ensuring that the rest of the primary survey is adequately and rapidly performed i.e. airway and breathing assessed and optimised (e.g. O_2 administered, patient intubated, chest tube inserted, as necessary).
- The patient should remain in three-point immobilisation of the C-spine.
- I would ensure that adequate, large-bore intravenous access is obtained using at least 2 x 14G cannulae and if the patient hasn't responded to 2 L of crystalloid, he requires a blood transfusion — possibly as part of a massive transfusion protocol.

- The most useful imaging studies in an unstable patient are chest and pelvic x-rays. It is important that pelvic fracture is excluded in cases of blunt trauma, as it may be pelvic bleeding.
- I would inform the anaesthetic team, theatre nurse in charge and ensure adequate assistance is available. Baseline bloods, in particular urgent group and hold will be made available. I would ensure that I am familiar with the mechanism of injury and examine the abdomen so I can anticipate the bleeding organ. An IDC would be inserted, a bair hugger used and ICU bed booked urgently.

Examiner question: okay, so what would you do when you arrive in theatre?

Candidate answer

Preparation:

- GA
- prophylactic antibiotics
- thromboprophylaxis
- IDC/NGT if not already inserted
- modified Lloyd-Davies to allow access to the pelvis with Trendelenburg tilt
- prep and drape.

The goals of a trauma laparotomy are to (in order):

1. arrest haemorrhage
2. control peritoneal contamination
3. definitive repair of injury (usually at a later stage when patient is stable).

The procedural steps involve:

1. entry/laparotomy
2. manual removal of clot/suction of free blood
3. four-quadrant packing
4. systematic inspection of abdominal contents, commencing with the quadrant *least* likely to be the source of haemorrhage
5. arrest haemorrhage and contamination control
6. temporary closure of abdomen.

- I would wear a head light and ensure that my scrub nurse has large suckers and multiple rolled large packs. Ideally, I would prepare cell savers, large-bore suckers, numerous packs and vascular instruments, haemostatic agents (surgicel/ flowseal/ etc).
- I would perform a midline laparotomy from xiphisternum to pubic symphysis, evacuating clots by hand into a kidney dish. I would pack all four quadrants of the abdomen using packs. Several packs may need to be placed in each quadrant to achieve adequate packing.
- I would use assistants to retract the abdominal wall with retractors.
- Next, I would assess each quadrant carefully by removing packs and methodically assessing all organs and vascular structures to find the source of bleeding, beginning with quadrant *least* likely to be source of haemorrhage.

- I would systematically assess the entire abdominal contents, paying particular attention to the liver, spleen, and small and large bowel in cases of blunt abdominal trauma.
- I would perform medial and lateral visceral rotation to access the major vessels and retroperitoneal structures, as indicated.
- In blunt abdominal trauma, the most common sites of injury would be solid organ injury (liver, spleen and kidneys). Initially, bleeding should be controlled by 'packing'.
- A patient who is unstable and bleeding from the spleen requires a splenectomy. Bleeding from the liver requires mobilisation of the liver and packing and return to theatre (once stabilised) for definitive management. Other hollow organ injuries would be closed but no anastomosis performed in acute setting.
- Definitive control of haemorrhage may require complete or partial (anatomical or extra-anatomical) removal of the 'offending' organ.
- 'Damage control' laparotomy to allow correction of the components of the lethal triad may be appropriate with return to theatre in 24 hours or sooner if necessary for definitive treatment.
- I would close the abdomen temporarily using an abdominal management system.

Post-operatively:

- transfer to ICU for monitoring
- the secondary survey is completed (if not already) or a tertiary survey performed to identify other missed injuries
- a definitive management plan should be formulated with ICU team
- DVT and stress ulcer prophylaxis.

Examiner question: what is meant by damage control laparotomy?

Candidate answer

- Damage control laparotomy is a well established method of managing a trauma patient with impending or established physiological derangement.
- It refers to early termination of surgical intervention before the development of irreversible physiological changes known as the lethal triad, namely: hypothermia, coagulopathy and metabolic acidosis.
- It refers to three phases of management: (i) volume resuscitation with rapid control of intra-abdominal bleeding and contamination followed by temporary closure of abdomen; (ii) establishment of normal physiology (in an ICU setting); and (iii) definitive operative management of intra-abdominal injuries.

Examiner question: how would you apply a supracoeliac clamp?

Candidate answer

- The goal of a supracoeliac clamp is to control major haemorrhage in an acute setting where the bleeding is arterial and originates below the thoracic aorta.
- The stomach is retracted caudally, the left lobe of the liver is retracted upwards and the lesser omentum (pars flaccida of gastrohepatic ligament) is opened to permit access to the lesser sac.

- The oesophagus is retracted to the left (the NGT can help in its identification) and the muscle fibres of the aortic hiatus of the diaphragm are separated digitally. An aortic clamp is then applied above the origin of the coeliac trunk.
- The clamp would then be removed as soon as definitive control is achieved.

4.4.13 Perforated peptic ulcer

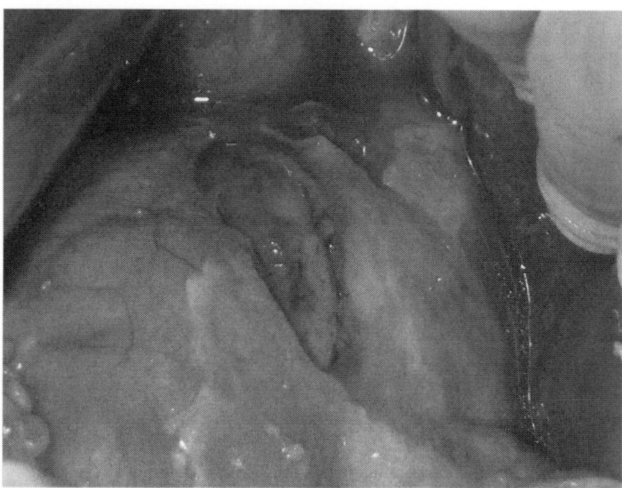

Figure 4.4.13
Perforated duodenal ulcer

Examiner question: you have diagnosed a patient in emergency with a perforated peptic ulcer. The patient has generalised peritonitis and you are taking the patient to theatre. The patient has been resuscitated and has received antibiotics. DVT prophylaxis is in place and the patient is under general anaesthetic, prepared and draped. Describe your operative management.

Candidate answer

The procedural steps involve:

1. entry/laparotomy
2. evaluate the size/extent/location of the ulcer
3. mobilisation and appropriate measures to deal with the ulcer (primary closure/omental patching/distal gastrectomy, as necessary)
4. generous peritoneal lavage and drainage
5. closure of abdomen.

- The patient should also have a nasogastric tube and I would make sure that suction and a self retaining retractor are available.
- I prefer to stand on the right-hand side of the patient with my assistant on the left.

- I would perform an upper midline incision and on entering the abdomen suction any free fluid and ligate the falciform ligament.
- I initially perform an exploratory laparotomy. I expect to find the perforated ulcer in the first part of the duodenum, the prepyloric region of the stomach or along the lesser curve of the stomach.

Examiner: there is a large perforated gastric ulcer just proximal to the pylorus.

Candidate response

- My concern regarding the presence of a gastric ulcer is the potential for malignancy (4% overall, 30% for ulcers greater than 3 cm).
- I complete my exploratory laparotomy inspecting the mesentery, peritoneum and liver for any evidence of metastatic disease.
- I then have to make a decision regarding management of the ulcer. The options to deal with the ulcer essentially include:
  - freshening the ulcer edges and primary closure
  - Graham Omental patch
  - distal gastrectomy.
- Because this is a large ulcer located close to the pylorus, it is not likely to be amenable to local excision and primary closure.
- I would take biopsies from the edge of the ulcer for histopathology.
- I would identify an appropriate piece of omentum and perform an omental patch. I may need to mobilise the right omentum from the transverse colon to achieve this.
- I would insert several interrupted 2-0 PDS sutures across the ulcer bed but leave them clipped. I position the omentum through the sutures and tie them gently over the omentum to secure the patch.

Examiner question: the sutures pull through the ulcer and patching the defect is impossible. How do you proceed?

Candidate answer

- I would perform a distal gastrectomy. The aim of my operation is to remove the antrum of the stomach and to perform an appropriate reconstruction.
- The landmark for my proximal resection is a line between the incisura of the lesser curve of the stomach and the terminal branches of the right gastroepiploic on the greater curve. The distal resection margin will be the pylorus/proximal D1. I need to take care not to injure the pancreas.
- I begin my dissection inferiorly, incising the gastrocolic omentum near the terminal branches of the right gastroepiploic to enter the lesser sac. First, I mobilise the greater curvature and ligating the branches of the right gastroepiploic until I reach the distal pylorus and the main trunk of the right gastroepiploic artery, which I ligate using 0 vicryl.
- My assistant now elevates the stomach carefully retracting it proximally while I divide any congenital adhesions between the stomach and pancreas.

- The lesser curvature is likewise mobilised to the incisura. I incise the lesser omentum near the incisura and dissect distally, ligating the descending branch of the left gastric artery and the right gastric artery. On reaching the pylorus my assistant elevates the distal stomach and I mobilise any final attachments between the pylorus/proximal D1 and the pancreas if it is safe to do so.
- Having confirmed the position of the NGT, I divide the stomach proximally (incisura to greater curve) with a linear cutting stapler. I underrun this staple line with 3-0 PDS for haemostasis.
- Next, I divide D1 just distal to the pylorus (linear cutting stapler). This allows removal of the specimen. I bury the staple line on the duodenal stump with 3-0 PDS if the duodenum isn't thickened/oedematous.
- At this point, I perform a thorough lavage of the abdomen.
- The next step is to perform a gastrojejunostomy reconstruction. I perform an inline reconstruction. If the jejunal mesentery is sufficiently long, I perform an antecolic gastrojejunostomy. I position stay sutures between the stomach (3 cm proximal to the staple line) and jejunum (afferent limb approx 20 cm long from DJ flexure — short but tension free) and the outer layer is performed by placing interrupted 3-0 PDS in a Lembert fashion. I then position sponges to prevent contamination before making a 5 cm gastrotomy and jejunotomy. The inner row of the anastomosis is performed using 3-0 PDS. This suture is continued anteriorly in a Connell fashion and the anastomosis completed anteriorly. I position the NGT in the jejunum just beyond the anastomosis.
- I perform a final lavage, position two 10 Fr drains (one adjacent to duodenal stump and second near the gastrojejunostomy) before closing the abdomen with 1 loop PDS and staples to skin.
- Post-operatively: HDU as indicated, especially if concern regarding sepsis. NBM 48 hours, NGT free drainage with 4-hourly aspirates, IV antibiotics, PPI bd, DVT prophylaxis. I would chase the histology and organise H. pylori eradication. I would perform a gastroscopy in 6 weeks to confirm no other disease.

Examiner question: what if the perforation was more distal involving the duodenum, the walls of which are thickened, distorted and friable by florid ulcer disease? How do you proceed?

Candidate answer

In such cases, it is difficult and hazardous to dissect out and close the duodenum. If the ulcer is in the second part of the duodenum, the ampullary region and structures will be endangered. I would consider three options.

1. Gently pinch off the duodenum at the distal ulcer edge, providing mobilisation of just enough cuff distally to close but leaving the ulcer crater undisturbed.
2. If the anterior duodenal wall is soft and pliable, the duodenum can be left attached to the ulcer posteriorly and the anterolateral duodenal wall mobilised (Kocher manoeuvre) so that it can be sewn down to the distal fibrotic edge of the ulcer crater (Nissen's manoeuvre). A second layer of Lembert sutures may

be inserted between the anterior wall of the duodenum and the proximal edge of the ulcer.

3. If neither can be accomplished, I would sew in a large tube (tube duodenostomy) that I would bring out to the anterior abdominal wall and leave for 10 days. I would then gradually withdraw it if the patient was well to create a controlled duodeno-cutaneous fistula which will heal spontaneously providing that there is no distal obstruction.

4.4.14 Intra-operative management of common bile duct stones

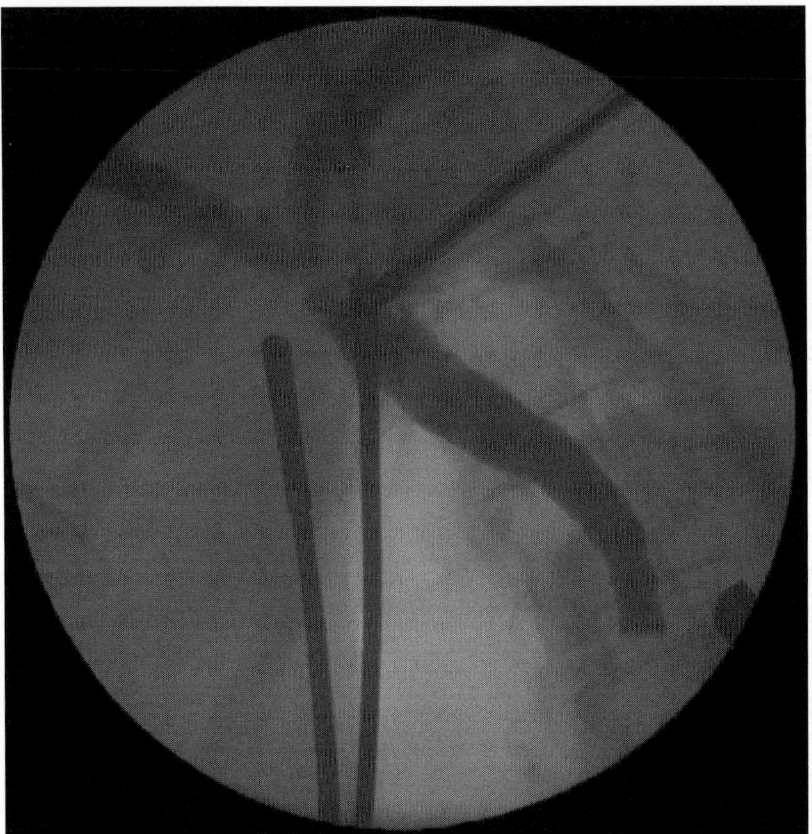

Figure 4.4.14
Cholangiogram with common bile duct stone

Examiner question: this 53-year-old man has had a Roux-en-Y gastric bypass as a treatment for morbid obesity some years ago. He presented with acute cholecystitis and underwent an urgent laparoscopic cholecystectomy. How would you proceed after finding this cholangiogram?

- Answering questions on bile duct stones is difficult because there are so many options, not all of which you have seen or done yourself. Often a number of different approaches are reasonable.
- There are certain factors/issues that will determine the safest and most appropriate course in individual cases and you should mention them to demonstrate awareness of the issues. These include:
  - general condition of the patient
  - anatomy of the biliary tree — the size of the cystic duct and common bile ducts (especially relative to size of stones) and whether contrast flows freely into duodenum
  - number/size/location of stones — especially if in the hepatic ducts.
- Generally, the following options should be considered and a decision regarding their appropriateness be made in individual cases:
  - additional clip or endoloop on the cystic duct, insertion of a large adjacent drain and subsequent ERCP
  - antegrade transcystic stenting
  - transcystic exploration using a basket
  - bile duct exploration — will usually require conversion to an open procedure, although can be laparoscopic in very expert (probably not your!) hands.
- Before launching into a description of a procedure or declaring that you always do ERCP, consider the information that you have in the scenario. The line of questioning is almost always heading to an open choledochotomy!

Candidate answer

- The bile duct has to be cleared during this procedure as endoscopic access is not likely to be possible after gastric bypass.
- The bile duct is dilated at about 10 mm.
- There appears to be a single large stone and there is no contrast flowing into the duodenum.
- I would attempt laparoscopic transcystic exploration first using a basket. If this is unsuccessful, choledochotomy would be feasible given the duct size. I would convert to an open procedure via a right subcostal incision to perform this and I would insert a T-tube afterwards.

Examiner question: okay. How would you perform your laparoscopic trans-cystic exploration?

Candidate answer

- I remove the cholangiogram catheter from the cystic duct. The x-ray and laparoscopic monitors should be positioned so they can be seen simultaneously and neither obscured by the C-arm.
- I squeeze the cystic duct from medial to lateral with Marylands forceps to clear stones or debris from the cystic duct.

- I dissect carefully down to the junction of the cystic duct and CBD.
- I use the Nathanson basket. I assemble the basket, its catheter and injection port and insert it down the Riddoch-Olsen clamp. I generally use the right mid-clavicular line port as this offers the best angle for entering the common bile duct.
- I withdraw the hard tip of the basket about 3 cm into the catheter. This protects the bile duct from the hard basket and allows the catheter (which has a softer tip) to thread past the spiral valves.
- I thread the catheter gently into the common bile duct.
- I advance the tip of the catheter (whilst screening) past the most distal stone.
- Under screening control, I then simultaneously withdraw the catheter and slowly advance the wire of the basket, aiming to place the stiff distal tip of the basket (the olive) just beyond the most distal stone.
- The basket is rigid and, when not constrained by the catheter, will expand into the duct.
- When the basket is fully opened, the whole device (basket and catheter) is withdrawn under laparoscopic vision.
- I don't attempt to close the basket around the stone as this usually breaks up the stone and makes more debris. This is repeated until the duct is clear on the cholangiogram.
- I clip the cystic duct long and then divide and secure below the clip with an 0 PDS endoloop.
- I complete the cholecystectomy.
- I place a subhepatic drain.

Examiner question: what if this fails to clear the stones?

Note: the examiner is only looking for the safety of your approach. There are no extra points for laparoscopic surgery, so perform an open procedure!

Candidate answer

I would complete the operation using an open choledochotomy.

- I use a supra-duodenal exploration.
- A right subcostal incision is made.
- I place fixed costal retractors to get good visualisation (e.g. omni-tract or Goligher frame, Doyen's blades and chains). My assistant stands on the left holding the duodenum down. A second assistant or fixed device allows anterior liver retraction at the base of Segment 4B to spread the hilum.
- Kocherization of the duodenum may help.
- I fenestrate the peritoneum of the hepatoduodenal ligament in the region of the junction of the cystic duct and CBD.
- When I have identified the CBD and the hepatic artery, I confirm the anatomy by aspiration of bile from the CBD using a 21 g needle and 5 ml syringe.
- I insert stay sutures in the supraduodenal CBD either side of the proposed choledochotomy.
- I open the duct longitudinally with a scalpel and extend the incision with Pott's scissors.
- First, I insert the Desjardin's forceps into the duct distally and remove whatever stones I can grab.

- Then I use a 3–4F Fogarty balloon catheter to trawl the duct.
- Finally, I then use a flexible choledochoscope with saline irrigation (usually an 8.5F flexible ureteroscope — such as the Olympus® URV-F which has a 3.6F working channel).
- Once the scope passes into the duodenum without seeing stones, I examine the upper system to the level of the second order ducts. Additional, smaller stones can be removed using a basket passed down the working channel of the choledochoscope.
- Once the duct is clear, I close the duct over a T-tube (10–16F depending on duct size) with fine interrupted absorbable sutures of 4-0 PDS.
- I score the tube with a scalpel to remove the silicon coating of the latex. I cut the back of the tube to ensure easy removal.
- I place all the sutures untied and then insert the tube to avoid suturing it in. I then tie all the sutures.
- The T-tube is brought out laterally. A 19F subhepatic Blake drain is inserted.
- A T-tube cholangiogram is performed.
- Post-operatively, I leave the T-tube on free drainage until a T-tube cholangiogram is arranged on days 3–5. If this confirms no obstruction or leak, I clamp the T-tube and remove the drain, if no bile leaks after 24 hours. I send the patient home with the tube (clamped) and remove it in 4 weeks.

4.4.15 Trauma splenectomy

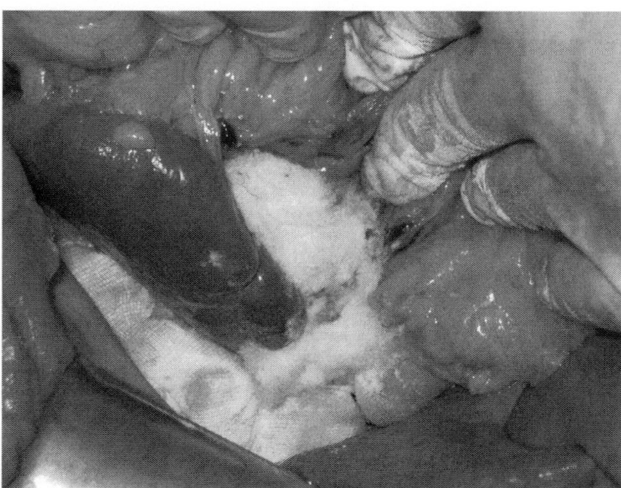

Figure 4.4.15
Traumatic splenic injury treated conservatively

Examiner question: what do you see here?

Candidate answer

This is an intra-operative image of a spleen which appears to be taken from the left at laparotomy. There are sponges under the spleen.

Examiner question: in this case the patient had a traumatic injury to the spleen and the conservation was attempted. If this is unsuccessful, can you describe how you would perform a splenectomy for trauma?

Candidate answer

Preparation:

- GA
- prophylactic antibiotics
- thromboprophylaxis
- IDC/NGT if not already inserted
- supine position with reverse Trendelenburg and left-side up tilt after entry
- prep and drape
- ensure that there are 20 large packs and two large suckers are available
- have a vascular tray with vascular clamps available
- also, if the patient is haemodynamically unstable, I will ensure that there are packed red blood cells available in the theatre or a multiple transfusion protocol has been activated if indicated
- have a good assistant.

The procedural steps involve:

1. entry/laparotomy
2. quadrant packing of the abdomen as necessary
3. mobilise the spleen by dividing the splenorenal, splenophrenic and splenocolic ligaments
4. ligation of splenic vessels
5. check for inadvertent injury/haemostasis
6. closure.

- I stand on the patient's right and make a midline incision from xiphisternum to past the umbilicus down to the linea alba with entry into the peritoneal cavity at the cicatrix by dividing the peritoneum between two artery clips.
- If there is a large amount blood in the abdomen, I will eviscerate the small bowel, evacuate as much blood and clots as possible and pack all four quadrants of the abdomen commencing in the left upper quadrant (LUQ) (see Chapter 4.4.12).
- I use a Gray's fixed abdominal wall retractor. I ask the anaesthetist to provide Trendelenburg and left-side up and I begin removing all abdominal packs, leaving the LUQ packs until last.
- Often, in the setting of significant splenic injury, haematoma around the spleen partially mobilises the spleen.
- My first step is to mobilise the spleen medially and caudally using my left hand and the lateral, posterior and superior retroperitoneal attachments are rapidly divided, whilst taking care not to injure adjacent structures (the tail of the pancreas and splenic flexure of the colon).
- I sharply divide the splenorenal, splenophrenic and splenocolic ligaments using Mayo scissors, bringing the spleen to the midline. Often the tail of the pancreas at the splenic hilum will come up at this stage. Haemorrhage control can be gained by compressing the splenic vessels manually (or with a straight soft bowel clamp) across the hilum of the spleen, taking care not to clamp the tail of the pancreas, to control bleeding.

- I place a large pack in the LUQ (behind the spleen), whilst I tend to the splenic vessels.
- I then identify and clamp the vessels at the hilum of the spleen with Roberts clamps and divide between the clamps, taking care to avoid injury to the tail of the pancreas. I ligate all vessels that are clipped using 0 vicryl ties.
- The short gastric vessels will probably need deliberate and formal division between clips or using an automated clip applicator, whilst protecting the greater curvature of the stomach from injury.
- I check the splenic bed for haemostasis and ensure that there has been no injury to the tail of the pancreas or greater curve of the stomach.
- I lavage the LUQ and abdomen and place a JP drain at the splenic bed.
- Mass closure of the laparotomy with 1 loop PDS and clips to close skin.

Post-operatively:
- ICU for monitoring
- NG decompression of the stomach to manage post-operative gastroparesis
- intravenous antibiotics
- check drain amylase prior to removal to exclude an unrecognised pancreatic tail injury
- the patient will need to be vaccinated against encapsulated organisms (pneumococcus, meningococcus and H. influenzae) 2 weeks post-operative and consideration for prophylactic amoxicillin in liaison with haematology/ microbiology
- the patient will need to be educated about lifetime risk of OPSI prior to discharge.

4.4.16 High ligation of the long saphenous vein

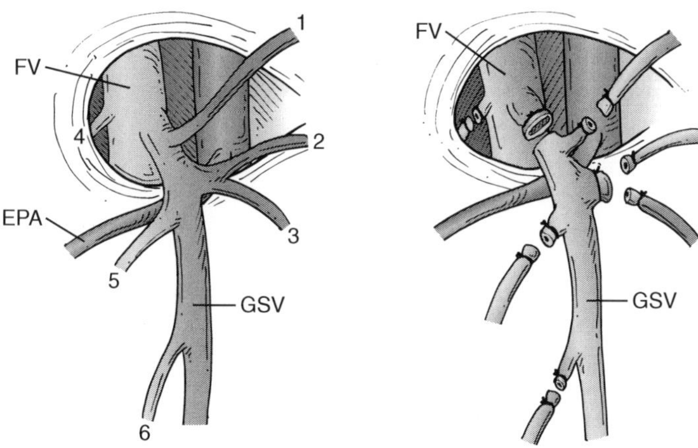

Figure 4.4.16
The most common arrangement of tributary veins at the left saphenofemoral junction. The external pudendal artery (EPA) usually runs between the great saphenous vein (GSV) and the femoral vein (FV), but it may pass above the GSV and is then more susceptible to injury during dissection. 1, inferior epigastric vein; 2, superficial circumflex iliac vein; 3, lateral accessory saphenous vein; 4, deep external pudendal vein; 5, superficial external pudendal vein; 6, medial accessory saphenous vein (Source: *Rutherford's Vascular Surgery*, 7th edn. Cronenwett J L, Johnston K W. 2010, Saunders: an imprint of Elsevier, Fig 55-5A, p 862.)

Examiner question: please discuss the anatomy relevant to high ligation of the long saphenous vein (LSV) and how you can try to prevent recurrence.

Candidate answer

- High ligation of the LSV refers to ligation and division of the LSV at the saphenofemoral junction (SFJ).
- The LSV provides superficial venous drainage of the lower limb, commences anterior to the medial malleolus, as a continuation of medial marginal vein of foot, passes up to medial aspect of the lower leg behind the tibia to the knee, passing a hands breath behind the medial border of patella, then passes the medial border of the thigh, through the cribriform fascia into the common femoral vein (CFV).
- The LSV receives a variable number of tributaries:
  - superficial and deep external pudendal
  - superficial circumflex iliac
  - superficial inferior epigastric
  - posteromedial and anterolateral 'accessory' branches
  - some tributaries drain directly into SFJ and CFV
  - can be duplicated (up to 30%).
- The external pudendal artery (EPA) usually runs between the LSV and CFV, but it may pass above the LSV and is then more susceptible to injury during dissection.
- Factors aiding identification of the LSV and SFJ:
  - placement of incision — groin crease medial to femoral artery pulse
  - the LSV enters the CFV on its anteromedial border at an acute angle
  - the LSV typically receives multiple tributaries
  - the LSV typically looks thin walled compared to the CFV
  - pre-operative marking with Duplex US can aid localisation of SFJ and significant tributaries
  - dissection of the CFV 2 cm proximal and distal to the SFJ ensures that the CFV continues down into the thigh.

Examiner question: how do you perform high ligation of the long saphenous vein?

Candidate answer

Preparation:

- GA
- prophylactic antibiotics
- thromboprophylaxis
- supine position with Trendelenburg tilt
- legs abducted (on leg board)
- prep and drape.

The procedural steps involve:

1. skin incision/initial dissection
2. dissection to identify all tributaries and SFJ

3. ligation and division of all tributaries and the SFJ
4. haemostasis
5. closure.

- I palpate the femoral pulse and imagine the femoral vein medial to it. I then make a 4 cm transverse incision in a skin crease centred over the femoral vein.
- I deepen the incision through the subcutaneous tissues and the superficial fascia of the thigh.
- I then continue the rest of the dissection very carefully as the tributaries will be encountered in this layer.
- Using a combination of blunt and sharp dissection, I sweep the fat away from the tributaries draining into the LSV so that they are easily identifiable.
- I then insert a self-retaining retractor and turn my attention to the LSV. I gently elevate it with atraumatic forceps and dissect it towards the SFJ, clearing it and its tributaries of fat. I do not cut any veins until I am satisfied that I have identified the CFV, the LSV and the SFJ (see above).
- Once I am happy, I apply small arterial clips to all the tributaries of the LSV as far away from their confluence as possible. I then place another arterial clip downstream on the LSV distal to where the tributaries enter it.
- I then apply a further clip approximately 0.5 cm away from the SFJ, cephaloid to where the tributaries join the LSV. I cut the tributaries to the LSV proximal to the clips (i.e. within the 'ring of clips') and individually ligate them with 2/0 vicryl.
- I then divide the distal end of the LSV cephaloid to the clip and tie or insert a stripper as appropriate.
- This gives me the opportunity to elevate the LSV stump as it heads towards the CFV to ensure that I have identified and ligate *all* tributaries. I then suture ligate the SFJ without narrowing the CFV using 0 vicryl, excising the segment of LSV in so doing.
- I check for haemostasis and close the wound in layers.

Chapter 4.5

Pathophysiology and critical care/clinical reasoning

What the mind can conceive and believe, the mind can achieve. (Napoleon Hill, 1883–1970)

The examination format

The pathophysiology and critical care and clinical reasoning viva consists of:

- two 10-minute scenarios with discussion
- five computer images of pathology specimens discussed during a 20-minute period.

After the bell rings, you walk in, sit down with the examiners and look at the computer screen. The scenario is summarised with supporting images and then you are asked a series of specific, structured questions. It is common for the examiners to interrupt the flow of your answer to stop you from talking and to move you on to the next topic.

If the examiners present you with an image(s) and remain silent and you know what it shows, you should state what is going on. Often, they will ask you something like '*what do you see here?*', '*what does this image show?*'. If you know the answer, you should state it, but if you don't know then you should be honest so that the examiners can help you out and progress with the viva. Remember, the image is only really serving as a basis for the subsequent discussion, which is where the real examination will take place. You may be asked about the pathogenesis or management of the condition; for example, '*what would you do?*', '*how do you stage this tumour?*'.

EXAMPLES

Acute pancreatitis

Candidate: 'this is an intraoperative image of pancreatic necrosis into the lesser sac'.
Examiner: 'what is the pathophysiology of acute pancreatitis?'

Melanoma

Candidate: 'this is an image of a nodular melanoma'.
Examiner: 'what types of melanoma are there and how is it staged?'

Perimenopausal single duct discharge

Questions may include: 'what would you ask in the history?', 'what would you examine?', 'what are your differential diagnoses?'

Exam technique

Remember: 'Listen, think, pause, speak'.

Start talking as soon as you are able to without interrupting the examiners, but make sure that you answer the question that has been asked. It sounds incredibly obvious but a common mistake made by candidates (much to the annoyance of the examiners) is failure to listen to the question or to answer the question that they *wished* they'd been asked rather than the actual question that they *have* been asked! The examiners are looking for specific answers — this is how points will be awarded. Do not waffle or ramble. Present clear, concise, considered responses.

Remember this is pathophysiology and critical care, but this does not mean that you don't include your clinical assessment and objectives. Let the examiners direct the depth of pathophysiology discussed. Your aim is to demonstrate that you are a safe and competent clinician with a robust but relevant pathophysiological knowledge.

If you have the opportunity to speak uninterrupted, we recommend the following schema:

1. recognise the organ/tissue/image being shown
2. describe your findings
3. offer a probable diagnosis if possible
4. describe the pathogenesis and potential complications of the underlying pathological process, irrespective of whether present in the image.

The picture is merely a primer. You are not being asked to make a histological diagnosis of the tumour from a single (and sometimes difficult to interpret) picture. Even if you guess correctly, a systematic approach to, for example, small bowel tumours is what is being sought by the examiners.

Do not panic if the diagnosis does not come to you straight away. You can simply describe what you see and begin listing differential diagnoses. The examiner will then probably lead you to the right diagnosis. It is crucial to listen to the scenario — there are always clues.

For all cancers encountered commonly in general surgical practice (e.g. melanoma, colorectal, breast, thyroid, stomach, head and neck), you must know:

- an appropriate staging system (e.g. TNM)
- data on 5-year (overall and stage specific) survival and recurrence
- the aetiology, spread and management.

Preparation and practising

As previously stated, frequent practise is imperative. Look at the list of common viva topics in Chapter 1.3, and add to it with reports from previous exam candidates of what they were examined on. Most of the questions that you will encounter within this section of the examination are predictable. Accordingly, there can be no excuse for not having thought about your answers ahead of the viva. We encourage you to think about, plan and prepare 'scripted' answers for common scenarios before the exam.

Try to talk to pathologists and anaesthetists about disease processes and their physiological consequences at every opportunity. As with each of the other *viva voce* examinations, how you present yourself in front of the examiners and how you structure your answers is critical in determining your performance within the exam. Only with regular practise will you be able to limit your responses to avoid verbose, irrelevant answers. Practise constructing *precise and concise* responses. Assembling material and drafting answers and plans really helps to this end. Importantly, get used to saying them out loud. Responses can very often sound different when said out loud, compared to how they look on the page.

Chapter 4.6

Pathophysiology and critical care/clinical reasoning viva topics: model answers

In this chapter, we have again provided 'model answers' to the commonest topics that are examined in the pathophysiology and critical care viva to help guide your revision. Capturing the realism of this viva is more challenging than with the anatomy and operative vivas, as the format often favours a series of short questions that require direct answers. Wherever possible, we have tried to capture this style within individual worked answers but again we are guilty of providing more complex answers than you would often be expected to provide within the time limits of the examination.

4.6.1 Synoptic breast pathology reporting

BREAST SYNOPTIC REPORT
Specimen: Wide local excision & sentinel lymph nodes
Site: right breast

Invasive carcinoma
- Size 12 mm
- Type: invasive ductal carcinoma
- Grade: II
- Tubules: 3/3
- Nuclei: 3/3
- Mitoses: 1/3

Peritumoural lymphovascular invasion: present (focal)
Margins:
- Superior: 1 mm
- Anterior: 2 mm
- Posterior: 4 mm
- Inferior: 5 mm
- Medial and lateral: 10 mm

Multifocal: No
Multicentric: No

***In-situ* carcinoma**
DCIS
- Size: 10 mm
- Site: Within IC
- Grade: low/intermediate
- Comedo Necrosis: Absent
- Architectural type: Clining, cribriform
- Margins: see invasive carcinoma

LCIS
- None

Lymph nodes
- Site: sentinel lymph node
- Total nodes: 1
- Involved nodes: 1
- Size of largest deposit: 4 mm
- Extracapsular invasion: none

Hormone status
- ER: positive – 3+ and 100% cells+
- PgR: positive – 2+ and 50% cells+

SUMMARY
1. Right breast wide local excision: invasive ductal carcinoma, 12 mm, Grade II, completely excised with close margins (please read above), focal lymphovascular invasion, ER+ and PR+, associated focal DCIS.
2. Right sentinel node: hot and blue and Lymph node status: 1N+/1 (SLN, 4 mm deposit).

Supplementary report
Immunhistochemistry for HER2
RESULT: negative (1+)
HER-2 immunohistochemistry has been performed using the Ventana PATHWAY Her-2/neu (4B5). Rabbit Monoclonal Primary Antibody.

SISH for HER2
RESULT: SISH negative
TUMOUR STATUS:
Mean copy no per cell: 2.75
Pattern: dots
Non-amplified: polysomy 2.4-4 copies
(Signal detection has been performed for the HER2 gene that maps to chromosome 17q21 using the Ventana INFORM Her2 Probe and Ventana UltraView SISH detection kit.)

Figure 4.6.1
Synoptic breast pathology

Examiner question: have a look at this pathology report. What is the important information in this report?

Candidate answer

- This is a synoptic report. The critical elements which determine prognosis and further treatment are summarised here. These are:
  - diagnosis of carcinoma of breast
  - type: invasive ductal carcinoma
  - size of primary
  - grade: this is reported using the Scarff-Bloom-Richardson grading system. This independently assesses tubule formation, nuclear pleomorphism, mitotic count (per 10 HPF). Grade is independently related to survival
  - presence of lymphovascular invasion
  - margin status and distance from margin to closest invasive or in situ cancer
  - presence of in situ disease
  - the estrogen and progesterone status of the cancer
  - assessment of HER2 status by immunohistochemistry and silver in situ hybridization (SISH)
  - lymph node assessment: details of harvest source are provided, i.e. axillary dissection or sentinel biopsy. The number of nodes examined and the number positive. The size of tumour deposits, the presence of extra-capsular extension of the metastasis.

Examiner question: what is HER2?

Candidate answer

- HER2 is Human Epidermal Growth Factor Receptor 2 and is also known as Neu, ErbB-2, CD340 or p185. It is a member of the epidermal growth factor receptor (EGFR/ErbB) family.
- HER2 is encoded by ERBB2, a known proto-oncogene located at the long arm of human chromosome 17 (17q12).
- The ErbB family is composed of four plasma membrane-bound receptor tyrosine kinases. All four contain an extracellular ligand binding domain, a transmembrane domain, and an intracellular domain that can interact with a multitude of signaling molecules and exhibit both ligand-dependent and ligand-independent activity.
- HER2 can heterodimerise with any of the other three receptors and is considered to be the preferred dimerisation partner of the other ErbB receptors. Dimerisation results in the autophosphorylation of tyrosine residues within the cytoplasmic domain of the receptors and initiates a variety of signaling pathways, which promotes cell proliferation and opposes apoptosis.

Examiner question: what its relevance to breast cancer?

Candidate answer

- The ERBB2 (c erbB2) gene is rarely, if ever, mutated. However, the HER-2 protein is over-expressed in 25–30% of breast cancers through gene amplification and transcriptional up-regulation.

- Over-expression results in a ligand-independent activation of the kinase and uncontrolled proliferative and anti-apoptotic signals. This is diagnosed by:
  - immunohistochemistry (qualitative measure of receptors)
  - Silver in situ hybridization (SISH)
  - FISH (fluorescence in-situ hybridisation) — measures the number of copies of the HER2 gene on Ch17. More than two copies per chromosome is counted as positive
  - HER2 over-expression is a marker of poorer prognosis and associated a with poor endocrine response
  - it is a predictive marker of good response to anthracycline chemotherapy.

Examiner question: how is HER2 targeted?

Candidate answer

- Via Trastuzumab (Herceptin).
- This is a humanised monoclonal antibody to the extracellular domain of the HER2 protein. The antibody reduces phosphorylation, Akt activity and angiogenesis factor levels.

Examiner question: what is the significance of estrogen receptor status?

Candidate answer

- If 10% or more of the tumour cells within the invasive component stain positive for ER, the cancer is ER+.
- PR expression requires the presence of intact ER machinery. Positive staining for PR serves as evidence of functional ER, and tumours which are ER– but PR+, display intermediate hormone responsiveness.
- Objective response rate to endocrine therapy in ER+/PR+ cancers is 80%. By contrast it is only 10% in ER–/PR– cases.

Examiner question: this cancer is positive for ER, PR and HER2. What is the prognostic implication?

Candidate answer

- Being ER+/PR+ predicts a better prognosis and responsiveness to endocrine therapy.
- Being HER2 *per se* is a poor prognostic maker. However, when Trastuzumab is used this effect is reversed.
- It is important to note that cancers which are ER/PR/HER2 negative are high grade, express molecular markers for basal or myoepithelial cells (called basal-like cancers) and carry a poor prognosis.

4.6.2 Colonic polyps

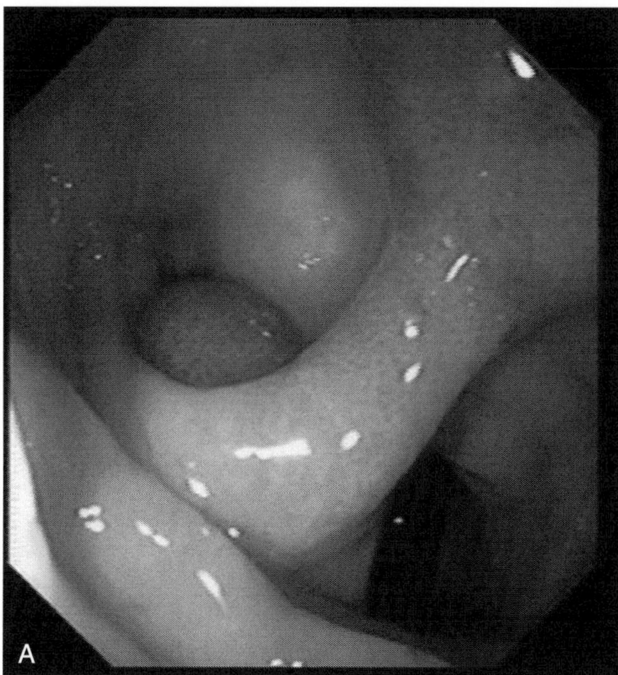

Figure 4.6.2A
Pedunculated colonic polyps.

Examiner question: what can you see here?

Candidate answer

It appears to be a pedunculated colonic polyp with another polyp behind it.

Examiner question: what is a polyp?

Candidate answer

- A polyp is an abnormal macroscopic projection of a soft tissue mass from the surface of an organ or tissue.
- In the context of the large bowel, a polyp is an abnormal macroscopic protrusion of colonic mucosa. This may result from either a mucosal or submucosal process.

Examiner question: how would you classify polyps?

Candidate answer

- There are numerous types of polyps which can be classified in a number of ways. One system is to classify polyps as mucosal or submucosal and neoplastic or non-neoplastic.

- Neoplastic mucosal polyps:
  - benign adenomatous (tubular, villous, tubulovillous)
  - serrated polyps
  - adenoma with intra-mucosal (in situ) carcinoma
  - adenomatous polyp containing invasive carcinoma.
- Non-neoplastic mucosal polyps include:
  - metaplastic/hyperplastic polyps
  - hamartomatous
  - inflammatory
  - Peutz-Jegher's polyps.
- Neoplastic submucosal polyps include:
  - lipomatous
  - leiomyomatous
  - lymphomatous
  - carcinoid
  - GIST polyps.
- Non-neoplastic submucosal polyps are most commonly caused by lymphoid aggregates.
- Neoplastic polyps account for about 70% of colonic polyps, most of which are adenomatous.

Examiner question: the polyp in the image proves to be an adenomatous polyp on histopathological analysis. How would you further classify such polyps?

Candidate answer

- They can be classified according to gross morphology into pedunculated and sessile polyps.
  - Pedunculated polyps are attached to the bowel wall by a stalk of submucosa lined by normal mucosa.
  - Sessile polyps have a broad base.
- Adenomatous polyps may also be classified histologically into tubular, villous and tubulovillous.
  - Tubular adenomas exhibit dysplastic tubules in ≥ 80% of the lesion.
  - Villous adenomas have dysplastic villous fronds in ≥ 80% of the lesion. The finger-like villi are actually elongated crypts.
  - Tubulovillous adenomas have >20% tubular and <80% villous formation.

Examiner question: what is the significance of this classification?

Candidate answer

- The risk of cancer is greater in villous adenomas compared with tubular.
- The differential risk between villous and tubular adenomas is greatest for smaller polyps. For polyps <10 mm, the risk of malignancy with tubular adenomas is 1%, but about 10% for polyps of villous morphology (i.e. 10x).
- When polyps are larger than 20 mm the risk of malignancy is high, irrespective of histological type. Accordingly, the differential risk between

villous and tubular adenomas is less with the risk of malignancy being 35% for tubular adenoma but 55% for villous lesions (i.e. 1.5x).

Examiner question: what is the cause of adenomatous colonic polyps?

Candidate answer

- Adenomatous polyps are multi-factorial in aetiology, including genetic predisposition (such as germ-line APC mutation, mismatch repair gene mutations) and environmental factors (principally dietary elements which for the most part are only associative rather than causative; e.g. increased saturated fat intake and reduced fibre intake).
- The occurrence of polyps increases with age.

Examiner question: what is the relationship of adenomatous polyps and colorectal cancer?

Candidate answer

- There is a step-wise change from normal colonic epithelium to adenomatous polyps with progressive proliferation and dysplasia and finally adenocarcinoma.
- These morphological changes are associated with progressive genetic change (2 hit hypothesis). APC (tumour suppressor gene) mutation is an early event, followed by k-ras (oncogene) mutation, then *DCC* (tumour suppressor gene) mutation, and finally p53 (another tumour suppressor gene) loss.

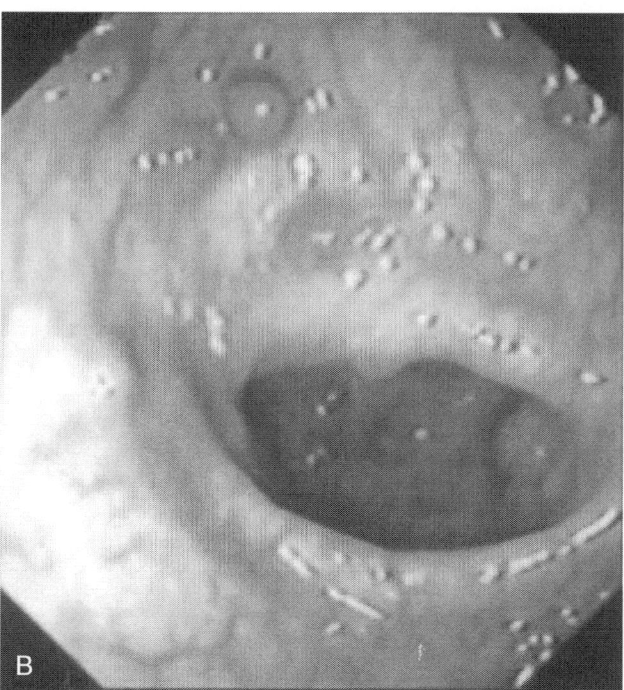

Figure 4.6.2B
Familial adenomatous polyposis

Examiner question: what can you see here?

Candidate answer

There are multiple colonic polyps evident.

Examiner question: if I told you that this patient has familial adenomatous polyposis (FAP), what would the genetic basis be and how is this gene relevant in colorectal cancer?

Candidate answer

- FAP is associated with germ-line mutations in the *adenomatous polyposis coli* (APC) gene.
- The clinical diagnosis requires >100 adenomatous polyps and carries a 100% life-time risk of developing colorectal cancer.
- Although autosomal dominant, about 30% of cases are new mutations.
- APC is a tumour suppressor gene located on chromosome 5. It is a normal cytoplasmic protein which appears to regulate the intracellular concentration of β-catenins. When APC is mutated, β-catenin levels rise leading to cell-cycle dysregulation and unchecked proliferation.
- As well as being germ-line (as in FAP), APC mutations can also occur sporadically. Most mutations create a premature stop codon in the gene leading to a truncated APC protein. Although only about 1% of colonic and rectal cancers are associated with germ-line APC mutations, 80% of sporadic colorectal cancer specimens harbour APC truncation mutations. Only 6% with UC-associated dysplasia and cancer have mutations in APC.

Examiner question: a healthy 70-year-old man has an 11 mm pedunculated polyp removed from his descending colon. Five days later the pathologist calls you to say that there is cancer in the polyp. What are the important determinants of how you would manage him?

Candidate answer

- The critical factors are:
  - completeness of excision (margins)
  - the risk of lymphatic metastasis. It is difficult to determine lymph node status clinically or radiographically, although risk can be estimated using histological features of the polyp, including:
    - differentiation (poorly differentiated increases the risk of LN metastases)
    - lymphovascular invasion
    - Haggitt's levels.

Candidate: let me draw you a polyp to explain Haggitt's levels

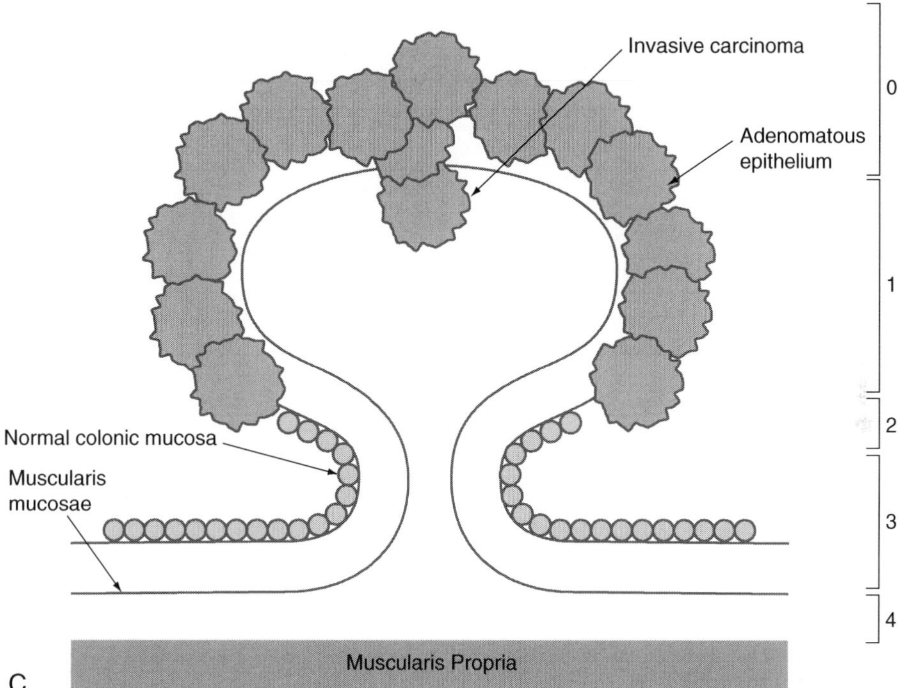

Figure 4.6.2C
Haggitt's levels

- In a pedunculated polyp, the muscularis mucosae is drawn up into the stalk, so that the submucosa is within the polyp.
- In adenomatous polyps of the colon, invasive carcinoma is defined as invasion through the muscularis mucosae into the submucosa. Before such invasion, it is known as carcinoma in situ.
- As the carcinoma penetrates the submucosa lower down the stalk, the risk of lymphatic metastasis increases. Levels were described by Haggitt.

Level 0: carcinoma in situ.
Level 1: head of pedunculated polyp.
Level 2: neck of pedunculated polyp.
Level 3: stalk of pedunculated polyp.
Level 4: base of pedunculated polyp.
For Haggitt, with levels 1–3 the risk of lymph node metastasis is less than 1%.
For Haggitt, with level 4 the risk of lymph node metastasis is 12–25%.

4.6.3 Crohn's disease

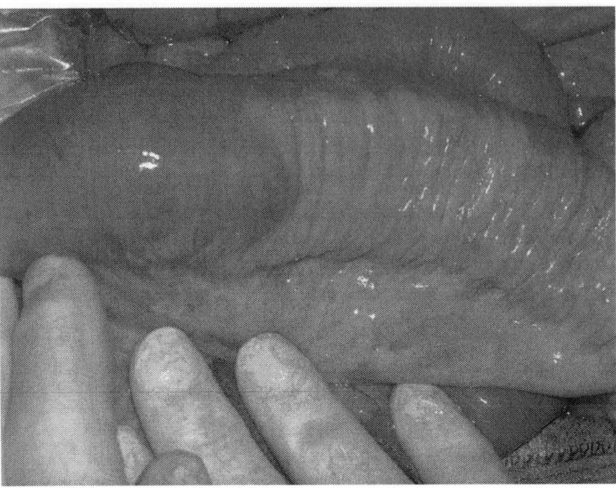

Figure 4.6.3
Small bowel Crohn's disease

Examiner question: please describe what you see in this image?

Candidate answer

- This is an intra-operative photo demonstrating a segment of small bowel.
- The bowel towards the right of the image displays fat wrapping and to the left the bowel appears mildly distended, suggesting obstruction possibly from a stricture. The finding of fat wrapping and stricture in the small bowel is suggestive of Crohn's disease (CD).
- The presence of a stricture may be due to previous ischaemia, malignancy (primary or metastatic) or radiation enteritis. Additional gross features that would further suggest CD include the presence of skip lesions. Changes occurring at the terminal ileum would also be consistent with CD as this is the most common site to be affected, although the whole GI tract may be involved.

Examiner question: describe the pathology of Crohn's disease.

Candidate answer

- Definition: Crohn's disease is a chronic transmural inflammatory disorder that can affect any site in the gastrointestinal tract and that is associated with extra intestinal manifestations.
- Demographics: the prevalence is approx 0.1%. The peak age of onset is 20–40 years and there is a second peak in the 60–70 age group. It occurs slightly more commonly in women.
- Aetiology: the cause of CD is not known but almost certainly involves an interaction between genetic and environmental factors. Genetic factors are implied by the fact ~15% of patients have a first-degree relative with CD. A potential role of an infective aetiology has been proposed

(e.g. paratuberculosis) but not substantiated. It is likely that the inappropriate immune response to the microbial flora of the gut has a role in CD and inflammatory bowel disease but this has not been proven.

- Smoking increases the relative risk of CD by 2–2.5x.
- Macroscopically: it most commonly affects the terminal ileum (~50%), colon (30%) and ileocolic region (20%). It is characterised by a full thickness inflammation of the bowel wall. Areas of inflammation are separated by normal bowel, which are known as a 'skip lesions'.
- Microscopically: it may be difficult to distinguish CD from ulcerative colitis (UC) leading to the diagnosis of indeterminate colitis. However, the typical microscopic features of CD are full thickness granulomatous inflammation with fissures. By contrast, UC is characterised by crypt abscesses, distorted crypt architecture and goblet cell depletion. Importantly, UC affects the colon and rectum in a continuous fashion and the small bowel is not affected unless 'backwash' ileitis is present.
- Clinically: CD most commonly presents with diarrhoea. Other symptoms include abdominal pain due to full thickness bowel wall inflammation and passage of blood or mucus PR. The bowel wall inflammation may result in stricturing, abscesses or fistulae. Less commonly, patients may present with complex fistulae-in-ano.

4.6.4 Carcinoid of the appendix

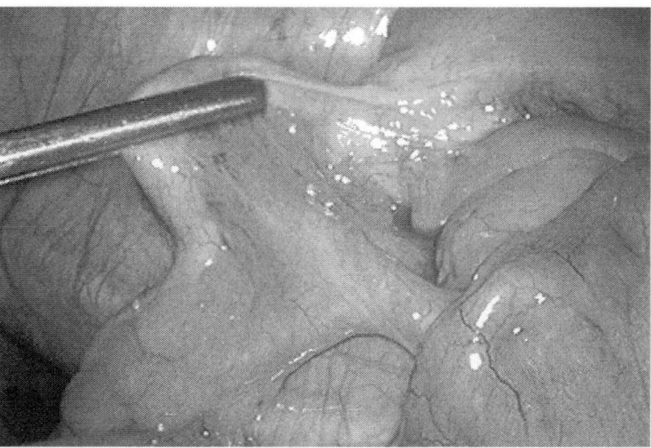

Figure 4.6.4
Laparoscopic view of a normal appendix (to discuss coincidental pathological finding of carcinoid)

Examiner question: you are going through the pathology results from the last week and find a report of an appendicectomy performed on a 23-year-old woman. The report indicates the presence of a carcinoid tumour. What would you need to know about the pathology to plan further treatment?

Candidate answer

- The features of the report which are critical are:
  - size of primary tumour
  - margin status either within the appendix wall (if at the base) or due to invasion of the mesoappendix
  - if the mesoappendix was excised, whether there were any lymphatic metastasis
  - lymphovascular invasion.

Examiner question: when would further treatment be required and why?

Candidate answer

- About 1:200 appendectomy specimens contain a carcinoid, usually as an incidental finding.
- The majority are located at the tip of appendix. About 10% are located at the base of the appendix where they may have caused the appendicitis.
- Tumour size is the most important predictor of metastasis. For lesions <1 cm, the risks of metastasis and recurrence are negligible.
- The indications for right hemicolectomy in an appendix carcinoid are:
  - lesion >2 cm (where the incidence of metastasis is 30–60%)
  - LN metastasis to mesoappendix
  - invasion of the base of the appendix with a positive margin
  - invasion of mesoappendix with positive margin (where appendix was skeletonised from mesoappendix).
- For tumours in the range 1–1.9 cm (where risk of lymph node metastasis is 11%), other factors should be taken into account, including:
  - patient wishes
  - fitness for surgery
  - pathological features particularly lymphovacular invasion.

Examiner question: what are the gross features of carcinoid tumours?

Candidate answer

- They represent a nodular growth in the mucosa or submucosa.
- They exhibit a bright yellow colour following fixation in formalin.
- There is often a mesenteric desmoplastic reaction.

Examiner question: what about the microscopic features?

Candidate answer

- The tumour consists of solid masses of monotonous-appearing cells with small round nuclei.
- The cells typically demonstrate a moderate amount of finely granular cytoplasm and fine nucleoli.

Examiner question: which cells are carcinoid tumours derived from?

Candidate answer

- The enterochromaffin-like cells of the neuroendocrine system of the GI tract.
- These are APUD (amine precursor uptake and decarboxylation) tumours.

4.6.5 Fistula-in-ano

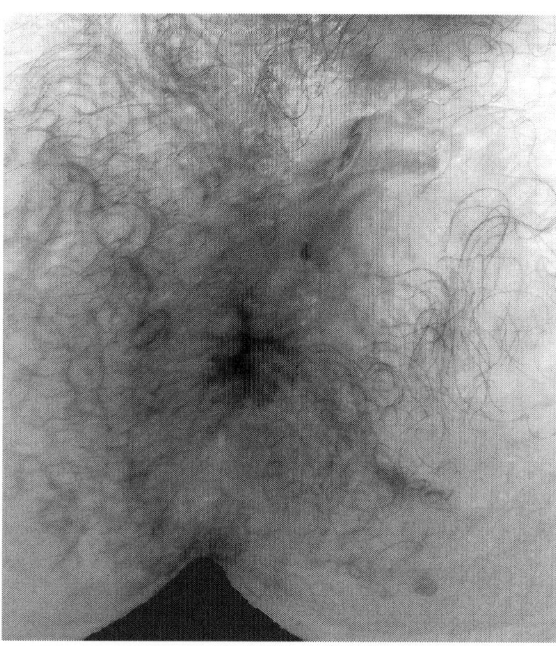

Figure 4.6.5
Fistula-in-ano in left anterior position

Examiner question: please discuss what you see.

Candidate answer

- This image displays an external opening about 2 cm from anal verge at about the one o'clock position.
- This clinical sign is most consistent with a fistula-in-ano.
- Importantly, there are no other obvious associated perianal/perineal abnormalities to suggest that it is secondary to other underlying aetiologies.
- I would assess this patient by taking a complete history, including:
  - local symptom assessment, especially pain/discharge/sepsis
  - GI symptom assessment to exclude underlying causes (e.g. diarrhoea/pain suggestive of Crohn's etc.)
  - previous history of fistula/perianal sepsis/anal surgery
  - details of previous investigations (e.g. colonoscopy)
  - risk factors for STI
  - FHx of IBD.
- On examination, I would look for:
  - associated sepsis — evidence of fluctuant perianal swelling, erythema or purulent discharge
  - information relating to the anatomy of the fistula if possible
  - clinical condition/function of the anal sphincters.

- After consideration for resuscitation and sepsis treatment if relevant, this patient will require a thorough examination of the anorectum under anaesthesia.
- The aim of which is to:
  1. incise and drain any sepsis
  2. confirm the presence of a fistula
  3. define the anatomy of fistula which will involve:
     i. location of the external opening
     ii. location of the internal opening
     iii. course of the primary track
     iv. presence of secondary extensions
     v. presence of other diseases complicating the fistula
  4. maintain continence.
- In the acute setting, my personal preference is to place a loose draining seton if there is an obvious fistula (as in this scenario).

Examiner: discuss the pathophysiology of fistula-in-ano.

Candidate answer

- A fistula-in-ano is an abnormal communication between the anoderm (epithelialised surface of anal canal) and the perianal skin.
- Aetiology:
  - primary (>90%): cryptoglandular hypothesis (obstruction of anal glands → sepsis/abscess formation within intersphincteric space → drainage of sepsis externally through a fistula tract)
  - secondary: traumatic, malignant, iatrogenic, STI, IBD (Crohn's disease).
- They can be classified according to Park's classification (BJS 1976) where 'sphincteric' relates to the *external* anal sphincter into:
  - intersphincteric
  - transphincteric (>50%)
  - suprasphincteric
  - extrasphincteric.
- Intersphincteric and transphincteric are the two most common.
- Superficial fistula (i.e. not related to the anal sphincters) is not part of Park's classification.
- Fistulas can further be classified as simple vs complex. Complex being regarded as the presence of:
  - >30% of the sphincter muscle involved by the track
  - recurrent disease
  - anterior fistula in women
  - multiple tracts
  - pre-existing incontinence
  - prior radiation
  - secondary (e.g. to Crohn's disease).

Examiner: describe the relevance of anal anatomy in management of fistula.

Candidate answer

- Defining the anatomy of fistula is an essential step in treatment.
- It is important to identify the relationship of the fistula track to the anal sphincter muscles. The amount of sphincter muscle involved in the fistula has implications on whether it can be safely laid open (fistulotomy) or not.
- Traditionally, most attention has focused on the relationship of the fistula and the external anal sphincter. However, it should be remembered that the internal anal sphincter may contribute up to 70% of the anal tone at rest and its division (which is inevitable during sphincterotomy, no matter how low) may result in incontinence to flatus and/or faecal soiling.
- If the fistula is simple or the underlying aetiology is cryptoglandular then by definition the internal opening should be at the dentate line.
- The further away the external opening is from the anal verge, the more likely that it is a complex fistula.

Examiner: what is Goodsall law?

Candidate answer

- This is a law that helps to predict the relationship of an external opening (within 3 cm of anal verge) to that of internal opening.
- An imaginary line drawn transversely through the anal canal is the reference point.
- External openings posterior to this line tend to have a semi-circular course and open in the midline of anal canal at the dentate line.
- External openings anterior to this line predict a radial tract.
- In selected cases, this law can provide clues to finding the internal opening and thus may prevent false passage creation.

Examiner question: how is the classification of an anorectal abscess different to that of a fistula?

Candidate answer

- Abscesses are classified according to their location within the anorectal space.
- Generally speaking, perineal abscess may represent simple skin appendage infection or occur secondary to an underlying fistula. Microbiology alone isn't specific/sensitive enough to confidently make the differentiation.
- Such abscesses may be:
  - perianal abscess (>60%)
  - ischiorectal (20%)
  - intersphincteric (5%)
  - supralevator (4%)
  - submucosal (1%).
- About 30% of abscesses drained will go on to reveal an underlying fistula. Abscesses other than the true perianal and ischiorectal may be difficult to appreciate clinically. Therefore, it is essential to perform an EUA of the anorectum to rule out an underlying intersphincteric abscess in patients with severe anal pain and sepsis. Imaging may be helpful in suspected cases of supralevator abscess formation.

4.6.6 Pilonidal sinus

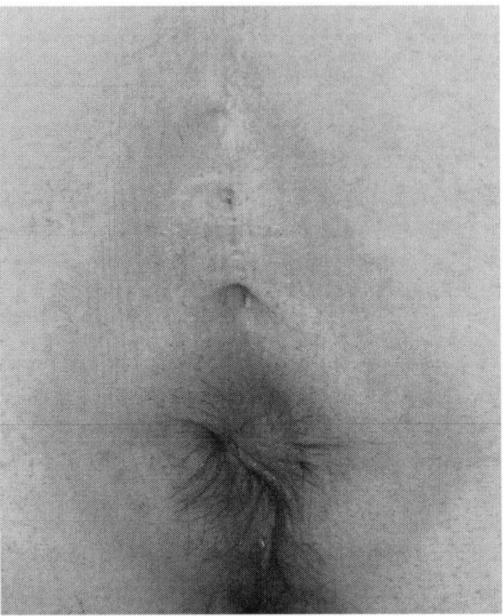

Figure 4.6.6
Pilonidal sinus

Examiner question: please discuss what you see.

Candidate response

- This is a clinical image of the natal cleft demonstrating a number of openings or pits in the midline of the skin, which are known as pilonidal sinuses.
- They likely communicate with a cavity beneath the skin.

Examiner question: what is the pathophysiology of this condition?

Candidate answer

- Pilonidal sinus is a chronic inflammatory disorder consisting of midline pits sited cephalad to the anal canal in the natal cleft with associated lateral secondary tracks.
- The term pilonidal refers to a nest of hairs. In this condition hair fragments are found within the sinuses, burrowing below through the skin of the natal cleft, although their role in the pathoaetiology isn't entirely clear.
- The proposed aetiologies include:
  - congenital hypotheses (medullary canal/dermoid theories)
  - acquired hypotheses (penetration of the skin by hairs)
  - combined congenital and acquired hypothesis (most intuitive in that a tendency exists for hairs to enter the skin in the natal cleft).
- This resulting sinus, which is an abnormal communication with the skin and the subcutaneous tissue, can lead to abscess formation in this region. Such abscesses are typically maximally fluctuant in a paramedian position and toward the superior aspect of the natal cleft.

- There are a number of factors which increase the chances of this condition occurring and they relate to hair factors, depth of the natal cleft and the condition of the skin in this region.
- The hair that causes this condition is believed to have fractured and lodged in the natal cleft. Individuals from racial backgrounds that have coarse, straight hair (e.g. Mediterranean) are at greater risk.
- A deeper, narrow natal cleft also increases risk of pilonidal sinus. Furthermore, skin that is macerated or has erosions/scars from previous of surgery and open wounds are more likely to permit passage of hair into the subcutaneous tissue.

Examiner question: what are the principles of management?

Candidate answer

- In the acute setting, the priority is to drain and eliminate sepsis by performing incision and drainage of abscesses.
- In individuals who remain relatively asymptomatic, it is justifiable to undertake conservative management with expectant treatment of minor sepsis, since the disease usually 'burns' out by the fourth decade.
- Definitive management involves surgery and procedures can be classified as:
  - conservative: excision of midline pits and clearing of tracks (Lord/Bascom procedures)
  - radical excision with:
    - primary closure
    - healing by secondary intention
    - flap closure (e.g. Karydakis/Rhomboid flaps).

4.6.7 Small bowel tumours

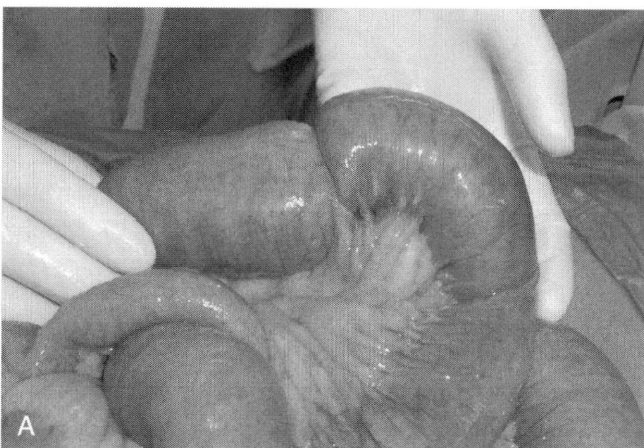

Figure 4.6.7A
Small bowel intussusception

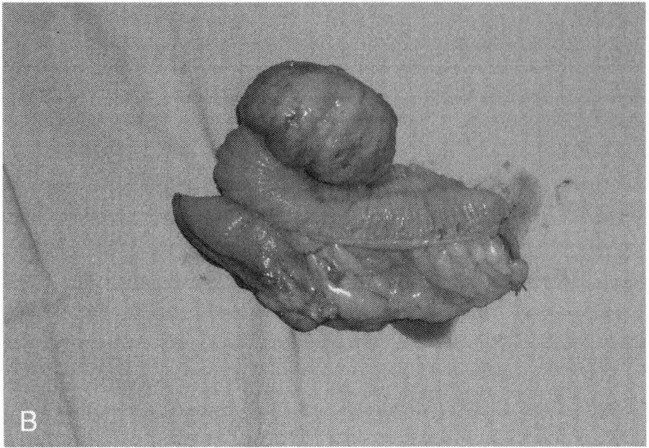

Figure 4.6.7B
Small bowel tumour

Examiner question: this is a tumour of the small bowel. What different pathologies might cause small bowel tumours?

Candidate answer

- Small bowel tumours may be non-neoplastic or neoplastic.
- Neoplasms may be benign or malignant and the latter may be primary or secondary.
- Non-neoplastic tumours:
  - haemangiomas
  - hamartoma
  - hyperplastic polyps
  - heterotopic tissue (in a Meckel's diverticulum)
  - endometriosis and dermoid cysts.
- Benign neoplasms:
  - lipoma
  - leiomyoma
  - adenoma
  - neurogenic tumours (neurofibroma and gangliocytic paragangliomas).
- There are neoplasms which display variable behaviour including:
  - carcinoid
  - GIST tumours.
- Primary malignant neoplasms include:
  - adenocarcinoma
  - gastrointestinal lymphoma
  - leiomyosarcoma
  - liposarcoma.
- Secondary malignant neoplasms include:
  - direct extension (from colonic, gastric, pancreatic or renal carcinoma)
  - metastatic small bowel tumour may include those from:
    - melanoma (most common in Australia)
    - lymphoma

- breast
- renal
- lung cancer.

Examiner question: which conditions are associated with an increased risk of small bowel malignancy?

Candidate answer

- There are a variety of genetic and acquired conditions associated with various types of small bowel cancer, all of them relatively uncommon.
- The congenital conditions include:
  - FAP: first develop adenomatous polyps of duodenum then adenocarcinoma. Lifetime risk of polyposis is 88% and cumulative cancer incidence 18% at 75 years of age (Bulow et al Colorectal Dis 2012)
  - Peutz-Jeghers syndrome: adenocarcinoma of small bowel
  - neurofibromatosis: leiomyosarcoma, adenocarcinoma and carcinoid.
- The acquired conditions include:
  - Crohn's disease: 100 fold increased risk of adenocarcinoma with areas affected with active disease (usually ileum)
  - coeliac disease: increased risk of lymphoma and adenocarcinoma. Unclear whether a gluten-free diet reduces this risk
  - immunosuppression (including biological agents e.g. infliximab): increased risk of non-Hodgkin lymphoma (post-transplant lymphoproliferative disorder, PTLD) after long-term immunosuppression; the greater the degree of immunosuppression the greater the risk of PTLD
  - HIV associated with lymphoma and Kaposi sarcoma.

4.6.8 Thyroid cancer

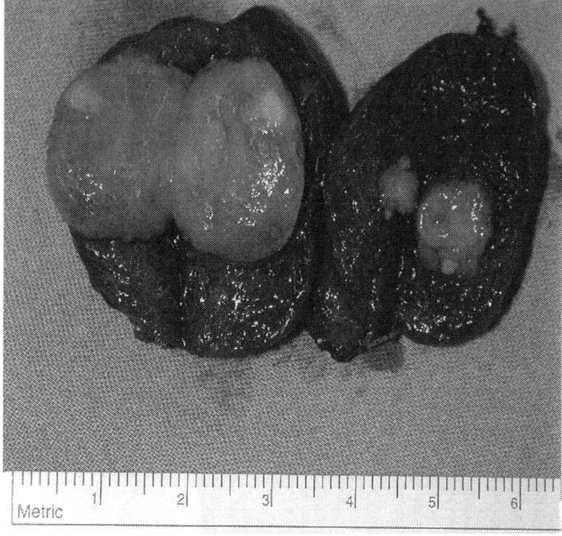

Figure 4.6.8
Bilateral medullary thyroid cancer

Examiner question: this patient had a medullary thyroid cancer. What can you tell me about thyroid cancer?

Candidate answer

- Thyroid cancer can be divided into papillary, follicular, medullary and anaplastic carcinoma. Other rarer cancers include lymphoma and metastatic carcinoma (from breast/kidney).
- Incidence: represents 1% of new cancer diagnosis each year. Female to male ratio is 3:1.
- Aetiology: familial (papillary, medullary), radiation exposure (papillary), low dietary iodine intake (higher proportion of follicular and anaplastic cancer).
- Presentation: varies depending on stage on presentation. Often presents as an asymptomatic nodule. Symptoms include hoarseness of voice, neck swelling, late feature is stridor (anaplastic). Presentation with symptoms of thyrotoxicosis is very rare.
- Assessment: triple assessment using clinical examination, imaging and pathology and staging investigations once diagnosis confirmed.

The pathological types

PAPILLARY THYROID CANCER (PTC)

- Accounts for 75–80% of thyroid cancer.
- Papillar**Y: p**aed = occurs in 20s; **Y** = **Y**ellow = lymph spread central ipsilateral then level 2–5 lateral neck.
- Micropapillary (< 1 cm), intrathyroidal, and extrathyroidal.
- Treatment:
  - due to multifocality, my approach to a diagnosis of PTC is to perform a total thyroidectomy and ipsilateral central neck dissection
  - I^{131} adjuvant treatment: for patients with high risk features (ages — age, tumour grade, tumour extent, tumour size; AMES — age, metastases, extent of primary cancer, tumour size) or close margins and central nodal involvement. Also allows for post-operative surveillance with thyroglobulin.

FOLLICULAR THYROID CANCER

- Accounts for 10–15% of thyroid cancer.
- Follicula**R: f**orties/**f**ifties; **R** = **R**ed = blood spread.
- Capsular invasion is the hallmark of malignancy, which cannot be determined on fine needle biopsy. Requires a hemithyroidectomy to provide a diagnosis and differentiate between adenoma and cancer.
- Treatment:
  - generally, surgery is the initial treatment modality. Given hemithyroidectomy is generally a diagnostic tool for follicular carcinoma, completion thyroidectomy is the operation of choice. Iodine ablation is adjuvant treatment for high risk patients (AGES >6).

MEDULLARY THYROID CANCER

- Accounts for 5% of thyroid cancer.
- Arises from parafollicular C cells.

- Two forms: sporadic and familial.
  - Sporadic: 80% of patients (40–50 years).
  - Familial: 20% of patients (younger age):
    - inherited autosomal dominant, almost complete penetrance
      - MEN 2a
      - MEN 2b.
- Treatment:
  - determined based on stage of cancer
  - total thyroidectomy and bilateral central neck dissection if incidental finding/impalpable
  - total thyroidectomy, bilateral central neck dissection and ipsilateral lateral neck dissection (level 2–5) if palpable (risk lateral node involvement ~15%)
  - excluded concomitant phaeochromocytoma
  - external beam treatment should be considered in patients with high risk of locoregional recurrence after maximal surgical treatment:
    - positive surgical margins
    - extranodal soft tissue extension
    - extensive mediastinal tumour extension.

ANAPLASTIC THYROID CANCER

- Generally occurs in the elderly.
- Associated with rapidly progressive thyroid lump.
- Poor prognosis with survival less than <1 year.
- Generally non-operative management.
- In certain cases, thyroidectomy can be performed for local control.

4.6.9 Multinodular goitre

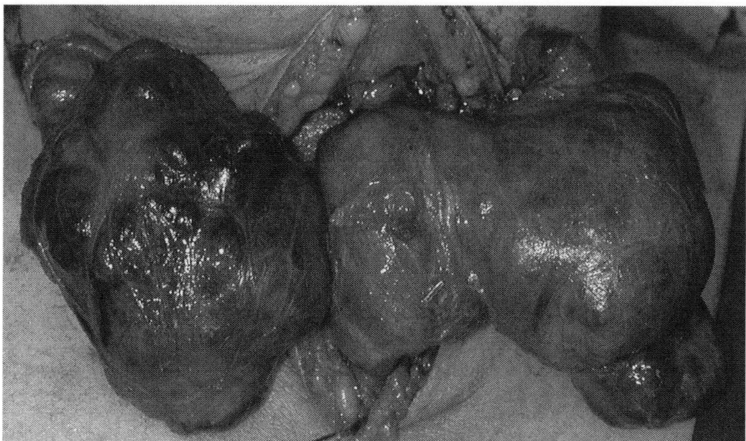

Figure 4.6.9
Multinodular goitre

Examiner shows the image in Figure 4.6.9 to the candidate.

Candidate begins speaking immediately.

- This is an operative image of a large multinodular goitre.
- Definition: a goitre refers to non-specific enlargement of the thyroid gland, whilst the term multinodular goitre indicates enlargement of the thyroid gland with multiple areas of nodularity.
- Aetiology: this is idiopathic, but associated with iodine deficiency and there is a high familial incidence.
- Pathogenesis: diffuse and multinodular goitres reflect impaired synthesis of thyroid hormone, most often caused by dietary iodine deficiency. Impairment of thyroid hormone synthesis leads to a compensatory rise in the serum TSH level which, in turn, causes hypertrophy and hyperplasia of thyroid follicular cells and, ultimately, gross enlargement of the thyroid gland. With time, recurrent episodes of hyperplasia and involution combine to produce a multinodular goitre.
- Sex: it occurs in females more than males.
- Macroscopic appearance: there is often asymmetrical nodularity. The nodules may be haemorrhagic and associated with fibrosis.
- Microscopic appearance: colloid filled nodules are evident with varying degrees of inflammation, haemorrhage, necrosis and fibrosis.
- Clinical presentation: varies depending on the size of the goitre and may be:
  - asymptomatic
  - mechanical symptoms of pressure (dyspnoea, stridor, dysphagia)
  - thyrotoxic symptoms.
- It can also be associated with an increased risk of cancer with nodules greater than 1 cm or irregular ultrasonographic features (incidence of cancer is 5–10%).
- Investigations:
  - TSH, T_3, T_4, thyroid autoantibodies, TSH receptor antibodies
  - diagnosis with ultrasound
  - isotope scans in thyrotoxic patient (*no* role diagnosing malignancy)
  - fine needle aspiration cytology (FNA) of dominant nodule
  - CT: assessment of retrosternal extension.
- Indications for surgery — manage jointly with endocrinologist — the 6Ms:
  1. **m**alignancy (or suspicious dominant nodule)
  2. **m**edical therapy failure
  3. **m**echanical compression
  4. **m**enacing consequences of radioactive iodine (pregnancy, allergy, severe eye disease)
  5. **m**ediastinal extension (unable to monitor changes clinical)
  6. **m**arred beauty (young/patients with large goitres).
- Benefits of surgery over radioablation:
  - pathological confirmation
  - avoidance of radiation
  - reduced risk of recurrence
  - one stage treatment.

4.6.10 Adrenal tumours

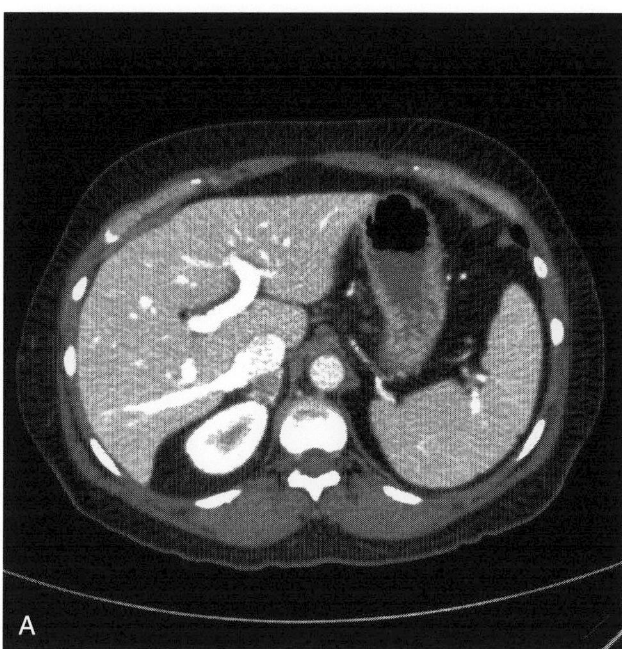

Figure 4.6.10A
Right adrenal tumour CT scan

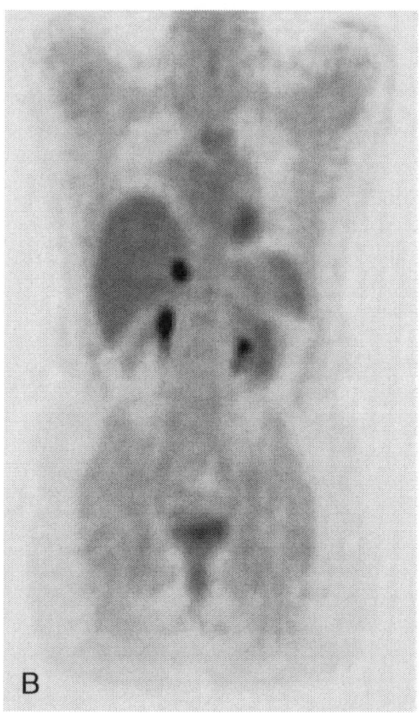

Figure 4.6.10B
Right adrenal tumour PET scan

Examiner question: this 56-year-old woman had lung cancer 3 years ago. She is asymptomatic. What are the potential causes of an adrenal mass?

Candidate answer

Adrenal lesions can be classified pathologically or physiologically.

The pathological classification includes neoplastic and non-neoplastic lesions.

- The neoplastic lesions may be primary or secondary.
  - Primary neoplastic lesions include:
    - cortical lesions (adenoma and carcinoma)
    - medullary lesions (phaeochromocytoma both benign and malignant, ganglioneuroma and neuroblastoma).
  - Secondary neoplastic lesions include metastasis from:
    - lung, breast, renal, colorectal cancer and melanoma.
- Non-neoplastic masses may be:
  - endothelial lined cysts (lymph angiomatous or angiomatous)
  - myelolipoma
  - haemorrhage (particularly after trauma).
- The physiological classification separates lesions into functioning or non-functioning.
  - Non-functioning lesions include:
    - non-functioning cortical adenoma (80%)
    - adrenocortical carcinoma (8%)
    - metastatic disease (3%)
    - myelolipoma (3%).
  - Functioning lesions include:
    - phaeochromocytoma (8%)
    - adrenocortical adenoma with subclinical Cushing's syndrome (6%)
    - adrenocortical adenoma producing aldosterone (2%).

Examiner question: what is phaeochromocytoma?

Candidate answer

- It is a functional adrenal tumour derived from the neuroectodermal cells of the adrenal medulla and certain extra-adrenal sites. It can be remembered as the disease of 10s:
  - 10% bilateral
  - 10% extra-adrenal
  - 10% familial
  - 10% occur in children
  - 10% multi-centric
  - 10% malignant.

Examiner question: which genetic syndromes are associated with an increased risk of phaeochromocytoma?

Candidate answer

- MEN: 2–50%.
- Von Hippel Landau syndrome: 10–20%.
- Neurofibromatosis type I: 2%.
- Mutations in the succinate dehydrogenase gene have also been found in association with familial paraganglioma syndromes:
  - germ-line mutations in the B and D subunits of succinate dehydrogenase gene have been associated with about 10% of sporadic phaeochromocytoma.

Examiner question: where are the sites of occurrence and what are the pathologic features of phaeochromocytoma?

Candidate answer

- 80–90% in adrenal medulla.
- Most extra-adrenal tumours are intra-abdominal, the majority arise in the region of the aortic bifurcation from the organ of Zuckerkandl or in region of urinary bladder.
- 3% are extra-abdominal, most in the paravertebral region in chest. Rarely, they arise in the neck from cervical ganglia.

Examiner question: what is the organ of Zuckerkandl?

Candidate answer

The organ of Zuckerkandl is a chromaffin body derived from neural crest and located at the aortic bifurcation or near the origin of the IMA.

Examiner question: what substances do pheochromocytomas produce?

Candidate answer

- Catecholamines are the major product.
- Noradrenaline, adrenalin or dopamine may predominate.
- Occasionally they produce other compounds — ACTH, CRH, IL-6, Neuron specific enolase, calcitonin, PTHrP and VIP.

Examiner question: what is the difference between secretion from adrenal and extra-adrenal tumours?

Candidate answer

- In the extra-adrenal lesions, NA is usually the only secreted catecholamine.
- In adrenal tumours, adrenaline is usually the predominantly secreted catecholamine. This is because the enzyme that converts NA to adrenaline, phenyl ethanolamine-N-Methyl-transferase (PNMT), is inducible by cortisol and so is not highly active outside the adrenal medulla.
- Therefore, only in tumours of the adrenal medulla, which has a high cortisol concentration form the surrounding cortex, is PNMT highly active and NA readily converted to adrenaline.

4.6.11 Systemic inflammatory response syndrome

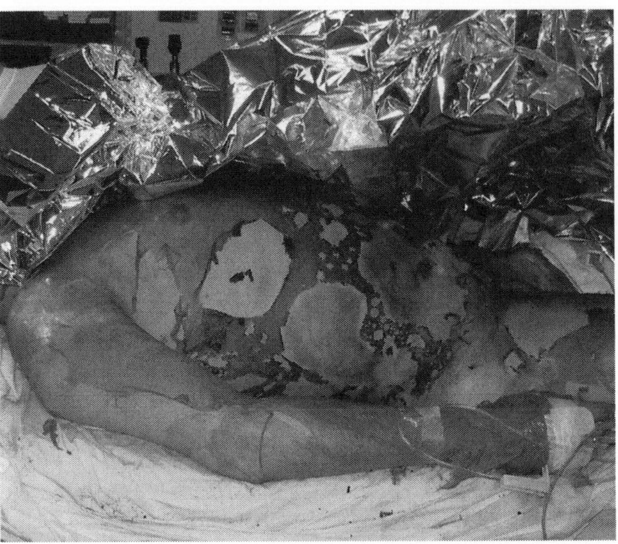

Figure 4.6.11
A male patient having sustained extensive burns

Examiner question: a 24-year-old man presents with extensive burns after a house fire. He is hypothermic, tachycardic and tachypnoeic. He has a WCC of 24. He is intubated because of airway burns. How do you explain the systemic response to burn injuries to skin?

Candidate answer

- Although there is loss of fluid and protein from burns to skin, much of the reaction described is an example of the systemic inflammatory response syndrome (SIRS).
- This is defined clinically by two or more of:
  - temp >38 or <36 °C
  - pulse rate >90bpm
  - WCC >12 x 10^9/L or <4 x 10^9/L
  - respiratory rate >20/min or $PaCO_2$ <32 mmHg.
- It is an endogenously generated response to an injury or infection.
- Non-infectious causes include:
  - inflammatory conditions (such as pancreatitis, anaphylaxis, transfusion reactions or vasculitis) or trauma (major injury to abdomen/chest/limbs, burns, even extensive surgery or haemorrhage).

Examiner question: what mediates this response?

Candidate answer

- It is initiated locally at the site of injury by the production of IL 1,2 and 6 and TNF-alpha from tissue macrophages, monocytes, mast cells and platelets.

- These cytokines are responsible for the fever, release of stress hormones (noradrenaline, vasopressin), renin-angiotensin system activation and hypotension.
- They also result in the activation of the coagulation and complement cascades and the release of nitric oxide, platelet-activating factor, prostaglandins and leukotrienes.
- The alternative pathway of the complement cascade leads to the production of C3a and C5a (potent vasodilators). These, in addition to prostaglandins and leukotrienes, cause endothelial damage and altered vascular permeability that leads to organ dysfunction (especially lung and kidney injury), which may progress to multi-organ dysfunction syndrome (MODS) (see 4.6.12).
- The body also initiates a compensatory anti-inflammatory response syndrome (CARS) through cytokines IL-4 and IL-10, in order to localise and control the effect of pro-inflammatory cytokines.

TOP TIP

There is almost invariably a SIRS question in the exam. Burns and pancreatitis are the exam archetypes of the systemic inflammatory response. When presented with such a scenario in this section, the examiner usually wants to talk about SIRS.

4.6.12 Multi-organ dysfunction syndrome

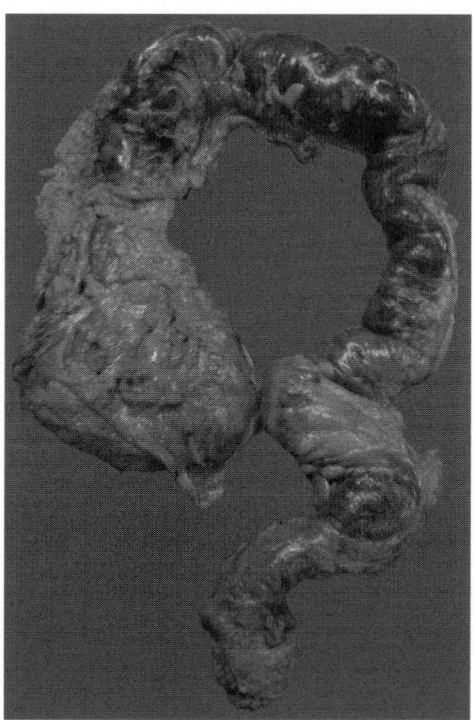

Figure 4.6.12
Infarcted colon

Examiner question: a 70-year-old patient presented 5 days ago with an acute abdomen and generalised peritonitis. At laparotomy, she was found to have an infarcted colon and underwent emergency colectomy with ileostomy formation. This is the specimen that was removed. Subsequently, she was managed on ICU. During the last 48 hours she has deteriorated and has refractory hypoxia, oliguria and hypotension requiring inotropes. How do you interpret this scenario pathophysiologically?

Candidate answer

- This is an example of multi-organ dysfunction syndrome (MODS).
- This is defined as alteration of organ function in an acute illness such that homeostasis cannot be maintained without intervention.
- Typically, it occurs on a background of SIRS, since progression from SIRS to severe sepsis is associated with organ dysfunction.
- MODS includes renal dysfunction (oliguria), cardiac dysfunction (hypotension), cerebral dysfunction (delirium), lung dysfunction (refractory hypoxia) and coagulation failure (often recognised as DIC).
- Of infectious causes, gram negative bacteraemia with endotoxaemia is the most commonly encountered. This is often a result of translocation of endogenous bacteria and/or endotoxin from the GI tract as a result of intestinal injury (such as ischaemia, or interruption of enteral feeding leading to loss of trophic enterocyte nutrition).
- The mainstay of management is supportive treatment for organ failure, with particular attention to control/eliminate any source of infection. Maintenance of tissue oxygenation is crucial and may require airway, ventilator and circulatory support.

Examiner question: what are the determinants of tissue oxygen delivery?

Candidate answer

- Tissue oxygen delivery is dependent on the oxygen content of arterial blood and cardiac output.
- The oxygen content of arterial blood is governed by the oxygen bound to haemoglobin (Hb concentration x oxygen saturation) plus the (less significant) amount dissolved in plasma (0.023 x PaO_2).
- Cardiac output is equal to heart rate x stroke volume.

4.6.13 Necrotising soft tissue infections

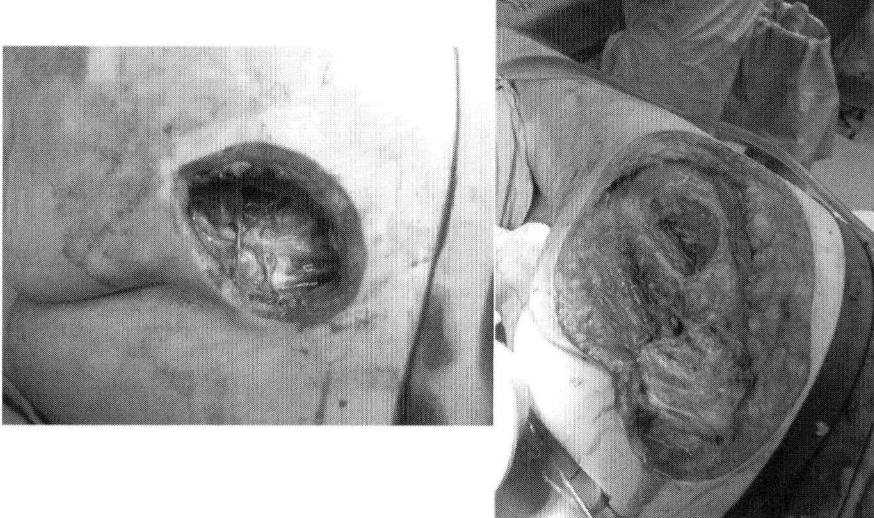

Figure 4.6.13
Necrotising fasciitis of the buttock

Examiner question: this 53-year-old woman with a history of alcoholism presented to the emergency department with hypotension, delirium and a WCC of 22. She had an indurated area on her buttock and was taken to theatre. What is the diagnosis?

TOP TIP

Most often you will be shown a picture of gangrene involving the scrotum, but be prepared for variations including the leg or abdominal wall.

Candidate answer

- This is a necrotising soft tissue infection (NSTI).
- These include infections of skin, subcutaneous fat, superficial fascia, deep muscular fascia or muscle or any combinations of these.
- NSTI are generally characterised by extensive soft tissue destruction, systemic toxicity and a high mortality.

Examiner question: how would you classify necrotising fasciitis (NF)?

Candidate answer

This is a deep-seated infection of subcutaneous tissue that results in destruction of fascia and fat but may spare the skin. It can be type I or type II.

- Type I (70–80%): mixed infection of aerobic and anaerobic bacteria, usually occurring after surgical procedures or in patients with diabetes and peripheral vascular disease. An average of 3–4 organisms are involved typically including: Clostridia, Streptococci, Enterococci, Coliforms (E.coli, Klebsiella, enterobacter), Pseudomonas, Acinetobacter, Staphylococci, Bacteroides and Corynebacteria.

- Type II (20–30%): mono-microbial. Organisms include:
  - Clostridium perfringens causing Clostridial myonecrosis (gas gangrene), usually post-trauma or surgery
  - Streptococcal necrotising fasciitis (usually community acquired):
    - group A β-haemolytic streptococci
    - subacute variety due to groups C and G
    - ± Strep toxic shock syndrome
  - Vibrionaceae: Vibrio vulnificus after contact with warm salt water
  - aeromonas hydrophilia (myonecrosis) (fresh or salt water).

Examiner question: what is the pathophysiology of this condition?

Candidate answer

- Complex interaction between the aerobic and anaerobic organisms and the host.
- Facultative anaerobic organisms lower the oxidation-reduction potential of the microenvironment and promote multiplication of anaerobes.
- The anaerobes interfere with host phagocyte function, allowing aerobes to proliferate. Some organisms (e.g. B. fragilis) produce B-lactamase to interfere with antibiotic activity.
- Bacterial exotoxins (C. perfringens — alpha toxin, S. pyogenes — haemolysin, Streptolysin O and S, Leukocidin) cause tissue digestion.
- The inflammatory process involves local blood vessels leading to necrosis of blood vessel walls and thrombosis of small blood vessels. Pressure increases due to the tissue oedema, further impairing blood supply. Ischaemia leads to liquefactive necrosis of fascia with concomitant breakdown to skin, muscle and surrounding tissue.

Examiner question: what features help to differentiate cellulitis or an abscess from NF?

Candidate answer

- It can be difficult to differentiate, especially in the early stage of the illness. Suggestive features include:
  - pain out of proportion to soft tissue findings
  - thin grey exudates
  - WCC >20
  - sepsis (tachycardia, hypotension, high fluid requirements)

- crepitus
- gas in soft tissues on x-ray
- marked induration or oedema of entire limb
- skin changes (especially sloughing, ecchymosis of skin, necrosis or bullae).

- If any of these features are present then NSTI should be suspected.

Examiner question: what conditions predispose to Fournier's gangrene?

Candidate answer

- It is more common in males (10:1) and with increasing age.
- In two-thirds of cases, a source can be identified including skin infections (24%), urinary infection (19%) (renal abscess, urethral stone, urethral stricture) or colorectal sources (21%) (ruptured appendicitis, colonic carcinoma, diverticulitis).
- In the one-third of cases where no source is found, there is usually an associated disease such as diabetes mellitus (10–60%), alcoholism, leukaemia, HIV. Recent surgery is sometimes a precipitant, typically hernia repair, haemorrhoid banding, urethral catheterisation or prostatic biopsy.

Examiner question: what are the principles of treatment of necrotising soft tissue infections?

Candidate answer

- Rapid clinical assessment and IV fluid resuscitation are essential.
- Vasopressors such as noradrenaline may be required to maintain BP.
- Broad spectrum IV antibiotics such as Ampicillin, gentamicin and metronidazole. For patients with prior hospitalisation use Tazocin (piperacillin with tazobactam). In communities where community acquired-MRSA is prevalent use Vancomycin.
- However, prompt and aggressive debridement is essential. This should involve:
  - wide excision of all infected tissue to margins with normal tissue both laterally and deep (*excise skin until it bleeds, fat until it glistens and muscle until it twitches*)
  - dress wounds with saline-soaked packs and return to operating room in 24 hours to ensure all necrotic material is removed; consider colostomy for patients with perineal gangrene
  - tissue should be sent for gram stain and culture
  - ICU support including nutrition.

4.6.14 Mesenteric ischaemia

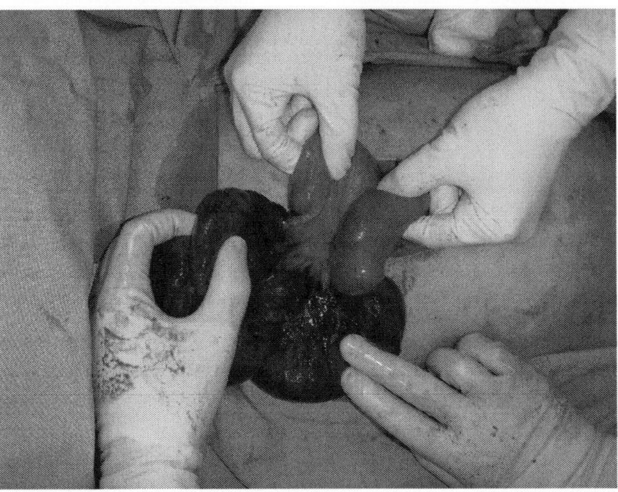

Figure 4.6.14
Small bowel mesenteric ischaemia

Examiner question: you take a patient to theatre for small bowel obstruction. This image reveals what you find at laparotomy. Please discuss.

Candidate answer

TOP TIP

Remember that this is a *pathophysiology* viva. Therefore, there is no need to describe in detail how you would do a small bowel resection. State the obvious diagnosis, differential diagnoses and the objectives of your surgery.

- This image illustrates mesenteric infarction with frank necrosis of small bowel.
- The objective of surgery in this setting is to resect the non-viable small bowel and resuscitate the patient in an ICU setting.
- The most likely aetiology is a band adhesion causing small bowel volvulus.
- Other causes of mesenteric infarction include:
  - occlusive (emboli to SMA and its branches from AF, recent infarct)
  - venous thrombosis (e.g. in hypercoagulable states)
  - non-occlusive (e.g. cardiogenic shock).
- I expect this patient to be critically unwell with evidence of systemic inflammatory response or septic shock.

Examiner question: please discuss the pathophysiology of mesenteric ischaemia.

Candidate answer

There are four stages of mesenteric ischaemia:

1. mucosal ischaemia, characterised by visceral pain without clinical signs
2. disruption of microvascular integrity — capillaries become damaged, increase mucosal permeability, blood may extravasate causing haemorrhagic foci and bowel wall thickening
3. progressive mucosal injury, leakage of protein, fluid and electrolytes — gas-producing organism, translocation of bacteria, pneumatosis, portal venous gas and peritonitis
4. reperfusion — more damaging production of free radicals, neutrophil infiltration, anaerobic metabolism leading to lactic acidosis.

Examiner question: what are the consequences if you were to resect a considerable length of this patient's small bowel?

Candidate answer

- I would be most concerned about the risk of short gut syndrome.
- This is when absorption of nutrients is less than that necessary for maintenance of the body due to loss of small bowel.
- This will result in maldigestion and malabsorption, resulting in deficiencies of macronutrients, minerals, vitamins, trace element and waters.
- Clinically, diarrhoea, weight loss, vitamin deficiencies, electrolyte derangements, etc. are evident.
- Such patients may become reliant on long-term TPN.

Examiner question: in general terms, how much small bowel is required for relatively normal function and avoidance of short gut syndrome and reliance on parenteral nutrition?

Candidate answer

- 100 cm in the absence of the colon.
- 50–60 cm if the colon is present.

4.6.15 Testicular tumours

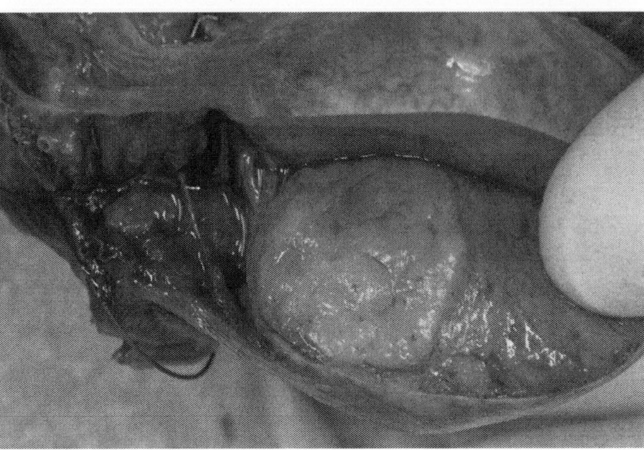

Figure 4.6.15
Testicular seminoma

Examiner question: could you tell me what this image shows?

Candidate answer

- This image shows a transected testicle.
- There appears to be an approximately 2.5 cm diameter, light brown colour tumour of the testicle.
- It is likely to be a seminoma given that they are the most common testicular tumours.

Examiner question: can you classify testicular tumours?

Candidate answer

I use the WHO (histological) classification of testicular tumours.

- Testicular tumours can be broadly classified into germ cell and non-germ-cell tumours.
- Germ-cell tumours are the most common type (approximately 95% of all testicular tumours) and are further subdivided into:
  - seminoma: from immature germ cells
  - non-seminomatous tumours: from mature germ cells:
    - embryonal carcinoma
    - yolk sac tumour (most common testicular tumour in infants and children)
    - trophoblastic tumours
    - teratoma (immature teratoma, malignant teratoma, dermoid cyst, mature teratoma).
- Non-germ-cell tumours are a diverse group and subdivided into:
  - tumours of sex cord/gonadal stroma (approximately 4%):
    - Leydig cell tumour (most common non-germ-cell tumour. Can be associated with androgen excess which is converted peripherally to oestrogen)
      - Sertoli cell tumour

- secondary tumours including lymphatogenous and metastatic tumours
- tumours of the collecting ducts and rete testis
- tumours of the testicular adnexa.

4.6.16 Tension pneumothorax

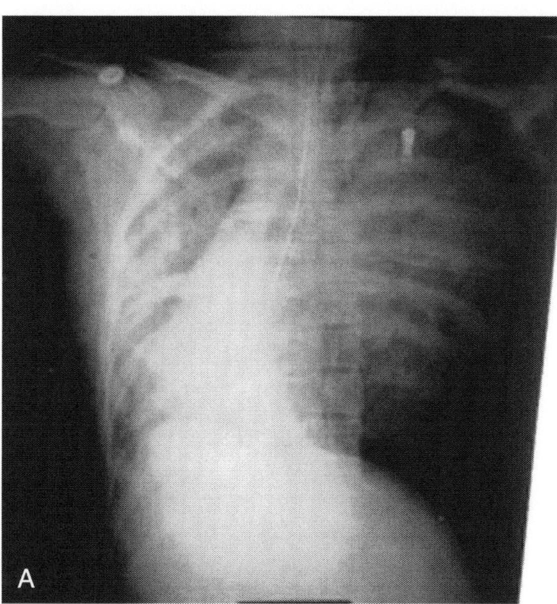

Figure 4.6.16A
Chest x-ray of a tension pneumothorax

Examiner question: please take a look at this chest x-ray and describe what you see.

Candidate answer

- This is a chest x-ray showing a left-sided tension pneumothorax.
- There is evidence of shift of the trachea and mediastinal structures across to the right.
- The left hemithorax appears radiolucent and devoid of lung markings on account of accumulation of air in the pleural space, with the left lung pushed across to the right.

Examiner question: please describe the pathophysiology of a tension pneumothorax.

Candidate answer

- The pathophysiology of a tension pneumothorax involves air from an injured lung or airway being trapped within the pleural cavity, resulting in loss of normal negative intrapleural pressure.
- A tension pneumothorax occurs when there is a valve mechanism at the site of the leak allowing air to enter but not escape from the pleural cavity.

- It is characterised by complete lung collapse, tracheal deviation and mediastinal shift leading to respiratory distress but also decreased venous return to heart, decreased cardiac output and hypotension.
- Respiratory decompensation occurs as a result of lung injury and changes in pulmonary blood flow and gaseous exchange resulting in hypoxaemia, hypercapnia and respiratory acidosis.
- The clinical features are dyspnoea, tachypnoea, hypotension, tachycardia and decreased PaO_2. There is usually asymmetrical expansion of the thorax, the percussion note on the side of the pneumothorax is hyper-resonant and the breath sounds markedly reduced/absent. The trachea and apex beat are deviated away from the side of the pneumothorax and there is often central cyanosis and distension of the neck veins.
- The diagnosis is *clinical* and x-ray confirmation should *not* be awaited before intervention.
- The management of a tension pneumothorax involves:
  - full resuscitation, including administration of maximal flow oxygen, followed by immediate decompression with a large bore needle inserted into the second intercostal space in the mid clavicular line on the ipsilateral side as the pneumothorax
  - subsequently, a 32F chest drain should be inserted on the ipsilateral side as the pneumothorax in the fifth intercostal space in the midaxillary line and connected to an underwater seal drain
  - clinical assessment and repeat CXR after insertion should confirm resolution.

Examiner question: can you explain how an underwater seal drain works, and can you draw its components?

Candidate answer

- An underwater seal drain (UWSD) allows drainage of hemopneumothorax and restores negative pressure in the pleural space to allow lung expansion.
- A UWSD has a three-chamber unit, including:
  - a collection chamber
  - an underwater seal which acts as a one way valve to allow air to escape but not return to the chest
  - a suction chamber that places –20 cmH_2O negative pressure to the pleural space. The depth of the water determines the negative pressure of the chamber
  - please allow me to draw a UWSD for you (see Fig 4.6.16B).

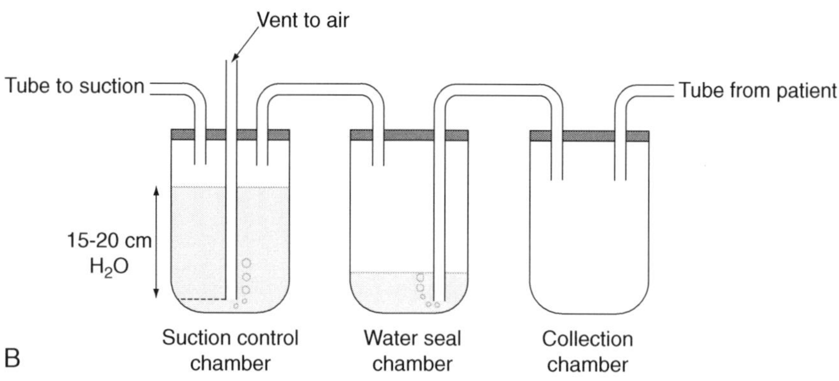

Figure 4.6.16B
Underwater sealed drain

4.6.17 Barrett's oesophagus

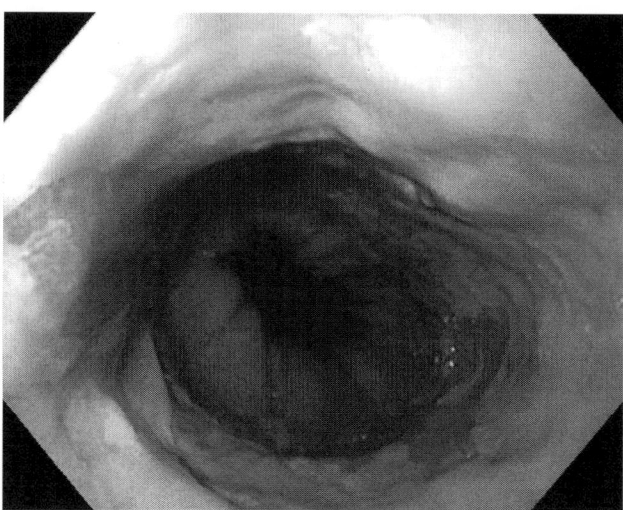

Figure 4.6.17
Barrett's oesophagus endoscopy image

Examiner: this is an endoscopic view of a 60-year-old man's distal oesophagus. He reports a history of reflux symptoms for many years. Please describe the picture.

Candidate answer

- This is an endoscopic view of the distal oesophagus and gastro-oesophageal junction.
- I can see a confluent tongue of red tissue extending proximally up the oesophagus. The gastro-oesophageal junction (represented by the most proximal gastric fold) and the Z line (squamocolumnar junction) don't seem to coincide spatially.

- Thus, I am most concerned here about the possibility of Barrett's oesophagus, although this will need to be confirmed by performing biopsies of the abnormal tissue.
- The other differential diagnosis includes severe oesophagitis (infective or inflammatory).

Examiner question: what is Barrett's oesophagus?

Candidate answer

- It is an acquired metaplastic abnormality in the distal oesophagus defined by two features:
  1. endoscopically: appearance of columnar mucosa within the tubular oesophagus
  2. histologically: intestinal metaplasia with Goblet cells or any epithelium that can predispose to adenocarcinoma.
- Columnar metaplasia of the distal oesophagus is a precursor of adenocarcinoma and the risk of oesophageal adenocarcinoma is increased by 100 fold (0.5–1% risk/year).
- Previously, it was classified as short and long segment. However, the severity of the dysplasia (no dysplasia, low grade and high grade dysplasia) is more useful. In addition, the Prague criteria, based on circumferential and vertical extent of the metaplasia, is used to classify the burden of disease.

Examiner question: what is the underlying pathogenesis?

Candidate answer

- Barrett's oesophagus represents the extreme end of the pathophysiological spectrum of gastro-oesophageal reflux disease (GORD), with a high prevalence of associated hiatal hernia, oesophageal dysmotility and high acid production compounded by impaired mucosal sensitivity.
- Longstanding exposure of the squamous epithelium of the distal oesophagus to gastric and bile acid results in trauma and mucosal injury. The stem cells then regenerate into intestinal type, as they are more acid-resistant.

Examiner question: how would you biopsy this area?

Candidate answer

- There are two principles to adhere to:
  1. biopsy any area suspicious of underlying cancer
  2. perform enough biopsies to sample the area to detect dysplasia/malignancy.
- I would perform four quadrant biopsies every 1–2 cm throughout the length of the segment, acknowledging the fact that underlying cancer can still be missed even with such sampling.
- I would accurately identify the site to record on the pathology form and obtain the biopsy using large endoscopic biopsy forceps.

Examiner question: what are the risk factors?

Candidate answer

- The prevalence increases with age.
- It is twice as common in men.
- Smoking, alcohol and obesity are risk factors for reflux disease, which will predispose to Barrett's oesophagus.

Examiner question: how would you treat this patient?

Candidate answer

- The goals of management are to:
  - modify risk factors (e.g. lose weight, stop smoking)
  - treatment of reflux symptoms/acid abolition with long-term maintenance
    - proton pump inhibitors (induce partial regression in RCTs)
    - (?) fundoplication (see below)
  - endoscopic surveillance of the oesophagus, the frequency of which is based on presence/severity of dysplasia.
- Endoscopic surveillance:
  - if no dysplasia, re-scope in 12 months then every 2 years, continue PPI
  - if low grade dysplasia, re-scope at 6 months x 2 and then yearly
  - the detection of high grade dysplasia usually signifies the end of surveillance and consideration for oesophagectomy if fit or ablative surgery if unfit. However, some patients may decline intervention and should continue with surveillance every 3 months.

Examiner question: what are the benefits of fundoplication?

Candidate answer

- Firstly, it ameliorates symptoms effectively.
- Secondly, it minimise both acid and bile reflux unlike medical therapy which only addresses acid reflux.
- It can potentially retard the progression of Barrett's oesophagus.
- However, there is *no* evidence to support the fact that fundoplication can reduce the risk of adenocarcinoma.

4.6.18 Oesophageal cancer

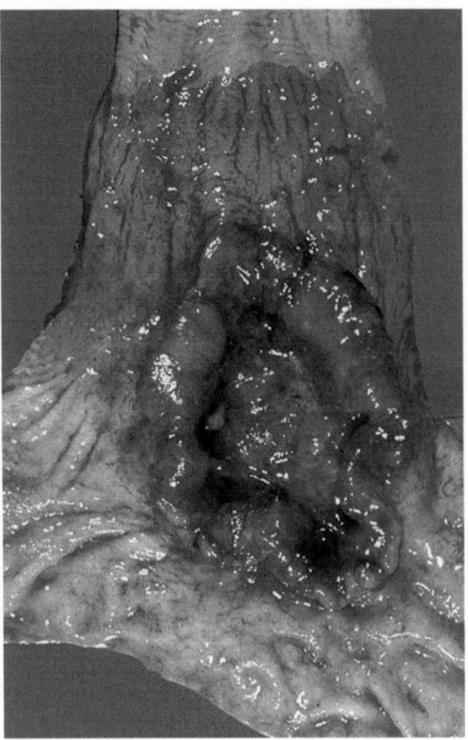

Figure 4.6.18
Oesophageal adenocarcinoma, resection specimen, with background of Barrett's oesophagus (Source: *Gastrointestinal and Liver Pathology*, 2nd edn. Iacobuzio-Donahue C A, Montgomery E. 2011, Saunders: an imprint of Elsevier, Fig 2-24, p 54.)

Examiner: this specimen was resected from a 70-year-old man who presented with dysphagia on a background of worsening symptoms of reflux. Please describe the picture.

Candidate answer

- This image shows the distal oesophagus at its junction with the stomach containing a large, ulcerative lesion suggestive of a primary oesophageal malignancy.
- More than 90% of oesophageal cancers are either squamous cell carcinomas or adenocarcinomas.
- About 75% of adenocarcinomas are located in distal oesophagus, whereas SCC is evenly distributed between the middle and lower third.

Examiner: what are the risk factors and pathogenesis of this disease?

Candidate answer

- Pathogenesis is thought to be due to mucosal injury in the form of oxidative damage from factors such as smoking, trauma and inflammation, which may initiate the carcinogenic process.

- Risk factors for SCC of the oesophagus include:
  - socioeconomic and dietary factors: smoking, alcohol abuse, hot beverages, low socioeconomic status
  - corrosive injury: ingestion of caustic agents
  - achalasia
  - history of head and neck/thoracic radiation
  - associated syndromes: Plummer-Vinson syndrome, palmoplantar keratosis.
- Risk factors for adenocarcinoma of the oesophagus include:
  - Barrett's oesophagus
  - GORD
  - smoking, obesity, race and gender.

Examiner: how would you stage a patient with an oesophageal cancer?

Candidate answer

- I would first confirm the diagnosis by taking adequate biopsies and complete the endoscopy.
- Oesophageal cancer is staged using the TNM system:
  - T is based on depth of invasion through the wall of the oesophagus (T1 submucosa; T2 muscularis propria; T3 adventitia; T4 adjacent structures)
  - N refers to the number of lymph nodes involved (N0 no nodes; N1 regional nodes)
  - M refers to the presence of distant metastasis (in lower oesophageal cancers, coeliac nodal involvement = M1a).
- I would stage this patient's cancer by:
  - clinical assessment:
    - cachexia
    - cervical lymphadenopathy
    - organomegaly
  - endoscopic assessment:
    - to confirm diagnosis
    - provides information re: position/size/morphology of cancer
  - imaging assessment:
    - CXR looking for a malignant effusion
    - CT chest/abdomen/pelvis (for N and M staging)
    - endoscopic ultrasound (for T staging)
    - PET scan (N and M staging especially if CT is negative)
  - laparoscopic assessment:
    - staging laparoscopy maybe useful in distal oesophageal cancers.

Examiner: how would you treat this patient?

TOP TIP

Be concise, this is not a long case. At times during this viva you may wonder what happened to the pathophysiology in this case! Remember that the examiners are assessing not only pathophysiology but also *critical care and clinical reasoning*. The latter is being tested with this and the previous question.

Candidate answer

- This patient would be discussed and managed in a multidisciplinary environment.
- The treatment offered depends on:
  - the site, type and stage of the cancer (will determine curative/palliative intent)
  - the fitness of the patient
  - the patient's wishes.
- Specific treatments offered will vary in individual cases. In general terms, treatment options for cancer of the oesophagus include:
  - not fit + no metastatic disease = definitive chemoradiotherapy
  - fit + no metastatic disease = oesophagectomy (+/– neoadjuvant treatment)
  - fit + metastatic = palliative chemoradiotherapy +/– stenting
  - frail + metastatic = palliative care
  - definitive chemoradiation has similar survival rate to oesophagectomy and neoadjuvant chemoradiotherapy for SCC of oesophagus (30–35%), but locoregional recurrence is higher in those with no surgery
  - the approach is similar for SCC and adenocarcinoma, although the data are limited on the role of definitive chemoradiotherapy in adenocarcinoma.

4.6.19 Stomach cancer

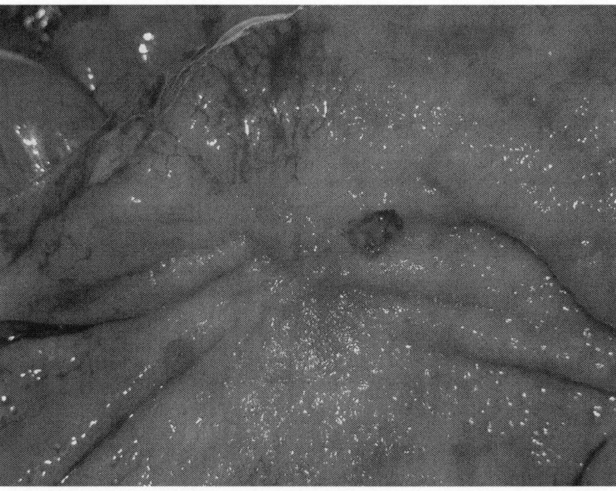

Figure 4.6.19
Stomach cancer, malignant ulcer

Examiner: this patient underwent surgery for a cancer of this organ. Tell me what you see.

Candidate answer

- This is an image of an operative specimen that looks like the stomach, given that I can see the rugae.

- There is a central ulcer of about 1 or 2 cm diameter.
- From the history you provided, this image most likely represents a gastrectomy specimen for gastric cancer.

Examiner: can you tell me about the aetiology of gastric cancer?

Candidate answer

- Gastric cancer is a relatively uncommon malignancy in Australia with an incidence of approximately 5/100 000. This is in contrast with countries such as Japan and Korea where the incidence is as high as 150/100 000.
- However, there has been a recent increase in the incidence of proximal gastric cancers and gastro-oesophageal junction cancers, associated with obesity and gastro-oesophageal reflux disease (GORD).
- Gastric cancer is more common in men and the incidence increases with age.
- The pathogenesis of gastric cancer is complex and multifactorial and involves a pathway of transformation from normal mucosa to gastritis to atrophic gastritis to metaplasia to dysplasia to cancer (Correa hypothesis).
- Inflammatory (acute then chronic) damage occurs in the mucosa as a result of bacterial infection (H. pylori), chemical irritants (ingested substances/reflux of duodenal contents) or as a consequence of autoimmune process (pernicious anaemia).
- Continuation of cellular destruction results in chronic atrophic gastritis and intestinal metaplasia.
- Environmental influences are required to effect this multistage transformation and include:
  - socioeconomic status: cancer more prevalent with lower status
  - dietary: high nitrates
  - infective: *Helicobacter pylori* induced atrophic gastritis, previous distal gastrectomy.
- Genetic factors can be relevant in the development of gastric cancer and include the autosomal dominant mutation seen in hereditary diffuse gastric cancer (*CHD1* — associated with lobular breast cancer and signet ring colonic malignancy) and gastric cancers occurring in the setting of HNPCC.

Examiner: how do you classify gastric cancer?

Candidate answer

- Of malignancies occurring in the stomach, 95% are adenocarcinomas.
- Other malignancies include: SCC, adenosquamous, carcinoid, GIST and lymphoma.
- There have been a number of systems proposed for the classification of gastric adenocarcinoma. Most useful is the classification of gastric cancers by the stage of presentation because it affects treatment.
- Early gastric cancers are those that are T1a (mucosal invasion only) or T1b (invasion into but not through submucosa), irrespective of lymph node status.
- All other presentations are considered as advanced gastric cancers, which is how most patients present in Australia.

- In addition, Borrman classified gastric adenocarcinoma based on macroscopic appearance:
  - type I: protruded
  - type 2: ulcerated with elevated borders
  - type 3: ulcerated with infiltrative margins
  - type 4: diffusely infiltrating
  - type 5: not fitting other types.
- The Lauren classification described two types of gastric cancer based on pathology, epidemiology, pathogenesis and prognosis.
  1. Intestinal type gastric cancers:
     - sporadic
     - occur in the setting of atrophic gastritis
     - M>F
     - older age
     - gland forming.
  2. Diffuse type gastric cancers:
     - familial
     - associated with blood type A
     - F>M
     - younger age group
     - poorly differentiated, signet ring cells
     - worse prognosis.

Examiner: you are referred a patient with a gastric cancer diagnosed by endoscopy and biopsy. How would you manage this patient?

Candidate answer

- Patient and disease factors need to be taken into account and a patient who is fit for any intervention needs to be accurately staged. Nutritional status should also be assessed and optimised.
- Staging involves:
  - repeat UGIT endoscopy to confirm size and location of the lesion and to take additional biopsies of the cancer and surrounding gastric mucosa
  - endoscopic ultrasound to assess T stage and N stage (approx 80% accurate for identification of T1 malignancies)
  - CT chest/abdo/pelvis — looking for evidence of hepatic metastases, ascites, peritoneal metastases
  - diagnostic laparoscopy looking for peritoneal disease and for cytology — alters management in approximately 30% of patients.
- Gastric cancer is staged using the AJCC TNM system:
  - T is based on depth of invasion through the wall of the oesophagus (T1 submucosa; T2 muscularis propria; T3 serosa; T4 adjacent structures)
  - N refers to the number of lymph nodes involved (N0 no nodes; N1: 1–2 nodes, N2: 3–6 nodes; N3: >7 nodes).
  - M refers to presence of distant metastasis (including positive peritoneal cytology).

- In Australia, the role of endoscopic mucosal resection is limited due to few patients presenting with T1 disease. Given a paucity of experience, it is best limited to patients medically unfit for open surgical resection. Otherwise, patients fit for surgery with T1 malignancies usually proceed to curative resection without neoadjuvant chemotherapy or radiotherapy.
- In fit patients with non-metastatic cancer, multimodality therapy provides the best prognosis.
  - The MAGIC trial showed an improvement in overall survival with pre- and post-operative ECF (epirubicin, cis-platin, 5FU) from 23% to 36%. Similarly, the Intergroup 0116 trial showed similar improvements with post-operative chemoradiation. The disadvantage of post-operative therapy is that patients with a prolonged recovery may miss the opportunity for adjuvant therapy.
  - In gastric cancer the quality of resection is important. This has been described as R0 (complete), R1 (microscopic residual), R2 (macroscopic residual). An R0 resection is necessary for curative resection. A total gastrectomy and appropriate lymphadenectomy is recommended for all patients except those with distal gastric cancers where a subtotal (80%) gastrectomy provides better functional outcome (margin must be at least 6 cm from tumour and frozen section negative).
  - The role of extended lymphadenectomy has been debated in Western countries. It is clear that at least a D1 resection (perigastric nodes) should be removed and removal of at least 15 nodes as recommended by the NCCN as being required for staging. Increased morbidity from D2 (along named vessels) resection has been demonstrated in some trials, although a D2 resection should be expected to improve outcomes in patients with metastases to D2 nodes in experienced hands.
- Patients who have metastatic disease have a poor prognosis and may be treated with:
  - systemic chemotherapy or palliation depending on patient fitness and the extent of metastatic disease
  - palliative surgery (gastrojejunostomy or more distal bypass) has a limited role and stents provide an alternative for the management of gastric outlet obstruction.

4.6.20 Hydatid cyst

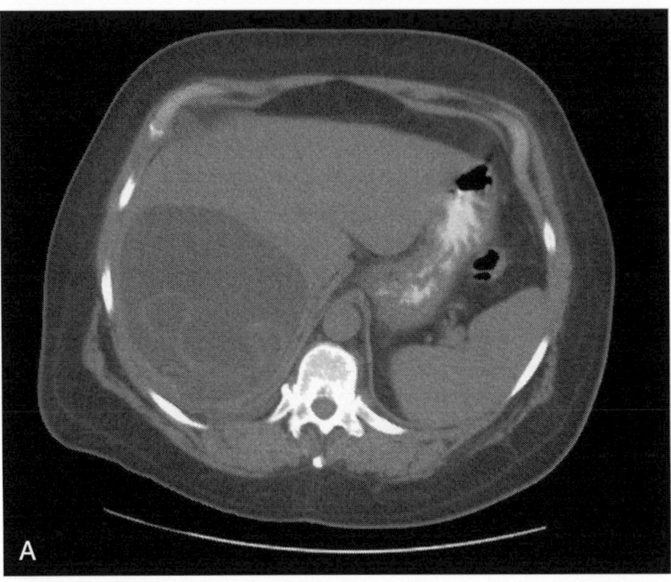

Figure 4.6.20A
Hydatid cyst CT scan

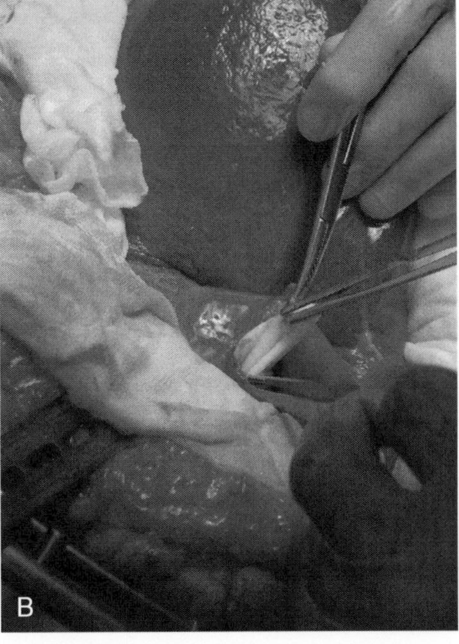

Figure 4.6.20B
Hydatid cyst operative image

Examiner question: please look at this CT scan and now this operative image. What is going on here?

Candidate answer

- The first image is a CT scan of what looks like a hydatid cyst, and the second image is taken intra-operatively and shows the liver walled off by white packs and an incision in the liver with forceps removing what looks like the whitish walls of a hydatid cyst.
- Hydatid disease is a zoonosis caused by a parasitic infestation by a tapeworm of the genus *Echinococcus*.
- The prevalence of human echinococcosis is directly related to contact with dogs and sheep.
- The lifecycle is as follows:
  - the *Echinococcus granulosus* tapeworm resides as an adult tapeworm in crypts of the small bowel of the definitive host, which is the canine
  - eggs are shed in faeces and infect an intermediate host (e.g. humans, sheep, pigs, cattle) when ingested
  - following ingestion by an accidental human host, an oncosphere larva is released from the egg due to interaction with bile salts and trypsin
  - larvae penetrate into the lamina propria in the jejunum and are transported via portal circulation to the liver or via lymphatics to the lung where oncosphere larvae develop into hydatid cysts
  - the hydatid cysts consist of three layers
    1. an inner nucleated germinal layer — responsible for production of hydatid fluid, brood capsules and daughter cysts
    2. an outer acellular laminated layer
    3. a host derived external fibrous capsule
  - the cyst enlarges asexually producing protoscolices (contained in brood capsules) and daughter cysts that fill the cyst interior. These protoscolices can form daughter cysts at distant sites upon rupture of the cyst
  - when cyst containing organs are ingested by the definite host, the protoscolices evaginate and the scolexes of the organisms attach to the intestine of the definite host and develop into adult tapeworms, completing the lifecycle.

Examiner: how does hydatid disease present?

Candidate answer

- Presentation may be:
  - asymptomatic (incidental finding on imaging/abnormal LFTs)
  - RUQ pain (distension of liver capsule)
  - hepatomegaly
  - hepatic abscesses may develop from secondary bacterial infection
  - obstructive jaundice or cholangitis from erosion or rupture of cysts into bile ducts
  - anaphylaxis can occur with rupture into the peritoneal cavity.

- Diagnosis is based on:
  - history suggestive of exposure
  - imaging with US and CT scanning
  - serology (arc 5 ELISA test as arc 5 is the main antigenic component of hydatid fluid, sensitivity 90%, specificity 90%).

Examiner question: how do you treat hydatid disease?

Candidate answer

- Treatment depends on the cyst size, location, complications and the overall health of the patient.
- Generally, surgery is required as the natural history of viable cysts is one of growth and complications, which carries significant morbidity and mortality.
- Surgery might be best avoided in elderly frail patients with small cysts. Non-operative management with percutaneous aspiration and injection with scolicidal agent (hypertonic saline/chlorhexidine) is possible, although has largely been abandoned as it carries a risk of anaphylaxis and developing sclerosing cholangitis.
- Surgical options include cystectomy or liver resection. The principles of surgical management are:
  - eradication of the parasite:
    - inactivation of scolices — pre-operative treatment with mebendazole/albendazole for 3 months
  - prevention of intra-operative spillage of cyst contents (spillage of infected scolices may induce an anaphylactic reaction or cause implantation in the peritoneal cavity):
    - surrounding area walled off with sponges soaked in hypertonic saline
  - elimination of all viable elements of the cyst
  - obliteration of the residual cavity:
    - can be marsupialised, packed with omentum or plicated
  - pericystectomy can be performed or formal liver resection performed.

4.6.21 Pancreatitis

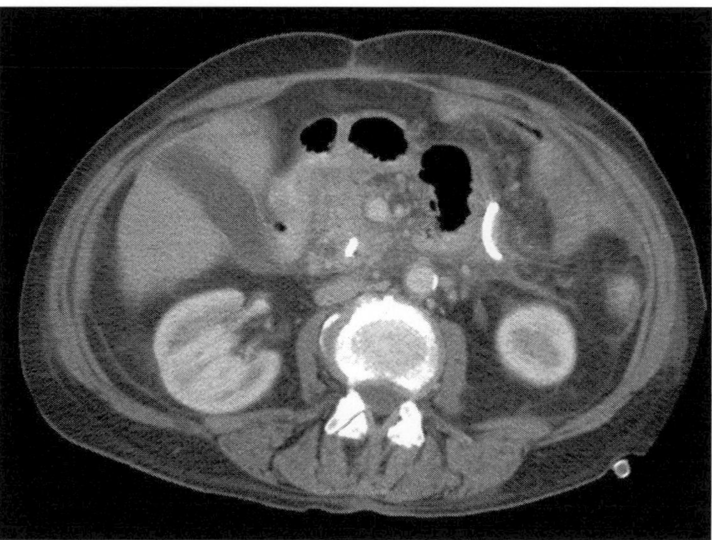

Figure 4.6.21
Pancreatitis CT scan

Examiner: a 56-year-old woman presents with abdominal pain radiating to the back, a serum bilirubin of 46umol/L and a serum lipase of 2450. A diagnosis of acute pancreatitis is made. This is her CT scan. What are the causes and natural history of acute pancreatitis?

> **TOP TIP**
>
> The acronym GET SMASHED is helpful when remembering the causes.

Candidate answer

- The commonest causes of acute pancreatitis are:
  - **G** — gall stones
  - **E** — ethanol abuse (a significant number with suspected alcohol aetiology will have coexistent cholelithiasis).
- Others include:
  - **T** — trauma
  - **S** — structural abnormalities (pancreas divisum)
  - **M** — mumps, malignancy
  - **A** — auto-immune
  - **S** — scorpion sting
  - **H** — hypercalcemia, hyperlipidemia
  - **E** — ERCP
  - **D** — drugs (especially azathioprine, steroids, diuretics).

- In terms of the natural history, acute pancreatitis varies from a mild, self-limiting attack to a severe, life-threatening illness.
- Approximately 25% of all cases will experience a severe attack (evidence of severe early organ dysfunction), the majority of whom will have pancreatic necrosis. Approximately 25% of these will develop infected pancreatic necrosis in the second to third week after admission, which has a poor prognosis when complicated by multi-organ failure.
- The majority of patients who develop severe acute pancreatitis have evidence of early systemic organ dysfunction. Most of these will be evident at the time of admission or shortly afterwards.

Examiner question: how does pancreatitis develop?

Candidate answer

- No matter what the inciting event, there is abnormal activation of proteolytic enzymes within the pancreatic acinar cell. There is abnormal co-localisation of lysozymes and zymogen granules allowing cathepsin B to hydrolyse trypsinogen.
- Acinar cell injury allows trypsin to be released into the pancreatic parenchyma where it activates more trypsinogen. These overwhelm the natural anti-proteases (pancreatic secretory trypsin inhibitor).
- Local inflammation causes monocytes and neutrophils to release IL1, IL6, TNF and PAF leading to SIRS.
- Hypoperfusion and erosion into vessels leads to necrosis.

Examiner question: how would you assess the severity of her disease?

Candidate answer

- It is incredibly important to identify those patients with severe acute pancreatitis as they are at highest risk of organ dysfunction, multi-organ failure and death.
- As stated above, most of these are identifiable at admission or shortly thereafter.
- Accordingly, a number of validated scoring systems, which correlate with mortality, have been developed to risk stratify patients into those with mild or severe acute pancreatitis.
- These include Ranson's score, the Imrie (Glasgow) score and APACHE II. The Ranson and Imre scores essentially rely on detecting features of SIRS (such as hypoalbuminaemia, fluid sequestration, renal impairment) and demographics (age). The sensitivity and specificity of these systems may be as low as 50–70%, meaning that some patients will be judged incorrectly to have severe disease and some with severe disease will be missed.
- One example of a multi-factorial scoring system is the modified Glasgow criteria:
  - **P** — P_aO_2
  - **A** — age
  - **N** — neutrophils (WCC) raised

- **C** — calcium reduced
- **R** — raised urea
- **E** — elevated liver enzymes (AST/ALT)
- **A** — albumin
- **S** — sugar (glucose).

- Although these are useful tools for stratifying patients retrospectively, it is the severity of organ dysfunction which is most critical in determining the level of critical care that is required and how to manage the patient. Patients who are hypotensive, hypoxic and oliguric need critical care. The Atlanta criteria for the classification of severity acknowledge this and shift the emphasis towards identification of organ dysfunction:
  - acute pancreatitis: an acute inflammatory process of the pancreas with variable involvement of other regional tissues or remote organs
  - mild acute pancreatitis: associated with minimal organ dysfunction and uneventful recovery
  - severe acute pancreatitis: associated with organ failure and/or other local complications such as necrosis (±infection), pseudocyst or abscess.
- Also the features of a CT at presentation correlate with outcome (Balthazar). Scores from the unenhanced CT are added to a CT necrosis score (based on an enhanced CT) to give a CT severity index.

Examiner question: the patient deteriorates progressively with oliguria, hypotension and worsening jaundice (serum bilirubin 102). She has gram negative rods in a blood culture. You perform a US showing intra-hepatic biliary dilatation and gallstones in the gallbladder. What is the pathophysiology of this and how would you manage it?

Candidate answer

- In this example, the patent has evidence of biliary obstruction (bilirubin >80 and intra-hepatic biliary dilatation).
- The presence of bactobilia alone does not cause cholangitis.
- Normal biliary pressure is 7–14 cmH_2O. Only when there is obstruction (pressure >20 cmH_20) is there cholangiovenous (into hepatic veins) and cholangiolymphatic (into perihilar lymphatics) reflux of bacteria and endotoxin. This elicits a systemic inflammatory response syndrome (SIRS). Unchecked SIRS results in multiple organ dysfunction syndrome (MODS).
- She requires immediate resuscitation, broad spectrum antibiotics (such as Imipenem) and supportive critical care (such as ventilation, haemofiltration) and relief of obstruction.
- Only biliary decompression will improve the patient's clinical course and prognosis in this scenario. In fact, in the randomised clinical trials of emergency ERCP for severe acute pancreatitis, it was only in the patients with ascending cholangitis (serum bilirubin >70–80 umol/L) that any survival benefit could be demonstrated. This illustrates the importance of 'source control' and differentiating infectious and inflammatory SIRS.

4.6.22 Anticoagulation

Examiner question: a 70-year-old women presents with an acute abdomen and evidence of a pneumoperitoneum and requires an urgent laparotomy. Her past history includes mitral valve replacement and she takes warfarin and aspirin. Her INR is 4. How would you prepare this patient for surgery?

Candidate answer

- This patient requires urgent surgery. I would start by resuscitating the patient (fluids, NG, IDC, cross match) and obtaining immediate consent. I would optimise her further by addressing the coagulopathy. Given the urgency of the operation, vitamin K will take too long to work. So I will organise Prothrombinex (PTX) and fresh frozen plasma (FFP) prior to surgery (in consultation with a haematologist).
- However, I will also give this patient low dose vitamin K so that the reversal continues post-operatively as PTX and FFP are short acting.

Examiner question: please tell us how warfarin works and the principles behind its reversal.

Candidate answer

- Warfarin acts by inhibiting vitamin K reductase and thus blocking synthesis of vitamin K dependent factors (factor II, VII, IX and X — hint: the original Australian TV channels) and thus prolongs prothrombin time.
- Its half life is 20–60 hrs, duration of action is 2–5 days and it is eliminated by the liver (cytochrome P450).
- The principle of reversing its action is to replace the deficient factors. This can be done in two ways, depending on the urgency of the situation:
  1. by supplementing vitamin K in the body in the form of oral or IV form (will take up to 12–24 hrs for the factors to regenerate)
  2. by replacing the factors in the form of prothrombinex and fresh frozen plasma.
- PTX is a freeze dried plasma containing factors II, IX and X but not much factor VII (thus the FFP). There is no need for ABO grouping. The vials contain 500 units, for effective reversal 25–50 units/kg are required.
- FFP contains all coagulation factors. It is available in 150–300 mls. It is stored at 2–6 degrees for up to 5 days once thawed. ABO grouping is required and thus there is the potential for transfusion reaction.
- These agents will work immediately but their effects last <12–24 hrs.

Examiner question: how would you manage this patient's anticoagulation post-operatively?

Candidate answer

- This patient is at high risk of thrombosis given her mechanical valve. I would observe this patient in an HDU or CCU setting in liaison with a cardiologist.

I would aim to reintroduce oral anticoagulation within 48 hrs if haemostasis is not an issue.

- I would bridge the therapy with either therapeutic doses of clexane or intravenous heparin. Heparin is preferable if bleeding might still be an issue and rapid reversal potentially required. Clexane can't be reversed but is easier to administer and no monitoring is required.
- I would restart warfarin once there is no evidence of bleeding with clexane/heparin.

Examiner question: imagine you are booking a patient for elective lap cholecystectomy. The patient is on plavix (clopidogrel) for cardiac stents. How would you prepare this patient?

Candidate answer

- There are two issues that need to be considered and risk/benefits need to be balanced:
  1. indication for antiplatelets/anticoagulation and risk of cessation
  2. potential for intra- and post-operative bleeding.
- In this case, considering the first issue, there is a risk of stent thrombosis and subsequent mortality on cessation of antiplatelet therapy. The surgery does carry a risk of bleeding intra- and post-operatively.
- The decision should be taken in consultation with the patient's cardiologist and involve a senior anaesthetist.
- I would assess this patient's risk by considering:
  - type of stent and date of placement
    - bare metal stents need lifelong aspirin and at least 4 weeks of clopidogrel (Note: data from the CREDO study showed a small but definite benefit from one year of dual antiplatelet therapy following elective bare metal stent implantation)
    - drug-eluting stents need life-long aspirin and at least 12 months of clopidogrel
  - urgency of LAP chole (e.g. urgent if gallstone pancreatitis); otherwise is it possible to wait?
  - other comorbidities: diabetes, hypertension and smoking (increase the risk of stent thrombosis).
- A possible approach (in consultation with a cardiologist) would be to continue aspirin and cease plavix 10 days prior (if high risk may need hospital admission for heparin cover peri-operatively). Post-operatively, I would undertake careful cardiac monitoring in a coronary care unit setting. Plavix will be restarted as soon as possible. Due attention to optimise myocardial oxygen supply/demand is imperative. For example, increase oxygen delivery by optimising Hb concentration and O2 saturation, as well as correcting haemodynamic derangements post-operatively and preventing tachycardia (due to pain or hypovolaemia) to minimise demand.
- It is important that the patient is well informed and appropriately consented to the real risk of myocardial infarct and its consequences compared to the risk of haemorrhage peri-operatively.

Examiner question: how does plavix (clopidogrel) work?

Candidate answer

- Clopidogrel binds irreversibly to the platelet receptor $P2Y_{12}$ thereby inhibiting platelet response to exogenous and endogenous adenosine phosphate (ADP).
- ADP is a platelet receptor which is important in the aggregation of platelets and x-linking of fibrin.
- Accordingly, its therapeutic effect and bleeding risk persists for 5–10 days (since the average lifespan of a platelet is normally 5–10 days) following cessation.

Index

Page numbers followed by 'f' indicate figures, 't' indicate tables, and 'b' indicate boxes.

M

T

CPI Antony Rowe
Eastbourne, UK
January 10, 2023